Advances in the Discovery of Novel Antimicrobial Agents in Nature and Their Applications

Advances in the Discovery of Novel Antimicrobial Agents in Nature and Their Applications

Guest Editors

Ana Tomić
Olja Šovljanski

MDPI

Basel • Beijing • Wuhan • Barcelona • Belgrade • Novi Sad • Cluj • Manchester

Guest Editors
Ana Tomić
Faculty of Technology
University of Novi Sad
Novi Sad
Serbia

Olja Šovljanski
Department of Biotechnology
University of Novi Sad
Novi Sad
Serbia

Editorial Office
MDPI AG
Grosspeteranlage 5
4052 Basel, Switzerland

This is a reprint of the Special Issue, published open access by the journal *Antibiotics* (ISSN 2079-6382), freely accessible at: https://www.mdpi.com/journal/antibiotics/special_issues/NO1R6W3900.

For citation purposes, cite each article independently as indicated on the article page online and as indicated below:

Lastname, A.A.; Lastname, B.B. Article Title. *Journal Name* **Year**, *Volume Number*, Page Range.

ISBN 978-3-7258-6037-1 (Hbk)
ISBN 978-3-7258-6038-8 (PDF)
https://doi.org/10.3390/books978-3-7258-6038-8

Contents

About the Editors

Ana Tomić

Ana Tomić is a Teachnig Assistant and Research Associate at the Faculty of Technology, University of Novi Sad. She has actively contributed to numerous national and international research projects, including those under the FP7, EUREKA, and COST frameworks. Her primary interests focus on natural products with antimicrobial potential, food safety, and both applied and environmental microbiology. To date, dr Ana Tomić has authored over 63 scientific papers and has presented more than 40 contributions at international conferences. According to the SCOPUS database, she has a Hirsch index of 19 and her work has been cited 1009 times.

Olja Šovljanski

Olja Šovljanski is a Research Associate at the Faculty of Technology Novi Sad, University of Novi Sad. She has participated in nine national and international projects and two COST actions. Her primary interests are natural products with antimicrobial potential, food safety, and both applied and environmental microbiology. Her research activities and scientific production are reflected in almost 80 papers and more than 40 contributions at international conferences. According to the SCOPUS database, she has a Hirsch index of 19 and her work has been cited 1037 times.

antibiotics

Article

Towards a Greener Approach for Biomass Valorization: Integration of Supercritical Fluid and Deep Eutectic Solvents

Jelena Vladić [1,2,*], Martina Jakovljević Kovač [3], Valentina Pavić [4], Stela Jokić [3], Siniša Simić [2], Alexandre Paiva [1], Igor Jerković [5] and Ana Rita Duarte [1,*]

1 LAQV/REQUIMTE, Faculdade de Ciências e Tecnologia, Universidade Nova de Lisboa, 2829-516 Caparica, Portugal; abp08838@fct.unl.pt
2 Faculty of Technology, University of Novi Sad, 21000 Novi Sad, Serbia; sinisa.simic@uns.ac.rs
3 Faculty of Food Technology, Josip Juraj Strossmayer University of Osijek, 31000 Osijek, Croatia; martina.jakovljevic@ptfos.hr (M.J.K.); sjokic@ptfos.hr (S.J.)
4 Department of Biology, Josip Juraj Strossmayer University Osijek, 31000 Osijek, Croatia; vpavic@biologija.unios.hr
5 Faculty of Chemistry and Technology, University of Split, 21000 Split, Croatia; igor@ktf-split.hr
* Correspondence: jelenavladic@fct.unl.pt (J.V.); ard08968@fct.unl.pt (A.R.D.)

Abstract: A green and sustainable procedure for obtaining *Lavandula stoechas* extracts with antioxidant and antimicrobial properties was investigated. Green solvents, supercritical CO_2, and natural deep eutectic solvents (NADES) together with ultrasound-assisted extraction were used for the sequential extraction of terpene and polyphenols fractions. After the CO_2 extraction of the terpene fraction, the residue material was used in an extraction with different NADES (betaine-ethylene glycol (Bet:EG), betaine-glycerol (Bet:Gly), and glycerol-glucose (Gly:Glu)), intensified with an ultrasound-assisted method (at 30 and 60 °C). In the CO_2 extract, the major group of components belonged to oxygenated monoterpenes, while the highest polyphenol content with the dominant rutin (438.93 ± 4.60 μg/mL) was determined in Bet:EG extracts (60 °C). Bet:EG extracts also exhibited the most potent antioxidant activity according to DPPH, ABTS, and FRAP assays. Moreover, Bet:EG extracts showed significant inhibitory activity against Gram-positive and Gram-negative bacteria, with minimum inhibitory activity of 0.781–3.125 and 1.563–6.250 mg·mL^{-1}, respectively. By comparing the polyphenolic content and antioxidant and antimicrobial activities of Bet:EG extracts with extracts obtained with conventional solvents (water and ethanol), the superiority of NADES was determined. The established environmentally friendly procedure unifies the requirements of green and sustainable development and modern pharmacognosy because it combines the use of safe alternative solvents, the absence of solvent waste generation, more rational use of resources, and the attainment of safe and quality extracts.

Keywords: *Lavandula stoechas*; supercritical CO_2; deep eutectic solvent; antibacterial activity; antioxidant activity

1. Introduction

Antimicrobial resistance (AMR) is a global concern, which is estimated to threaten the lives of millions of people around the world (by increasing mortality and morbidity). In 2019, the deaths of 4.95 million people were associated with drug-resistant bacterial infections, while 1.27 million deaths were directly caused by AMR [1]. Additionally, foodborne pathogens affect millions of people annually, and many foodborne diseases can result in very serious and fatal consequences. The World Bank estimated that if AMR is not addressed, it would lead to an increase in healthcare costs of up to 25% in low-income countries and 8% globally. Therefore, this situation could push up to 28 million people into poverty by 2050 [2]. Due to such extensive consequences, AMR has significant effects on a range of Sustainable Development Goals (SDG); hence, without overcoming AMR, it is not possible to achieve the SDGs. Multisectoral and coordinated cooperation on the identification of new antimicrobials and the reduction of uncontrolled and excessive use of antibiotics is one of the primary goals in the strategy to combat AMR. Due to their diverse chemical profile and significant antimicrobial potential, medicinal plants can be a promising resource and part of the strategy for overcoming AMR.

Aromatic medicinal plants have a long tradition of use around the world. This presence and the increasing preference of consumers for natural products were the drivers behind the commercial recognition of aromatic medicinal plants. Therefore, there is a large number of products based on medicinal plants present in the market. However, for medicinal plant-based products to remain relevant, it is necessary that research in the field of natural product development keep pace with the needs of modern development and aim to create green innovation and sustainable development, as defined within the SDGs.

Therefore, research in the field of medicinal plants includes (i) the development of products that target global problems such as AMR, (ii) the use of safe green solvents, (iii) the use of renewable materials, (iv) the reduction of harmful waste generation, and (v) the reduced use of energy, in line with the SDGs.

Among the species whose traditional use is very widespread and diverse is *Lavandula stoechas* L., which belongs to the family Lamiaceae and the genus Lavandula. The chemical profile of *L. stoechas*, rich in different classes of compounds, such as terpenes, phenols, flavonoids, and coumarins, is responsible for numerous biological actions, including antioxidant, anti-inflammatory [3], antimicrobial, antispasmodic [4], insecticidal, and larvicidal activities [5].

Isolation of bioactive compounds and production of *L. stoechas* products are most often carried out using conventional extraction methods: terpene fraction hydrodistillation or steam distillation [6–8], while the phenolic fraction is obtained by solid–liquid extraction with organic solvents, such as methanol [3,9], aqueous–methanolic mixture [4], and ethanol [5]. The mentioned conventional methods for obtaining essential oil and extracts of *L. stoechas* do not fit into modern production procedures because they do not ensure a safe product profile and a green sustainable production process. Namely, they are characterized by low extraction efficiency and lack of selectivity, as well as a large environmental footprint due to the use of toxic solvents that must be removed from the final product, which increases the cost of the entire process. Therefore, alternative extraction technologies and solvents have been developed which, compared to conventional methods and solvents, are safer to work with and offer the possibility of changing selectivity and adjusting the final quality of the product.

Among alternative solvents, supercritical CO_2 has emerged as a successful alternative for the extraction of lipophilic components from materials, which ensures obtaining a clean and safe extract of high quality. Due to its characteristics, which include inertness, non-toxicity, mild conditions (31.1 °C and 73.8 bar) to reach the supercritical state, and the possibility of recirculation, it has already been implemented in commercial large-scale production in several applications, including pharmaceutical and food, and industrial-scale biochemical and chemical reactions [10]. Additionally, apart from extraction, it has been shown that the use of supercritical CO_2 can also play a role in the pretreatment of biomass before further extractions [11,12]. As a result of the exposure of the material to pressurized CO_2, there is a loosening of the cell walls which facilitates mass transport and the extraction of non-polar components by CO_2. The hypothesis behind this work is that due to the potential physical change in the structure of the material, the matrix can be more permeable and thus facilitate the subsequent extraction of the polar fraction and achieve a more rational use of the material [13]. It was previously shown that supercritical CO_2 can be used for the extraction of non-polar components from *L. stoechas* [14–17]. However, none of the works investigated the possibility of a more efficient use of the material. For this purpose, two green technologies, namely supercritical fluids and natural deep eutectic systems (NADES), were coupled.

NADES represent a new generation of alternative solvents characterized by low cost, easy synthesis, non-flammability, chemical and thermal stability, tunability, and versatility [18]. Due to their low toxicity and natural origin, they are considered environmentally safe and biodegradable solvents. NADES represent a mixture of natural components whose melting point is lower than the melting points of individual components when at a particular molar ratio [19]. They are usually prepared by mixing and stirring the components until a liquid is formed, therefore 100% atom economy is achieved and further purification is not necessary [20].

This work investigated the sequential extraction of non-polar and polar fractions and more efficient utilization of *L. stoechas* material, using green solvents supercritical CO_2 and NADES, to obtain potent antioxidant and antimicrobial extracts (Figure 1). In the first step, supercritical CO_2 extraction was performed for the extraction of lipophilic components, while the exhausted raw material (residue) was used in the next step for the extraction of polar compounds using NADES and ultrasound-assisted extraction. In addition, in order to determine whether the CO_2 extraction can play the role of pretreatment and help the release of polar components, extraction with NADES was performed with both, the raw material after CO_2 extraction (residue), and the raw material not subjected to CO_2 extraction (non-residue; control). The obtained extracts were examined in terms of chemical composition and their potential as antibacterial and antioxidant agents was investigated.

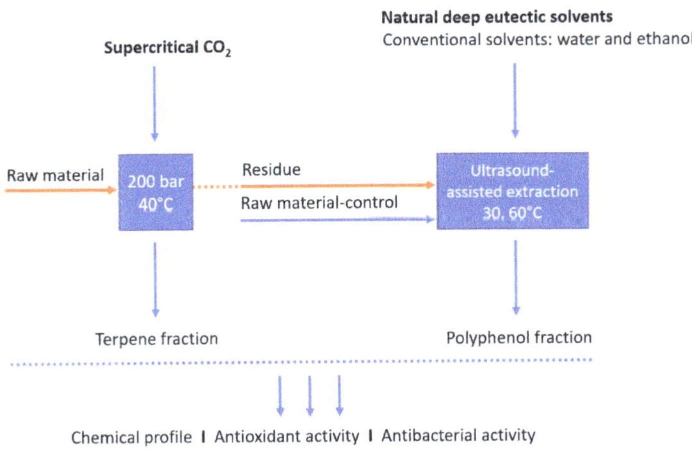

Figure 1. Schematic diagram of the sequential extraction procedure of *Lavandula stoechas*.

2. Results

2.1. Chemical Profile of *L. stoechas* Extract Obtained by Supercritical CO_2 Extraction

In our previous study based on which the conditions for the supercritical extraction were selected, the obtained extracts were analyzed by the GC-MS method. Therefore, to confirm the chemical composition of the extract obtained in this study (conditions 200 bar, 40 °C, and 3 h), GC-MS was also applied, and the results were similar to the ones reported (Figure 2), where the total extraction yield was 1.99% (*w/w*) [21] In the GC-MS profile of the extract, oxygenated terpenes were the most abundant with 72.21%. Within oxygenated terpenes, monoterpenes were more dominant (55.41%) with major components fenchone (12.93 ± 2.94%) and verbenone (12.08 ± 1.27), followed by camphor (7.80 ± 2.46) and 1,8-cineole (7.51 ± 2.02%). From the group of oxygenated sesquiterpenes, the most represented was α-cadinol 8.31 ± 1.88%, while viridiflorol and ledol were present with 2.64 ± 0.46% and 1.98 ± 1.01%, respectively. Moreover, minor oxygenated terpene compounds characteristic of the species *L. stoechas* were identified, such as borneol, bornyl acetate, lavandulyl acetate, linalool, α-cyclogeraniol, and others. Terpene hydrocarbons, monoterpenes 0.76%, and sesquiterpenes 2.61% were significantly less represented. Additionally, non-terpene components such as fatty alcohol and acids, alkanes, carboxylic acids, and esters (9.26%) were identified.

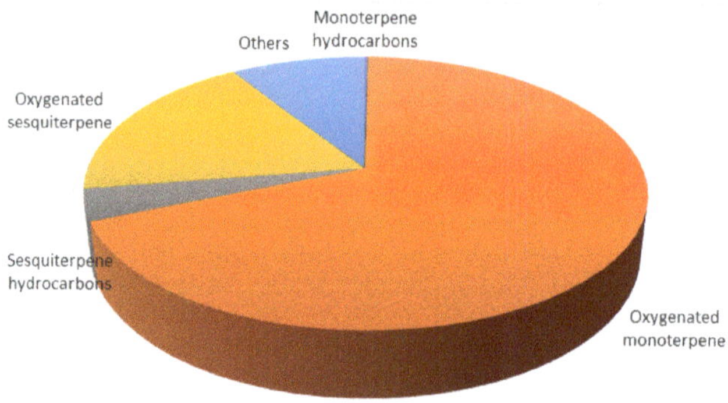

Figure 2. GC/MS analysis of *L. stoechas* supercritical extract (200 bar, 40 °C, and 3 h) [21].

2.2. *Chemical Profile of L. stoechas Extracts Obtained by Ultrasound-Assisted NADES Extraction*

After the CO_2 extraction of the non-polar fraction, the residue material was further used for ultrasonic-assisted NADES extraction, which was performed at 30 and 60 °C for 30 min. In order to establish if the supercritical CO_2 extraction can intensify the sequential extraction of polar compounds, ultrasound-assisted NADES extraction was also performed with non-residue material (control). Additionally, to evaluate the potential of NADES as solvents, conventional solvents, namely ethanol and water, were used. All obtained NADES and conventional extracts were examined in terms of chemical composition using HPLC analysis (Figure 3; Supplementary Materials, Table S1).

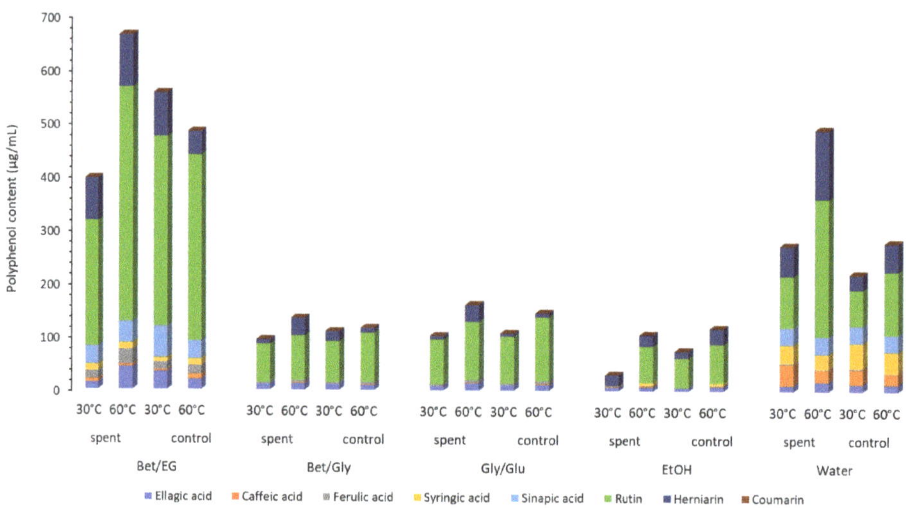

Figure 3. Content of polyphenols in NADES extracts.

The presence of different classes of components, including flavonoids, hydrolyzable tannins, derivatives of hydroxycinnamic and hydroxybenzoic acids, and coumarins was identified in the extracts. Observing the total sum of identified components (Figure 3, Supplementary Materials, Table S1), the highest phenolic content was recorded in the extracts obtained with Bet:EG (residue, 60 °C) and accounted for 664.19 μg/mL, while the second highest content was in the extract obtained from the extraction with the control material at 30 °C (555.43 μg/mL). Bet:EG extracts proved to be several times richer in polyphenols compared to Bet:Gly and Gly:Glu. Furthermore, ethanol extracts had the lowest polyphenol content, while the water extracts were richer in polyphenols than ethanolic, Bet:Gly, and Gly:Glu extracts. Extraction of non-residue material with Bet:EG and residue material with water (60 °C) had approximate values of 483.78 and 489.80 μg/mL, respectively.

At a higher temperature of 60 °C, a positive effect of the CO_2 treatment was observed, so NADES and water extracts with a higher polyphenolic content were obtained compared to the control samples. During CO_2 extraction, the material is exposed to high pressure and saturated with CO_2, as a result of which there is a weakening of the material structure and disruption of glandular structures where non-polar components are located, and their extraction. At the end of the CO_2 extraction, depressurization is performed, and there is a sudden drop in pressure which may affect the structure of the plant material. Due to pressure changes, the resistance of the material further weakens, potentially facilitating solvent penetration and access to polar components in a subsequent step. In order to further intensify the NADES extraction, UAE was used, where the pressure is transmitted as a series of compressions and decompressions, resulting in cavitation. As a consequence of collapsing cavitation bubbles, various effects on the material occur, such as fragmentation, pore formation, erosion of the material, shear force, and swelling, which, due to the increase in permeability of the material, facilitate the penetration of solvents into the material and intensifies the extraction [22,23]. The interaction between ultrasonic extraction conditions, solvent, and material characteristics determines the efficiency and selectivity of component extraction. Due to CO_2 exposure, as well as the effect of UAE, the permeability of the material and surface area increases, and there is more effective solubilization of components in the solvent and improved mass transfer in the boundary layer of solid material. It was previously reported that the use of CO_2-treated microalga biomass improved the yield of ultrasound-assisted, microwave-assisted, and subcritical water extraction, compared to CO_2-untreated microalga biomass [13]. Also, the pretreatment with high pressure has been shown to be effective in improving the yield of CO_2 extraction of *Origanum virens* and *Hypericum perforatum* [11,12].

The higher temperature was more effective in terms of polyphenolic content compared to the lower one at 30 °C. Increasing the temperature increases the solubility and desorption of target components in the solvent, but temperature also affects the characteristics of the solvent, reducing its viscosity and thus improving diffusivity into the material [22]. Additionally, the viscosity of NADES is one of the parameters that can significantly limit extraction. Due to the lowering of the temperature (30 °C), the viscosity increases, and the solvent penetration is aggravated; thus, the interaction with the analyte and its transition into the solvent is reduced. Viscosity values of NADES solvents were Bet:EG 18.27 ± 0.21 (60 °C) and 48.63 ± 0.42 (30 °C); Bet:Gly 227.33 ± 4.66 (60 °C) and 1250.10 ± 0.0028 (30 °C); Gly:Glu 525.37 ± 28.76 (60 °C) and 5443.90 ± 46.53 (30 °C) [24]. Bet:EG proved to be the most efficient NADES for the extraction of polyphenols, which is correlated with the lowest viscosity among the NADES used.

Observing the effect of temperature on the control material, it was noted that increasing the temperature from 30 to 60 °C led to an increase in polyphenolic content in all samples, except for Bet:EG control, where a decrease was observed with increasing temperature. Namely, although the viscosity decreases and penetration of the solvent increases with temperature, weakening of the cavitation effect can also occur. The potential explanation can be that due to the sequential collapse of cavitation bubbles at high temperature, shear stress increases and this can further cause degradation of the target component [22]. Additionally, the decrease in surface tension of the solvent at higher temperatures may lead to a decrease in the intensity of the collapse of cavitation bubbles, which further lowers the mass transfer and extraction efficiency [22].

The flavonoid rutin was the most abundant in extracts in the range from 55.53 μg/mL (ethanol extract, control, 30 °C) to 438.93 ± 4.60 μg/mL (Bet:EG, residue, 60 °C). Moreover, the extract obtained by extracting the CO_2-treated material with Bet:EG at 60 °C had the highest content of ferulic acid and ellagic acid (27.84 ± 0.60 μg/mL and 42.21 ± 2.63 μg/mL, respectively). Sinapic acid was identified only in Bet:EG and water extracts, while syringic acid was detected in Bet:EG and water extracts, and alcoholic extracts obtained at 60 °C. Significantly higher viscosity values of Bet:Gly and Gly:Glu were the most likely cause of the less efficient extraction of polyphenols.

For the extraction of caffeic acid and syringic acid, the most adequate solvent was water in combination with low temperature (40.64 ± 0.16 μg/mL). Low viscosity, high polarity, and high affinity to caffeic acid were previously established [25]. Additionally, water was the most adequate for the extraction of herniarin at 60 °C.

The polyphenolic profile of *L. stoechas* extracts varies in the literature depending on the applied extraction technique, solvents, and material characteristics. The presence and different presence of polyphenolic components may be due to different stages of development and environmental conditions that dictate the development of different adaptive mechanisms to different environmental conditions, such as air humidity, light, temperature, presence of nutrients, pathogen attacks, and others [26]. Ceylan et al. [9] reported caffeic acid, rutin, and rosmarinic acid as major components of the methanol extract of *L. stoechas* from Turkey. Epicatechin was found to be the major compound in ethyl acetate and acetone extracts, while sinapic acid was the major compound in methanolic and ethanolic extracts [26].

2.3. Antioxidant Activity of *L. stoechas* Extracts

Different tests were used for the analysis of antioxidant activity due to the differences in the properties of the extracts, their constituents, and the possibility of different interactions with the used radicals. Free radical scavenging activity assays DPPH and ABTS, and ferric-reducing antioxidant power FRAP assay were applied. DPPH is based on the color change of the stable violet DPPH radical into yellow diphenyl picryl hydrazine, due to the acceptance of electrons. The ABTS assay is based on the reduction of ABTS+• radicals by antioxidants present in extracts. FRAP method is based on the reduction of a colorless complex Fe^{3+}-tripyridyltriazine to a blue-colored complex Fe^{2+}-tripyridyltriazine by the action of electron-donating antioxidants.

The supercritical extract showed antioxidant activity measured by DPPH-IC_{50} and ABTS-IC_{50} tests of 2.34 mg/mL and 1.73 ± 0.12 mg/mL, respectively. However, high FRAP-IC_{50} (18.58 ± 3.09 mg/mL) indicated low ferric-reducing ability. Therefore, the antioxidant activity of supercritical extracts was manifested more significantly through the scavenging of free radicals. A significantly lower ferric-reducing capacity of essential oil compared to the extract rich in phenolic components was also observed in the study by Beghlal et al. [27] and was attributed to the greater antioxidant potency of polyphenols. The reducing power of phenol is probably due to the presence of hydroxyl groups, which may serve as electron donors [27]. Additionally, the FRAP test is more adequate for hydrophilic components, while DPPH and FRAP enable the determination of the antioxidant capacity of hydrophilic and lipophilic compounds [28].

By analyzing the antioxidant activity of NADES extracts of *L. stoechas*, the DPPH-IC_{50} values were in the range of 0.25 ± 0.08–5.31 ± 0.99 mg/mL, ABST-IC_{50} in the range of 0.47 ± 0.03–11.14 ± 1.56 mg/mL, and FRAP-EC_{50} varied between 0.52 ± 0.04–8.60 ± 0.88 mg/mL (Table 1). According to all three antioxidative tests, Bet:EG extracts were the most potent among the NADES extracts. Compared to Gly/Glu and Bet:Gly extracts, Bet:EG extracts exhibited approximately 7–10 times stronger antioxidant activity, which corresponds to the significantly lower polyphenol contents in Gly/Glu and Bet:Gly extracts. Gly:Glu extracts showed higher antioxidant activity than Bet:Gly extracts. Considering the effect of the temperature on the IC_{50} value, Bet:EG extracts obtained at 60 °C presented a slightly lower value than those at 30 °C, although not statistically significant. Compared to supercritical extract, Bet:EG demonstrated stronger antioxidant activity. On the other hand, the supercritical extract was on par with Gly/Glu extracts.

Table 1. Antioxidant activity of extracts determined using DPPH, ABTS, and FRAP assays (expressed as IC_{50} values; mg/mL).

Solvent	Material	Temperature (°C)	DPPH-IC_{50}	ABTS-IC_{50}	FRAP-IC_{50}
Betaine/ethylene glycol	residue	30	0.60 ± 0.02^{h}	0.96 ± 0.13^{ef}	1.14 ± 0.07^{gh}
		60	0.36 ± 0.03^{h}	0.58 ± 0.01^{f}	0.60 ± 0.02^{h}
	fresh	30	0.43 ± 0.04^{h}	0.76 ± 0.02^{ef}	0.79 ± 0.00^{gh}
		60	0.35 ± 0.04^{h}	0.50 ± 0.02^{f}	0.70 ± 0.01^{h}
Betaine/glycerol	residue	30	$3.20 \pm 0.23^{b\text{–}e}$	3.32 ± 0.19^{b}	3.30 ± 0.14^{cd}
		60	3.38 ± 0.52^{bcd}	3.36 ± 0.02^{b}	3.29 ± 0.07^{cd}
	fresh	30	$3.00 \pm 0.05^{c\text{–}f}$	3.02 ± 0.00^{b}	3.20 ± 0.05^{cd}
		60	$2.52 \pm 0.29^{d\text{-}g}$	2.60 ± 0.11^{bc}	3.18 ± 0.26^{cd}
Glycerol/glucose	residue	30	2.35 ± 0.09^{efg}	2.48 ± 0.04^{bcd}	2.65 ± 0.03^{de}
		60	1.81 ± 0.28^{g}	1.73 ± 0.11^{cde}	1.39 ± 0.15^{fg}
	fresh	30	2.73 ± 0.11^{def}	3.08 ± 0.10^{b}	1.93 ± 0.18^{f}
		60	2.13 ± 0.08^{fg}	1.37 ± 0.07^{def}	2.05 ± 0.03^{ef}
Ethanol 96%	residue	30	3.72 ± 0.08^{bc}	11.14 ± 1.56^{a}	8.60 ± 0.88^{a}
		60	3.98 ± 0.21^{b}	3.43 ± 0.22^{b}	4.50 ± 0.07^{b}
	fresh	30	5.31 ± 0.99^{a}	3.37 ± 0.12^{b}	4.80 ± 0.09^{b}
		60	3.29 ± 0.25^{bcd}	3.25 ± 0.05^{b}	3.77 ± 0.04^{c}
Water	residue	30	0.25 ± 0.08^{h}	0.51 ± 0.02^{f}	0.63 ± 0.03^{h}
		60	0.30 ± 0.03^{h}	0.47 ± 0.03^{f}	0.52 ± 0.04^{h}
	fresh	30	0.47 ± 0.01^{h}	0.62 ± 0.01^{ef}	0.55 ± 0.02^{h}
		60	0.43 ± 0.01^{h}	0.50 ± 0.00^{f}	0.72 ± 0.01^{gh}
Supercritical extract			2.34 ± 0.21	1.73 ± 0.12	18.58 ± 3.09

Means followed by different letters differ significantly, based on Tukey's HSD test at $p < 0.05$.

Ethanol extracts presented the lowest antioxidant activity, while water extracts showed an antioxidant activity similar to Bet:EG extracts, with no statistically significant differences. The obtained IC_{50} values were similar to the values (0.3 ± 0.010 mg/mL) obtained by Ceylan et al. [9] where the extract was obtained by extraction with methanol at 35 °C using a magnetic stirrer for 6 h (20 g/500 mL).

Pearson correlation test was used to determine the correlation between the antioxidant activity of extracts and the content of polyphenolic components (Table 2). Total phenol content and sinapic acid exhibited a very strong negative correlation with antioxidant activity determined using the DPPH test, with very high statistical significance ($p < 0.0001$). Additionally, herniarin had a strong correlation ($p < 0.001$), while the other components (except coumarin) had a moderate-to-strong negative correlation with antioxidant activity (DPPH) with statistical significance ($p < 0.05$), which means there is a tendency for low IC_{50} (high antioxidant activity) to associate with high polyphenolic scores (and vice versa). The antioxidant capacity of the extracts determined by the other two tests, ABTS and FRAP, had a weaker correlation with the total and individual components compared to the DPPH test.

Table 2. Pearson's correlation coefficient analysis between phenolic compounds and antioxidant activity in *L. stoechas* NADES extracts.

Assay	Total Phenol Content	Ellagic Acid	Caffeic Acid	Ferulic Acid	Syringic Acid	Sinapic Acid	Rutin	Herniarin	Coumarin
					DPPH				
r	−0.7864	−0.5971	−0.6416	−0.4748	−0.6946	−0.8458	−0.6702	−0.6905	0.1582
R squared	0.6184	0.3566	0.4117	0.2254	0.4825	0.7154	0.4491	0.4768	0.02502
p (two-tailed)	<0.0001	0.0054	0.0023	0.0344	0.0007	<0.0001	0.0012	0.0008	0.5054
p value summary	****	**	**	*	***	****	**	***	ns [1]
					ABTS				
r	−0.6045	−0.438	−0.4378	−0.3491	−0.4967	−0.5783	−0.5568	−0.454	−0.00847
R squared	0.3654	0.1919	0.1917	0.1219	0.2467	0.3345	0.31	0.2061	7.17×10^{-5}
p (two-tailed)	0.0048	0.0534	0.0535	0.1314	0.0259	0.0076	0.0108	0.0444	0.9717
p-value summary	**	ns	ns	ns	*	**	*	*	ns
					FRAP				
r	−0.6791	−0.5246	−0.5101	−0.4028	−0.5691	−0.6743	−0.613	−0.5348	0.1185
R squared	0.4611	0.2752	0.2602	0.1623	0.3239	0.4547	0.3758	0.286	0.01405
p (two-tailed)	0.001	0.0176	0.0216	0.0782	0.0088	0.0011	0.0041	0.0151	0.6187
p-value summary	***	*	*	ns	**	**	**	*	ns

Correlation is significant at the 0.05 level (2-tailed); [1] ns—not significant. **** $p < 0.0001$; *** $p \leq 0.001$; ** $p < 0.01$; * $p < 0.05$.

Therefore, the established correlation clearly indicates that extracts with a higher polyphenolic content exhibited more pronounced DPPH and ABTS scavenging capacities and reducing power, that is, antioxidant activity depended on the quantitative content of polyphenolic components. However, the antioxidant activity was also conditioned by the qualitative aspect of the identified polyphenols, that is, by their individual antioxidant capacity.

In the case of phenolic acids, the antioxidant activity is conditioned by the number and position of hydroxyl groups attached to the aromatic ring of the benzoic or cinnamic acid [29]. For instance, caffeic acid, due to the free phenolic group, has a significantly higher antioxidant activity than ferulic acid, whose antioxidant properties are significantly reduced due to the presence of the methoxyl group. This was confirmed according to different methods and tests, ferric reducing power [29], scavenging the free radical [30], and inhibiting peroxidation of LDL [31]. In our work, the most prominent presence of caffeic acid was determined in the water extract obtained at 30 °C, which corresponded to the lowest measured DPPH-IC_{50} value of 0.25 ± 0.08 mg/mL (DPPH), followed by the samples extracted with Bet:EG.

Syringic acid, derivate benzoic acid, due to the presence of a methoxy group attached to the aromatic ring exhibits considerable antioxidant activity [32]. However, derivatives of cinnamic acids are more active antioxidants than the derivatives of benzoic acid. The presence of the CH=CH–COOH group in cinnamic acid derivatives ensures a greater efficiency than the COOH group in benzoic acids [33]. In our study, a significantly higher content of cinnamic acid derivates in the Bet:EG extracts matched the stronger antioxidant activity of these extracts compared to other NADES extracts.

Ceylan et al. [9] reported that phenolic acids and flavonoids of *L. stoechas*, such as rutin and caffeic acid are responsible for the antioxidant activity and according to Sanchez-Moreno et al. [34] rutin was more potent than ferulic acid and its antioxidant capacity is due to its flavonoid structure. Bet:EG extracts were multifold richer in rutin compared to remaining NADES extracts, which could be the reason behind the more potent antioxidant capacity of these extracts. Furthermore, extracts the most abundant in herniarin, Bet:EG and water extracts, exhibited the strongest antioxidant effect. Herniarin belongs to the class of coumarins and its significant antioxidant activity is related to its benzopyrone structure, which is chemically analogous to flavonoids [35].

However, in most cases, the antioxidant activity is considered to be the result of the synergistic effect of all the components present in the mixture. Hence the cumulative presence of polyphenolic compounds observed in the Bet:EG extracts rendered more powerful antioxidant extracts.

2.4. Antibacterial Activity of *L. stoechas* Extracts

Antibacterial activity of the supercritical extract, NADES extracts, and control extracts (ethanolic and water) was tested against Gram-positive bacteria, *B. subtilis* and *S. aureus*, and Gram-negative bacteria, *E. coli* and *P. aeruginosa* (Table 3).

Table 3. Antibacterial activity of *L. stoechas* extracts expressed as minimum inhibitory concentrations (MIC) (mg·mL^{-1}).

Solvent	Material	Temperature (°C)	Gram-Negative Bacteria		Gram-Positive Bacteria	
			Escherichia coli	*Pseudomonas aeruginosa*	*Bacillus subtilis*	*Staphylococcus aureus*
Betaine/ethylene glycol	residue	30	6.250	6.250	3.125	3.125
		60	3.125	3.125	1.563	1.563
	control	30	3.125	3.125	1.563	1.563
		60	1.563	1.563	0.781	0.781
Ethanol 96%	residue	30	3.125	3.125	1.563	1.563
		60	1.563	1.563	0.781	0.781
	control	30	3.125	3.125	1.563	1.563
		60	1.563	1.563	0.781	0.781
Water	residue	30	1.563	3.125	1.563	1.563
		60	1.563	3.125	1.563	1.563
	control	30	1.563	3.125	1.563	1.563
		60	1.563	3.125	1.563	1.563
Supercritical CO_2	200 bar/40 °C/20 g/L		3.39	6.775	3.39	3.39
Control ciprofloxacin *			3.13	7.89	1.56	3.13

* µg/mL.

Supercritical extract showed antibacterial activity, with MIC 3.39 mg·mL^{-1} against *E. coli*, *B. subtilis*, and *S. aureus*, while the least resistant was *P. aeruginosa* with MIC 6.775 mg·mL^{-1}. Greater resistance of *P. aeruginosa* to essential oil *L. stoechas* was also reported in the study by Bouyahya et al. [36]. Additionally, the stronger antibacterial activity of L. *stoechas* against Gram-positive bacteria compared with Gram-negative bacteria is in accordance with the literature [36–38].

Among NADES extracts, Bet:EG were selected for antibacterial activity testing because they were significantly richer in polyphenols and with more pronounced antioxidant activity compared to other NADES extracts. Compared to the supercritical extract, Bet:EG extracts exhibited a stronger antibacterial activity. Gram-positive bacteria were more susceptible to Bet:EG extracts, so lower MIC values were achieved, 0.781–3.125 mg·mL^{-1}, compared to Gram-negative MIC between 1.563 and 6.250 mg·mL^{-1}. Bet:EG extracts obtained at 60 °C (residue or non-residue) exhibited stronger antibacterial activity against the pathogens than extracts at 30 °C, which is consistent with the antioxidant activity of these extracts. The most active extract was obtained from the control material at 60 °C, while the activity of the control at 30 °C and residue extract at 60 °C was equal.

No clear correlation was observed between the inhibitory effect on bacteria and the content of polyphenols. At both temperatures, extracts obtained from the control material showed stronger antibacterial activity compared to the residue. The reason may be an additive or synergistic antimicrobial effect due to the presence of other polyphenolic components with antimicrobial activity that were extracted using NADES, but which were not detected in the extracts. The effect of natural extracts is commonly the result of the synergistic effect, where minor compounds can play a very important role in enhancing the antimicrobial effect of the major component [39].

Water extracts exhibited activity against *E. coli* that was equal to Bet:EG extracts (control, 60 °C). However, for the other tested bacteria, Bet:EG samples (control, 60 °C) were more effective than water extracts. Additionally, the activity of water extracts did not depend on either the extraction temperature or the type of raw material used. Ethanol extracts obtained at high temperatures were more effective than water extracts and had the same activity as NADES extracts. Additionally, in the case of ethanol extracts, the type of raw material used had no influence on their activity at both temperatures.

Ez Zoubi et al. [40] investigated the antimicrobial activity of hydro-ethanolic, flavonoid, and tannin *L. stoechas* fractions/extracts against pathogenic bacteria *P. aeruginosa* and *S. aureus*. They determined that the hydro-ethanolic extract exhibited antibacterial activity with a MIC value against *P. aeruginosa* of 40 mg/mL, while it was 80 mg/mL against *E. coli* and *S. aureus*, while the MIC of flavonoid fractions, which showed the highest effect against bacteria, was from 10 to 40 mg/mL. Additionally, testing aqueous and methanol extracts of *L. officinalis* against Gram-positive and Gram-negative pathogenic multiresistant bacterial strains, Al-Niaame and Aziz [41] found that methanol extracts are active towards all bacteria with MICs of 25 mg/mL, while aqueous ones were not potent and did not inhibit bacteria.

In relation to ciprofloxacin, the antibacterial activity of the extracts was low, but in comparison with the literature data on the activity of *L. stoechas* extracts, NADES, and supercritical extracts showed significant potency. It has been clearly demonstrated that using green solvents and techniques can achieve a more efficient and rational use of materials in a green manner without generating solvent waste, and ensure obtaining extracts rich in bioactive components with antioxidant and antimicrobial capacity. Taking into account the wide variety of natural compounds and the possibility of system customization, it would potentially hinder the development of bacterial resistance [42].

The approach investigated in this work allows for the selective extraction of components. Moreover, the obtained extracts were of different chemical profiles and could, therefore, be used for different applications. NADES extracts were rich in polar polyphenolic compounds which possess significant antioxidant and antimicrobial properties. The antimicrobial activity of the extracts makes them potential constituents in the production of cosmetic, health, food, and veterinary-related products. Due to their antioxidant activity, the NADES extracts can be used for attenuating oxidative stress processes that are in the pathogenesis of many diseases.

On the other hand, supercritical extracts were rich in non-polar terpenic compounds which have numerous confirmed biological properties and potential applications. Due to their aromatic properties, they are very important constituents in the fragrance and perfume industries. Oxygenated terpenes are a parameter of the quality of extracts because highly active functional groups are considered responsible for numerous biological properties, such as antimicrobial activity [43]. Therefore, the prevalence of oxygenated components in supercritical extracts makes them potentially good antimicrobial agents and of great importance in health, food, and cosmetic-related areas. Additionally, the identified terpenes are attributed to numerous medically important properties. Verbenone in vivo antidiabetic activity was reported together with the conclusion that it could reduce diabetes-associated complications such as cardiovascular disease, by enhancing lipids' metabolism [44]. Fenchone exhibited an antidiarrheal effect [45], as well as a significant analgesic activity without inducing motor incoordination [46]. Borneol showed promising results as an effective adjuvant for improving drug delivery to the central nervous system [47], while Kong et al. [48]'s in vivo study determined that borneol possessed an anti-cerebral ischemia effect. Yang et al. [49] suggested the anti-inflammation potentials of bornyl acetate in patients with osteoarthritis, while viridiflorol exerted anti-mycobacterial, anti-inflammatory, and antioxidant activities [50].

In addition, the advantage of NADES extracts compared to the control extracts (ethanol and water) was confirmed and it can be seen in several aspects. Water was more efficient than ethanol for the extraction of polyphenols, but higher polyphenolic contents were achieved in NADES (Bet:EG) extracts. Although the higher antioxidant activity of water extracts was determined, it was not statistically different from Bet:EG, which exerted a more prominent antimicrobial activity. NADES extracts represent ready-to-use products, hence, additional purification steps are not required. Conversely, water extracts are susceptible to microbiological contamination and to preserve their stability, water removal is required representing an additional step that increases the process costs. Lastly, due to its low selectivity, water can extract non-bioactive components, thereby producing bioactive extracts of lower purity [51].

3. Materials and Methods

3.1. Material and Chemicals

L. stoechas L. ssp. *stoechas* flowers were commercial samples purchased in Celeiro, Lisbon, Portugal. Particle size reduction was performed using IKA Tube Mill 100 control (Staufen, Germany) at 20,000 rpm for 30 s. The mean particle size (0.31 ± 0.05 mm) of the material was determined using the vibration sieve sets (CISA, Cedaceria, Spain). The moisture content of the plant material (7.24 ± 0.18%) was determined with a moisture analyzer DAB (Kern, Balingen, Germany), equipped with a halogen quartz glass heater (400 W) and set at 105 °C.

Glycerol (99.5% purity) was purchased from Scharlau (Barcelona, Spain). Betaine (≥99% purity) and D-glucose monohydrate (≥97.5% purity) were purchased from Sigma-Aldrich (St. Louis, MO, USA). Ethylene glycol (≥99.5% purity) and ethanol (99% purity) were purchased from Carlo Erba (Val-de-Reuil, France).

3.2. Preparation and Characterization of NADES

NADES mixtures were prepared by mixing components in the adequate molar ratio and then heated (40 °C) and stirred until a clear liquid was formed. The NADESs and the molar ratio which were applied were betaine/ethylene glycol (Bet:EG) (1:3), betaine/glycerol (Bet:Gly) (1:2), and glycerol/glucose (Gly:Glu) (4:1). The water content of NADES was determined using Karl-Fischer titration using an 831 KF Coulometer with generator electrode (Metrohm, Herisau, Switzerland) and it was below 1% for all NADES. Measurements were conducted in triplicates.

3.3. Extraction Procedure

3.3.1. Supercritical Carbon Dioxide Extraction

Supercritical CO_2 extraction was carried out in a lab-scale apparatus with the following specifications: pneumatic pump (Williams P250V300), mass flow meter (Rheonik RHM 007), tubular extractor (316SS; 570 mm length, 24 mm I.D.; HiP), back-pressure regulator (Tescom Europe, model 26–1700, Selmsdorf, Germany), and separator (Swagelok 316L-HDF4-500). The extractions were performed using 30 g of plant material under the following conditions: pressure 200 bar, temperature 40 °C, extraction time 3 h, and CO_2 flow 20 g/min (total amount of used CO_2 4470.87 ± 31.85 g). All experiments were performed in triplicates. The parameters of extraction were selected based on the previously conducted experimental work [21]. The obtained extracts were stored at 4 °C until further analysis.

3.3.2. Ultrasound-Assisted Extraction with Deep Eutectic Solvents

Plant material after supercritical CO_2 extraction (residue) and non-residue material (control) were used for ultrasound-assisted NADES extraction. The material was mixed with different NADES in a ratio of 1:20 (plant material:NADES; *w/w*). Ultrasound-assisted extractions were carried out at temperatures 30 and 60 °C, for 30 min, with an ultrasonic power of 100 W, and frequency of 50–60 Hz (Grant XUB5, UK). Extractions were conducted in cycles of 15 min, with stirring in a vortex for 1 min between cycles to speed up the extraction, according to Vieira et al. [52]. Flasks were positioned in the same position in the ultrasound bath during each extraction. After extraction, filtration was performed, and the obtained extracts were stored at 4 °C until further analyses. Extractions were performed in triplicates.

3.4. Gas Chromatography-Mass Spectrometry (GC-MS) Analysis

An Agilent 8890 gas chromatograph (Agilent Technologies, Palo Alto, CA, USA) connected to a mass spectrometer (series 5977E, Agilent Technologies, Palo Alto, CA, USA) was used for the analysis. The components of *L. stoechas* lipophilic extracts were separated on an HP-5MS capillary column (30 m × 0.25 mm, 0.25 μm, Agilent Technologies, Palo Alto, CA, USA). The injector temperature was set at 250 °C with the injected sample of 3 μL in a split mode of 1:50. Helium of 99.99% purity was used as a carrier gas in a constant flow regime of 1 mL/min. The following temperature program was set at 70 °C (2 min) which was increased by 3 °C/min to reach 200 °C and maintained at constant temperature for 15 min. The separated components were analyzed with mass spectrometry (70 eV) with a scanning m/z range of 30–300. The injector and detector temperatures were 250 °C and 300 °C, respectively. Qualitative identification of the compounds was performed using Wiley 9 (Wiley, New York, NY, USA) and NIST 17 (National Institute of Standards and Technology, Gaithersburg, MD, USA) mass spectral libraries as well as literature data of retention indices calculated with C9–C25 alkanes. The analysis of each sample was performed in three replicates and the results are expressed as mean data.

3.5. High-Performance Liquid Chromatography (HPLC)

Determination of polyphenolic components was performed by high-performance liquid chromatography (HPLC) method with UV detection, on Cosmosil 5C18-MS-II column (Nacalai Tesque, Inc., Kyoto, Japan), 250 mm long with an internal diameter of 4.6 mm, filled with 5 μm particles. The HPLC system used for the analysis (Agilent, 1260 Infinity II series) consisted of a quaternary pump (G7111A), a column chamber (G7116A), a photodiode array detector (G7115A), an autosampler (G7157A), and a fraction collector (G1364E). The system was operated using the computer program Prep LC Online.

The separation of analyzed compounds was performed by using gradient elution for 50 min with 1% CH_3COOH (in Milli-Q water) as phase A and methanol as phase B, with an initial ratio of A:B as 80:20. The gradient conditions were: 0–5 min 80% of A, 5–15 min 80–40% of A, 15–35 min holding 20% of A, 35–40 min 20–40% of A, 40–50 min 40–80% of A. During the analysis, the flow rate was 1.0 mL min^{-1}, temperature at 25 °C, and detection at 250, 300, 320, and 360 nm. The injection volume of samples was 20 μL.

The standard stock solution for components (ellagic acid, ferulic acid, syringic acid, sinapic acid, caffeic acid, gallic acid, chlorogenic acid, neochlorogenic acid, cryptochlorogenic acid, rutin, myricetin, kaempferol-3-rutinoside, quercetin, luteolin, herniarin, coumarin) was prepared in methanol. The compound ellagic acid was calibrated at 250 nm, compounds ferulic acid, syringic acid, sinapic acid, and coumarin were calibrated at 300 nm, while caffeic acid and herniarin were detected at 320 nm and rutin at 360 nm. The calibration for ellagic acid was obtained at seven concentrations (5–100 mg/L), for caffeic acid at seven concentration (10–1000 mg/L), for ferulic acid at seven concentrations (10–500 mg/L), for syringic acid at eight concentrations (10–1000 mg/L), for sinapic acid at seven concentrations (10–500 mg/L), for rutin at seven concentration (10–500 mg/L), for herniarin at eight concentrations (10–200 mg/L) and for coumarin at eight concentrations

(10–150 mg/L). The linearity of the calibration curve was confirmed by R^2 = 0.99850 for caffeic acid, R^2 = 0.99993 for syringic acid, R^2 = 0.99922 for sinapic acid, R^2 = 0.99975 for ferulic acid, R^2 = 0.99665 for coumarin, R^2 = 0.99842 for rutin, R^2 = 0.99796 for ellagic acid, and R^2 = 0.99991 for herniarin. The retention time for caffeic acid was 14.376 min, for syringic acid 14.500 min, for sinapic acid 17.300 min, for ferulic acid 17.500 min, for coumarin 18.085 min, for rutin 19.034 min, for ellagic acid 19.726 min, and for herniarin 19.931 min. The limit of detection (LOD) was as follows: caffeic acid 0.15 mg/L, syringic acid 0.71 mg/L, sinapic acid 0.45 mg/L, ferulic acid 0.34 mg/L, coumarin 0.62 mg/L, rutin 0.30 mg/L, ellagic acid 1.63 mg/L, and herniarin 1.40 mg/L. The limit of quantification (LOQ) was for caffeic acid 0.46 mg/L, syringic acid 2.17 mg/L, sinapic acid 1.37 mg/L, ferulic acid 1.03 mg/L, coumarin 1.88 mg/L, for rutin 0.91 mg/L, for ellagic acid 4.95 mg/L, and for herniarin 5.31 mg/L. The sample analysis was performed in duplicate, and two injections were performed from each prepared solution. The compounds contained in the analyzed samples were expressed in μg/mL of extract. Gallic acid, chlorogenic acid, neochlorogenic acid, cryptochlorogenic acid, myricetin, kaempferol -3-rutinoside, quercetin, and luteolin were not identified in the extracts.

3.6. Determination of Antioxidant Activity

3.6.1. DPPH Assay

The antioxidant activity of extracts was analyzed using the 2,2-diphenyl-1-picrylhydrazyl (DPPH) assay [53]. Different volumes of extracts were mixed with 95% methanol solution and 90 μM DPPH solution. After the 60-min incubation period at room temperature, absorption was measured at a wavelength of 515 nm (6300 Spectrophotometer, Jenway, Dunmow, UK). The antioxidant activity was expressed as IC_{50} (mg/mL) value which represents the concentration of the extract which inhibits 50% DPPH radicals. All measurements were performed in triplicate.

3.6.2. ABTS Assay

The 2,2′-azino-bis(3-ethylbenzothiazoline-6-sulfonic acid (ABTS) assay was performed according to Miller et al. [54] method. ABTS and potassium persulfate were dissolved in distilled water to a final concentration of 7 mM and 2.45 mM, respectively. These two solutions were mixed and the mixture was left at room temperature in a dark space for 12 h. The ABTS+ solution was diluted with distilled water to an absorbance of 0.700 ± 0.02 at 732 nm. Samples were added to diluted ABTS+ solution and the absorbance was measured at 3 min (732 nm) after mixing using a spectrophotometer (6300 Spectrophotometer, Jenway, Dunmow, UK). All measurements were performed in triplicates and the results were expressed as IC_{50} (mg/mL).

3.6.3. FRAP Assay

The ferric ion-reducing antioxidant power (FRAP) of the samples was determined according to the assay based on the reduction of Fe^{3+} [55]. Different dilutions of liquid extract were mixed with phosphate buffer (0.2 M, pH 6.6) and 1% potassium ferricyanide in glass tubes. Tubes were incubated at 50 °C for 20 min. After incubation, 10% trichloroacetic acid solution was added to the reaction mixture. Tubes were then centrifuged at 3000 rpm for 10 min and supernatant was further mixed with double distilled water and 0.1% ferric chloride solution. Absorbance was measured at 700 nm (6300 Spectrophotometer, Jenway, Dunmow, UK). Antioxidant activity was further expressed as IC_{50} value (mg/mL), which causes a reduction of 50% Fe^{3+} ions. All experiments were performed in triplicates, and the results are expressed as mean values.

3.7. Determination of Antibacterial Activity

The determination of minimal inhibitory concentrations (MIC) of obtained extracts was performed by modified broth microdilution method in Mueller Hinton Broth (Fluka, BioChemica, Germany) according to Clinical Laboratory and Standard Institute (CLSI)

M7-A7 document [56]. Bacteria were collected from different clinical samples obtained from the Microbiological Service of the Public Health Institute of Osijek-Baranja County, Croatia. *Bacillus subtilis*, *Staphylococcus aureus*, *Escherichia coli*, and *Pseudomonas aeruginosa* previously cultured on Mueller Hinton agar were suspended in saline at a density standardized to 0.5 McFarland standard turbidity and added to 100 μL of two-fold serially diluted obtained extracts. Each plate contained a growth control (bacterial inoculum without extracts), background control (broth and ethanol), and the antibacterial standard ciprofloxacin (Hospira, Hurley, Maidenhead, Berkshire, England, UK). After incubation at 37 °C for 24 h, another incubation at 37 °C for three hours was performed using triphenyltetrazolium chloride as a reducing agent indicator for microbial growth. The MIC was defined as the lowest extract concentration at which no color change due to microbial growth occurred, derived from triplicate analyses and normalized against the negative control.

3.8. Statistical Analysis

All analyses were carried out in triplicate and the results were expressed as means ± standard deviation (SD). Mean values were considered significantly different at a $p < 0.05$ confidence level, after the performance of the one-way ANOVA statistical analysis followed by Tukey's HSD post hoc test. Pearson's correlation coefficients (0.05 level; 2-tailed) were calculated in GraphPad Prism 8.0.1.

4. Conclusions

In this study, a sustainable procedure for using the plant resource *L. stoechas* was established. By combining the sequential application of supercritical CO_2 and NADES with ultrasound-assisted extraction, the attainment of extracts rich in terpenes and polyphenols with significant antioxidant and antibacterial activity was achieved. Among NADES extracts, the highest polyphenolic content, as well as antioxidant activity, were determined in Bet:EG extracts. These extracts further exhibited significant antibacterial activity against bacteria, with the inhibitory activity being more pronounced against Gram-positive bacteria compared to Gram-negative. In comparison with conventional solvents, water, and ethanol, Bet:EG proved to be superior in terms of polyphenolic content as well as biological activities. Additionally, the supercritical extract, rich in oxygenated terpenes, also exhibited significant activity. Furthermore, the components identified in the obtained extracts also possess other confirmed biological properties and potential applications, hence these extracts can be used in other pharmaceutical, food, and cosmetic-related products. Due to their aromatic properties, they are very important constituents in the fragrance and perfume industries. The approach established in this study to obtain *L. stoechas* extracts represents the development of products in line with the principles of green and sustainable development and can successfully respond to the increased green consumerism. Extracts have the potential in the strategy of sustaining life and promoting good health, through roles in addressing AMR, as well as controlling foodborne diseases.

Supplementary Materials: The following supporting information can be downloaded at: https://www.mdpi.com/article/10.3390/antibiotics12061031/s1, Table S1: HPLC analysis of *Lavandula stoechas* extracts obtained with NADES. Results are expressed in μg/mL.

Author Contributions: Conceptualization, J.V. and A.R.D.; methodology; software, J.V. and I.J.; validation I.J.; formal analysis, J.V. and S.J.; investigation, J.V., I.J., M.J.K., V.P. and S.S.; resources, J.V., S.J. and V.P.; writing—original draft preparation, J.V.; writing—review and editing, I.J., A.R.D. and A.P.; visualization, J.V.; supervision, A.R.D.; project administration, J.V. and A.R.D.; funding acquisition, J.V. and A.R.D. All authors have read and agreed to the published version of the manuscript.

Funding: This project has received funding from the European Union's Horizon 2020 research and innovation program under the Marie Sklodowska-Curie grant agreement No 101003396. The biological activity has been supported by research ID: 3105-12-21.

Institutional Review Board Statement: Not applicable.

Informed Consent Statement: Not applicable.

Data Availability Statement: Not applicable.

Acknowledgments: The authors would like to thank Ana Jovanoski for her editorial support.

Conflicts of Interest: The authors declare no conflict of interest.

References

1. The Lancet. Antimicrobial resistance: Time to repurpose the Global Fund. *Lancet* **2022**, *399*, 335. [CrossRef] [PubMed]
2. WHO; FAO; OIE. *Antimicrobial Resistance and the United Nations Sustainable Development Cooperation Framework: Guidance for United Nations*; World Health Organization (WHO): Geneva, Switzerland; Food and Agriculture Organization of the United Nations (FAO): Rome, Italy; World Organisation for Animal Health (OIE): Paris, France, 2021.
3. Algieri, F.; Rodriguez-Nogales, A.; Vezza, T.; Garrido-Mesa, J.; Garrido-Mesa, N.; Pilar Utrilla, M.; González-Tejero, R.; Casares-Porcel, M.; Molero-Mesa, J.; Mar Contreras, M.; et al. Anti-inflammatory activity of hydroalcoholic extracts of *Lavandula dentate* L. and *Lavandula stoechas* L. *J. Ethnopharmacol.* **2016**, *190*, 142–158. [CrossRef] [PubMed]
4. Gilani, A.H.; Aziz, N.; Khan, M.A.; Shaheen, F.; Jabeen, Q.; Siddiqui, B.S.; Herzig, J.W. Ethnopharmacological evaluation of the anticonvulsant, sedative and antispasmodic activities of *Lavandula stoechas* L. *J. Ethnopharmacol.* **2000**, *71*, 161–167. [CrossRef] [PubMed]
5. Ezzoubi, Y.; Bousta, D.; Lachkar, M.; Farah, A. Antioxidant and anti-inflammatory properties of ethanolic extract of *Lavandula stoechas* L. from Taounate region in Morocco. *Int. J. Phytopharm.* **2014**, *5*, 21–26.
6. Angioni, A.; Barra, A.; Coroneo, V.; Dessi, S.; Cabras, P. Chemical composition, seasonal variability, and antifungal activity of *Lavandula stoechas* L. ssp stoechas essential oils from stem/leaves and flowers. *J. Agric. Food Chem.* **2006**, *54*, 4364–4370.
7. Dob, T.; Dahmane, D.; Agli, M.; Chelghoum, C. Essential oil composition of *Lavandula stoechas* from Algeria. *Pharm. Biol.* **2006**, *44*, 60–64. [CrossRef]
8. Gören, A.C.; Topçu, G.; Bilsel, G.; Bilsel, M.; Aydoğmusç, Z.; Pezzuto, J.M. The chemical constituents and biological activity of essential oil of *Lavandula stoechas* ssp. stoechas. *Z. Nat. C* **2002**, *57*, 797–800. [CrossRef]
9. Ceylan, Y.; Usta, K.; Usta, A.; Maltas, E.; Yildiz, S. Evaluation of antioxidant activity, phytochemicals and ESR analysis of *Lavandula stoechas*. *Acta Phys. Pol. A* **2015**, *128*, 483–487. [CrossRef]
10. Knez, Ž.; Markočič, E.; Leitgeb, M.; Primožič, M.; Hrnčič, M.K.; Škerget, M. Industrial applications of supercritical fluids: A review. *Energy* **2014**, *77*, 235–243. [CrossRef]
11. Gaspar, F.; Santos, R.; King, M.B. Disruption of glandular trichomes with compressed CO_2: Alternative matrix pre-treatment for CO_2 extraction of essential oils. *J. Supercrit. Fluids* **2001**, *21*, 11–22. [CrossRef]
12. Meyer, F.; Jaeger, P.; Eggers, R.; Stamenic, M.; Milovanovic, S.; Zizovic, I. Effect of CO_2 pre-treatment on $scCO_2$ extraction of natural material. *Chem. Eng. Process.* **2012**, *56*, 37–45. [CrossRef]
13. Gouveia, L.; Jazić, J.M.; Ferreira, A.; Maletić, S.; Cvetković, D.; Vidović, S.; Vladić, J. Green approach for the valorization of microalgae *Tetradesmus obliquus*. *Sustain. Chem. Pharm.* **2021**, *24*, 100556. [CrossRef]
14. Topal, U.; Sasaki, M.; Goto, M.; Otles, S. Chemical compositions and antioxidant properties of essential oils from nine species of Turkish plants obtained by supercritical carbon dioxide extraction and steam distillation. *Int. J. Food Sci. Nutr.* **2008**, *59*, 619–634. [CrossRef]
15. Akgün, M.; Akgün, N.A.; Dinçer, S. Extraction and modeling of lavender flower essential oil using supercritical carbon dioxide. *Ind. Eng. Chem.* **2000**, *39*, 473–477. [CrossRef]
16. Akgün, N.A.; Akgün, M.; Dinçer, S.; Akgerman, A. Supercritical fluid extraction of *Lavandula stoechas* L. ssp. cariensis (Boiss.) Rozeira. *J. Essent. Oil Res.* **2001**, *13*, 143–148. [CrossRef]
17. Marongiu, B.; Piras, A.; Porcedda, S.; Falconieri, D.; Maxia, A.; Frau, M.A.; Molicotti, P.; Zanetti, S. Composition and biological activity of supercritical CO_2 extract of some Lamiaceae growing wild in Sardinia (Italy). *J. Essent. Oil Bear. Plants* **2010**, *13*, 625–632. [CrossRef]
18. Li, G.; Row, K.H. Utilization of deep eutectic solvents in dispersive liquid-liquid micro-extraction. *TrAC Trends Anal. Chem.* **2019**, *120*, 115651. [CrossRef]
19. Liu, Y.; Friesen, J.B.; McAlpine, J.B.; Lankin, D.C.; Chen, S.N.; Pauli, G.F. Natural deep eutectic solvents: Properties, applications, and perspectives. *J. Nat. Prod.* **2018**, *81*, 679–690. [CrossRef]
20. Cao, J.; Su, E. Hydrophobic deep eutectic solvents: The new generation of green solvents for diversified and colorful applications in green chemistry. *J. Clean. Prod.* **2021**, *314*, 127965. [CrossRef]
21. Vladić, J.; Jerković, I.; Svilović, S.; Pavić, V.; Pastor, K.; Paiva, A.; Jokić, S.; Rebocho, S.; Duarte, A.R. Evaluation of the volatiles' chemical profile and antibacterial activity of *Lavandula stoechas* L. extracts obtained by supercritical carbon dioxide. *Sustain. Chem. Pharm.* **2023**, *33*, 101126. [CrossRef]
22. Kumar, K.; Srivastav, S.; Sharanagat, V.S. Ultrasound assisted extraction (UAE) of bioactive compounds from fruit and vegetable processing by-products: A review. *Ultrason. Sonochem.* **2021**, *70*, 105325. [CrossRef] [PubMed]
23. Lavilla, I.; Bendicho, C. Fundamentals of ultrasound-assisted extraction. In *Water Extraction of Bioactive Compounds*; Dominguez González, H., González Muñoz, M.J., Eds.; Elsevier: Amsterdam, The Netherlands, 2017; pp. 291–316.

24. Vladić, J.; Kovačević, K.; Rebocho, S.; Paiva, A.; Jokić, S.; Duarte, A.R.; Jerković, I. Towards a new approach for green aroma stabilisation: Supercritical CO_2 extracts of *Lavandula stoechas* dispersed in natural deep eutectic solvents. *Sci. Rep.* 2023; *submitted*.
25. Mansinhos, I.; Gonçalves, S.; Rodríguez-Solana, R.; Ordóñez-Díaz, J.L.; Moreno-Rojas, J.M.; Romano, A. Ultrasonic-assisted extraction and natural deep eutectic solvents combination: A green strategy to improve the recovery of phenolic compounds from *Lavandula pedunculata* subsp. *lusitanica* (chaytor) franco. *Antioxidants* **2021**, *10*, 582. [CrossRef] [PubMed]
26. Fadil, M.; Lebrazi, S.; Aboulghazi, A.; Guaouguaou, F.E.; Rais, C.; Slimani, C.; Es-safi, N.E. Multi-response optimization of extraction yield, total phenols-flavonoids contents, and antioxidant activity of extracts from Moroccan *Lavandula stoechas* leaves: Predictive modeling using simplex-centroid design. *Biocatal. Agric. Biotechnol.* **2022**, *43*, 102430. [CrossRef]
27. Beghlal, D.; El Bairi, K.; Marmouzi, I.; Haddar, L.; Mohamed, B. Phytochemical, organoleptic and ferric reducing properties of essential oil and ethanolic extract from *Pistacia lentiscus* (L.). *Asian Pac. J. Trop. Dis.* **2016**, *6*, 305–310. [CrossRef]
28. Munteanu, I.G.; Apetrei, C. Analytical methods used in determining antioxidant activity: A review. *Int. J. Mol. Sci.* **2021**, *22*, 3380. [CrossRef]
29. Pulido, R.; Bravo, L.; Saura-Calixto, F. Antioxidant activity of dietary polyphenols as determined by a modified ferric reducing/antioxidant power assay. *J. Agric. Food Chem.* **2000**, *48*, 3396–3402. [CrossRef]
30. Brand-Williams, W.; Cuvelier, M.E.; Berset, C. Use of a free radical method to evaluate antioxidant activity. *LWT Food Sci. Technol.* **1995**, *28*, 25–30. [CrossRef]
31. Wang, W.; Goodman, M.T. Antioxidant property of dietary phenolic agents in a human LDL-oxidation ex vivo model: Interaction of protein binding activity. *Nutr. Res.* **1999**, *19*, 191–202. [CrossRef]
32. Srinivasulu, C.; Ramgopal, M.; Ramanjaneyulu, G.; Anuradha, C.M.; Kumar, C.S. Syringic acid (SA)—A review of its occurrence, biosynthesis, pharmacological and industrial importance. *Biomed. Pharmacother.* **2018**, *108*, 547–557. [CrossRef]
33. Marinova, E.M.; Yanishlieva, N.V. Antioxidant activity and mechanism of action of some phenolic acids at ambient and high temperatures. *Food Chem.* **2003**, *81*, 189–197. [CrossRef]
34. Sánchez-Moreno, C.; Larrauri, J.A.; Saura-Calixto, F. A procedure to measure the antiradical efficiency of polyphenols. *J. Sci. Food Agric.* **1998**, *76*, 270–276. [CrossRef]
35. Borges Bubols, G.; da Rocha Vianna, D.; Medina-Remon, A.; von Poser, G.; Maria Lamuela-Raventos, R.; Lucia Eifler-Lima, V.; Cristina Garcia, S. The antioxidant activity of coumarins and flavonoids. *Mini Rev. Med. Chem.* **2013**, *13*, 318–334.
36. Bouyahya, A.; Et-Touys, A.; Abrini, J.; Talbaoui, A.; Fellah, H.; Bakri, Y.; Dakka, N. *Lavandula stoechas* essential oil from Morocco as novel source of antileishmanial, antibacterial and antioxidant activities. *Biocatal. Agric. Biotechnol.* **2017**, *12*, 179–184. [CrossRef]
37. Bouzouita, N.; Kachouri, F.; Hamdi, M.; Chaabouni, M.M. Volatile constituents and antimicrobial activity of *Lavandula stoechas* L. oil from Tunisia. *J. Essent. Oil Res.* **2005**, *17*, 584–586. [CrossRef]
38. Cherrat, L.; Espina, L.; Bakkali, M.; Pagán, R.; Laglaoui, A. Chemical composition, antioxidant and antimicrobial properties of *Mentha pulegium*, *Lavandula stoechas* and *Satureja calamintha* Scheele essential oils and an evaluation of their bactericidal effect in combined processes. *Innov. Food Sci. Emerg. Technol.* **2014**, *22*, 221–229. [CrossRef]
39. Burt, S. Essential oils: Their antibacterial properties and potential applications in foods—A review. *Int. J. Food Microbiol.* **2004**, *94*, 223–253. [CrossRef]
40. Ez zoubi, Y.; Farah, A.; Zaroual, H.; El Ouali Lalami, A. Antimicrobial activity of *Lavandula stoechas* phenolic extracts against pathogenic bacteria isolated from a hospital in Morocco. *Vegetos* **2020**, *33*, 703–711. [CrossRef]
41. Al-Niaame, A.E.; Aziz, R.A. Study of *Lavandula officinalis* L. buds of flowers extracts activity against some species of multi-drug resistant clinical isolates of bacteria. *Iraqi J. Biotechnol.* **2013**, *12*, 82–91.
42. De Oliveira, F.S.N.; Duarte, A.R.C. A look on target-specificity of eutectic systems based on natural bioactive compounds. In *Advances in Botanical Research*; Kuete, V., Ed.; Academic Press: Cambridge, MA, USA, 2021; Volume 97, pp. 271–307.
43. Guimarães, A.C.; Meireles, L.M.; Lemos, M.F.; Guimarães, M.C.C.; Endringer, D.C.; Fronza, M.; Scherer, R. Antibacterial activity of terpenes and terpenoids present in essential oils. *Molecules* **2019**, *24*, 2471. [CrossRef]
44. Tijjani, H.; Danyaro, A.M.; Olatunde, A.; Kura, A.U. Antihyperglycemic activity of verbenone and L-arginine in nicotinamide-streptozotocin-induced diabetic mice: In vitro and in vivo studies. *Beni Suef Univ. J. Basic Appl. Sci.* **2022**, *11*, 94. [CrossRef]
45. Souza Pessoa, M.L.; Silva, L.M.O.; Araruna, M.E.C.; de Lima Serafim, C.A.; Júnior, E.B.A.; Silva, A.O.; Pessoa, M.M.B.; Neto, H.D.; Oliveira Lima, E.O.; Batista, L.M. Antifungal activity and antidiarrheal activity via antimotility mechanisms of (-)-fenchone in experimental models. *World J. Gastroenterol.* **2020**, *26*, 6795. [CrossRef]
46. Him, A.; Ozbek, H.; Turel, I.; Oner, A.C. Antinociceptive activity of alpha-pinene and fenchone. *Pharmacologyonline* **2008**, *3*, 363–369.
47. Zhang, Q.L.; Fu, B.M.; Zhang, Z.J. Borneol, a novel agent that improves central nervous system drug delivery by enhancing blood–brain barrier permeability. *Drug Deliv.* **2017**, *24*, 1037–1044. [CrossRef] [PubMed]
48. Kong, Q.; Wu, Z.; Chu, X.; Liang, R.; Xia, M.; Li, L. Study on the anti-cerebral ischemia effect of borneol and its mechanism. *Afr. J. Tradit. Complement. Altern. Med.* **2014**, *11*, 161–164. [CrossRef]
49. Yang, H.; Zhao, R.; Chen, H.; Jia, P.; Bao, L.; Tang, H. Bornyl acetate has an anti-inflammatory effect in human chondrocytes via induction of IL-11. *IUBMB Life* **2014**, *66*, 854–859. [CrossRef]
50. Trevizan, L.N.F.; do Nascimento, K.F.; Santos, J.A.; Kassuya, C.A.L.; Cardoso, C.A.L.; do Carmo Vieira, M.; Moreira, F.M.F.; Croda, J.; Formagio, A.S.N. Anti-inflammatory, antioxidant and anti-*Mycobacterium tuberculosis* activity of viridiflorol: The major constituent of *Allophylus edulis* (A. St.-Hil., A. Juss. & Cambess.) Radlk. *J. Ethnopharmacol.* **2016**, *192*, 510–515.

51. Lefebvre, T.; Destandau, E.; Lesellier, E. Selective extraction of bioactive compounds from plants using recent extraction techniques: A review. *J. Chromatogr. A* **2021**, *1635*, 461770. [CrossRef]
52. Vieira, C.; Rebocho, S.; Craveiro, R.; Paiva, A.; Duarte, A.R.C. Selective extraction and stabilization of bioactive compounds from rosemary leaves using a biphasic NADES. *Front. Chem.* **2022**, *10*, 954835. [CrossRef]
53. Espín, J.C.; Soler-Rivas, C.; Wichers, H.J. Characterization of the total free radical scavenger capacity of vegetable oils and oil fractions using 2,2-diphenyl-1-picrylhydrazyl radical. *J. Agric. Food Chem.* **2000**, *48*, 648–656. [CrossRef]
54. Miller, N.J.; Rice-Evans, C.; Davies, M.J.; Gopinathan, V.; Milner, A. A novel method for measuring antioxidant capacity and its application to monitoring the antioxidant status in premature neonates. *Clin. Sci.* **1993**, *84*, 407–412. [CrossRef]
55. Oyaizu, M. Studies on products of browning reaction: Antioxidant activities of products of browning reaction prepared from glucosamine. *Jpn. J. Nutr.* **1986**, *44*, 307–315. [CrossRef]
56. Weinstein, M.P.; Patel, J.B. *Methods for Dilution Antimicrobial Susceptibility Tests for Bacteria That Grow Aerobically: M07-A11*, 11th ed.; Clinical and Laboratory Standards Institute: Wayne, PA, USA, 2018.

antibiotics

MDPI

Article

Artificial Neural Network Prediction of Antiadhesion and Antibiofilm-Forming Effects of Antimicrobial Active Mushroom Extracts on Food-Borne Pathogens

Jovana Vunduk [1], Anita Klaus [2], Vesna Lazić [2], Maja Kozarski [2], Danka Radić [1], Olja Šovljanski [3] and Lato Pezo [1,*]

[1] Institute of General and Physical Chemistry, Studenski trg 10-12, 11 158 Belgrade, Serbia
[2] Institute for Food Technology and Biochemistry, Faculty of Agriculture, University of Belgrade, Nemanjina 6, 11 080 Belgrade, Serbia
[3] Faculty of Technology Novi Sad, University of Novi Sad, Bulevar Cara Lazara 1, 21 000 Novi Sad, Serbia
* Correspondence: latopezo@yahoo.co.uk

Abstract: The problem of microbial biofilms has come to the fore alongside food, pharmaceutical, and healthcare industrialization. The development of new antibiofilm products has become urgent, but it includes bioprospecting and is time and money-consuming. Contemporary efforts are directed at the pursuit of effective compounds of natural origin, also known as "green" agents. Mushrooms appear to be a possible new source of antibiofilm compounds, as has been demonstrated recently. The existing modeling methods are directed toward predicting bacterial biofilm formation, not in the presence of antibiofilm materials. Moreover, the modeling is almost exclusively targeted at biofilms in healthcare, while modeling related to the food industry remains under-researched. The present study applied an Artificial Neural Network (ANN) model to analyze the anti-adhesion and anti-biofilm-forming effects of 40 extracts from 20 mushroom species against two very important food-borne bacterial species for food and food-related industries—*Listeria monocytogenes* and *Salmonella enteritidis*. The models developed in this study exhibited high prediction quality, as indicated by high r^2 values during the training cycle. The best fit between the modeled and measured values was observed for the inhibition of adhesion. This study provides a valuable contribution to the field, supporting industrial settings during the initial stage of biofilm formation, when these communities are the most vulnerable, and promoting innovative and improved safety management.

Keywords: antiadhesion; antibiofilm; food-borne pathogens; mushroom extracts; artificial neural network; model

1. Introduction

In December 2021 the Dole company from the USA recalled its iceberg lettuce and any finished products containing it. A Food and Drug Administration (FDA) and Center for Disease Control (CDC) investigation showed that 18 people from 13 states ended up infected with *L. monocytogenes* found in Dole's salad [1]. The traces led to the harvesting equipment. The same company has been involved in *L. monocytogenes* outbreaks in the past because the biofilm this food-borne pathogen produces enables it to stick to processing equipment. Hudson Valley Farms recalled their nuts and nut butter products because of the same problem of *Listeria* biofilm [2]. Although both companies practiced HACCP, which recognizes bacteria-connected critical points, this safety system does not necessarily include biofilm prevention measures or eradication. Similarly, most of the research focuses on species that form biofilms within the food industry, leaving the associated biofilm out of the investigations [3]. It has been pointed out that there is an existing gap between industrial practices and academic research on biofilms [4]. The focus has been mainly on fundamental knowledge regarding biofilms, while applicable solutions (beyond physico-chemical measures) for the industry are lacking. Biofilms are a common enemy across the food industry; they can be encountered in dairy, meat, ready-to-eat food, baby food, water, juices, or product manufacturing facilities. Nutrients; moisture; hard-to-reach, clean, and sanitize areas; and cross-contamination enable the growth of pathogenic bacteria followed by their adhesion to surfaces, biofilm-formation, maturation, and dispersal [5]. One outcome of this is bacterial infections, intoxications, food safety and quality deterioration, and manufacturing equipment corrosion [6]. The most common sanitation measures include different chemical agents such as chlorine-based sanitizers, hydrogen peroxide, ozone, quaternary ammonium compounds, salicylate-based polyanhydride esters, and synthetic brominated furanone [7]. However, they are not effective enough at all times because bacteria develop resistance. The presence of biofilms within meat processing facilities has been assessed previously, and it has been discovered that among 108 samples collected during processing and after cleaning and disinfection, 10 were biofilm hotspots [3]. Three originated after the cleaning and disinfection. This proves that innovation is urgently needed in this sector. It has also been emphasized that society needs to move toward "green" antibiofilm agents because conventional methods of biofilm control can cause the emergence of resistance and are costly and have low efficiency, while at the same time they can have a negative impact on human health and the environment [8]. Novel approaches consider the use of bacteriophages, bacteriocins, enzymes, essential oils, and substances known as quorum-sensing inhibitors [9]. There are even fewer compounds that can inhibit biofilm formation without exhibiting antimicrobial activity at the same time. Among substances of natural origin, most are phytochemicals such as carvacrol, hordenin, ginkgolic acid, epigallocatechin-3-gallate, isosteviol, phytol, curcumin, tannic acid, and 3,3′-diindolylmethane, to name a few [10–12].

Plants are already well-known and traditionally used sources of antimicrobial and antibiofilm compounds. Different parts, such as leaf, root, fruit, or peel, are rich in antibiofilm compounds, as has been demonstrated recently using the simple and cheap crystal violet staining method [13]. Recently, mushrooms became an interesting source of antimicrobial compounds, though only a few papers have dealt with the antibiofilm activity of mushroom-derived agents [14]. A pioneer work dealing with several methanol–water wild mushroom extracts against biofilms of selected clinical isolates of pathogenic bacteria was published in 2014 [15]. All tested samples exhibited some degree of antibiofilm activity, while at the same time they expressed no cytotoxicity on porcine liver cells. Another group of authors examined aqueous extracts of wild mushrooms and reported antiadhesion activity in the range of 26.6 to 73.7% against several pathogenic bacteria and fungi [16]. Two different groups of researchers isolated several low-molecular-mass compounds from shiitake mushroom and demonstrated their antibacterial and antibiofilm activity (mainly in the adhesion phase) against bacteria involved in caries and gingivitis [17,18]. When it comes to more commercially sustainable materials of mushroom origin, such as mycelium, Vunduk et al. [19] applied submerged cultivation technology to obtain exo- and endo-polysaccharides from *Pleurotus flabellatus* strain Mynuk, which expressed antiadhesion and antibiofilm activity against ATCC and the clinical isolates of several pathogens. Chlorinated orcinol derivate, a compound from the mycelial culture of North American *Hericium* sp. has been demonstrated as an effective agent in the prevention of pathogenic fungi biofilm formation [20]. One should remember that to be applied in the food industry, the substance must not be toxic or poorly soluble [21]. Thus, materials such as polysaccharides from mushrooms, which have been proven as non-cytotoxic against normal human cell lines, whose extracts are water-soluble, or solubility can be improved, are promising antibiofilm agents for the food industry.

As recently cited here, there are several promising compounds of natural origin, and only a scarce number of them have been tested in a clinical setting. According to the database of [22], only a frankincense extract (derived from *Boswellia sacra* Flueck.) got to the clinical trial phase for periodontal diseases [23]. This implies that the path from initial screening to commercial product is long, requires robust analysis, and is costly. On the other hand, the industry needs easy-to-apply, cheap, and innovative solutions. As an outcome of a series of academic–industry knowledge exchange workshops, a number of key challenges have been identified, and improved biofilm analysis methods including artificial intelligence and machine learning are one of them [6]. Shaban and Alkawareek [24] presented a machine learning-based predictive modeling approach for a qualitative prediction of the in vitro antibiofilm activity of antibiotics. However, there are no studies examining the other machine learning options, as well as those for mushroom-derived compounds, which are of interest to the food industry.

Thus, the goal of this study was to apply ANN as a good mathematical tool when there is a high variability of the variables and the nonlinear behavior of process parameters [25], which are all characteristics of bacterial biofilms. Furthermore, ANN systems are successively used in a novel study of the antimicrobial potential of natural-based agents with a high possibility of predicting all connected characteristics of the antimicrobial pathways [26–28].

It should be of significant use in the industrial setting, such as food manufacturing, which cannot deal with time- and resources-consuming assays. The ANN model does not need physical model parameters, but still encompasses a capacity to obtain results from the experimental data and is able to handle the complex system with nonlinearities and to elaborate the interactions between variables [29,30].

2. Results

Considering the aim of testing, a high number of different mushroom extracts was involved in antimicrobial and antibiofilm activity assays; the list of mushroom species, specific extracts, and their abbreviations are given in Table S1 from supplementary materials.

2.1. Antimicrobial Activity

The majority of tested samples exhibited antimicrobial activity toward both strains of food-borne bacteria, with minimal inhibitory concentrations (MIC) being mainly in the range of 10–20 mg/mL (Table 1). Specific sensitivity to mushroom extracts was not observed according to Gram-positive or Gram-negative bacteria. However, none of the samples showed a bactericidal effect when incubated with *S. enteritidis*, while the alkali extract of *Meripilus giganteus* and *Ganoderma lucidum* killed Gram-positive *L. monocytogenes* when the maximal tested concentration (20 mg/mL) was applied. In all cases, except one, the MIC of alkali-extracted samples was lower than the MIC of water extracts. In several cases, there was no difference concerning the method of extraction and antibacterial effect. The strongest inhibition of bacterial growth was recorded in the case of *S. enteritidis* and alkali extracts of *Trametes versicolor* and *Picipes badius* (2.5 mg/mL), while the water extract of *Cratherellus cornucopioides* had the lowest MIC against *L. monocytogenes* (2.5 mg/mL). Extracts derived from polypore species were not more effective than those extracted from the other groups.

2.2. Antiadhesion and Antibiofilm-Forming Activity

Mushroom extracts were able to prevent both bacterial strains' adhesion to a polystyrene surface. The effect was stronger against *L. monocytogenes*, usually between 50 and 60% (Table S2 from supplementary materials). The type of extraction was also significant in several cases where alkali extraction usually gave around 10% better results when applied in the presence of Gram-positive bacteria. In the case of *S. enteritidis*, the % of adhesion inhibition mostly went up to 30. The significant effect of mushroom species was not observed in this case. The effect was concentration-dependent. However, the dependency was not regular; lower concentrations, 0.312–0.625 mg/mL, were the most effective. In general, all extracts had strong activity when incubation took a longer time (48 h), so they expressed biofilm formation inhibition, while antiadhesion activity evolved; approximately 50% antibiofilm-forming effect went up to approximately 100%. Gram-positive bacteria were again slightly more sensitive. Alkali extracts (over 90% of samples) mostly had higher antibiofilm-forming activity, and the effect was concentration-dependent in the same manner as with the antiadhesion activity. The highest tested concentration was the least effective, or even had no effect, while the concentrations in the range of 0.312–0.625 mg/mL had the strongest antibiofilm-forming effect.

Table 1. Antimicrobial activity of mushroom extracts toward *L. monocytogenes* ATCC 19111 and *S. enteritidis* ATCC 13076, expressed as minimal inhibitory concentration (MIC) and minimal bactericidal concentration (MBC) expressed in mg/mL.

	L. monocytogenes		*S. enteritidis*		A Sample	*L. monocytogenes*		*S. enteritidis*	
	MIC	MBC	MIC	MBC		MIC	MBC	MIC	MBC
MgV	20	/	20	/	MgA	10	20	5	/
AsV	/	/	20	/	AsA	10	/	10	/
CcV	10	/	10	/	CcA	2.5	/	10	/
GaV	20	/	20	/	GaA	10	/	5	/
PbV	/	/	/	/	PbA	20	/	10	/
LsV	20	/	/	/	LsA	20	/	20	/
ScV	/	/	/	/	ScA	/	/	/	/
FpV	/	/	20	/	FpA	10	/	10	/
BeV	20	/	20	/	BeA	20	/	20	/
CgV	/	/	/	/	CgA	/	/	20	/
LbV	10	/	20	/	LbA	10	/	10	/
PsV	20	/	/	/	PsA	10	/	5	/
ChcV	/	/	10	/	ChcA	20	/	5	/
AaV	20	/	20	/	AaA	20	/	10	/
TvV	/	/	/	/	TvA	20	/	2.5	/
DqV	20	/	5	/	DqA	10	/	5	/
AmV	20	/	20	/	AmA	10	/	5	/
PibV	10	/	/	/	PibA	5	/	2.5	/
GlV	10	/	20	/	GlA	20	20	5	/
FhV	20	/	20	/	FhA	10	/	10	/
Gentamicin	*L. monocytogenes* MIC < 0.0024 and MBC < 0.0024 *S. enteritidis* MIC < 0.0024 and MBC < 0.0024								

All experiments were performed in triplicate. Standard deviations are not presented because all the repetitions were the same. V—water extract; A—alkali extract.

2.3. *Artificial Neural Network Model*

With an intention to study the non-linear relationship between the anti-adhesion and anti-biofilm-forming effects of 40 extracts from 20 mushroom species against two very important food-borne bacterial species, the ANN technique was used in building the models. The ANN structure (including the biases and weight coefficients) and results depend on the initial presumptions of the matrix parameters, which are vital for ANN building and fitting to experimental data. In addition, the number of neurons in the hidden layer can change the conduct of the ANN model. In order to avoid this issue, each topology was run 100,000 times to avoid random correlation due to initial assumption and random initialization of the weights. According to this approach, the highest r^2 value throughout the training cycle was obtained when the nine hidden neurons were used to build the ANN model (Figure 1a).

The model was trained for 100 epochs, and the training results, i.e., train accuracy and error (loss), are presented in Figure 1b. The training accuracy increased with the number of training cycle increments until the 70–80th epoch, when it reached almost constant value. The highest train accuracy and lowest train loss were detected for the 70–80th epoch, after which a slight train accuracy increase and a train loss decrease were observed due to overfitting. More than 80 epochs for training would possibly cause high overfitting, and 70 epochs would be enough to achieve high model accuracy without any risk of overfitting (Figure 1b).

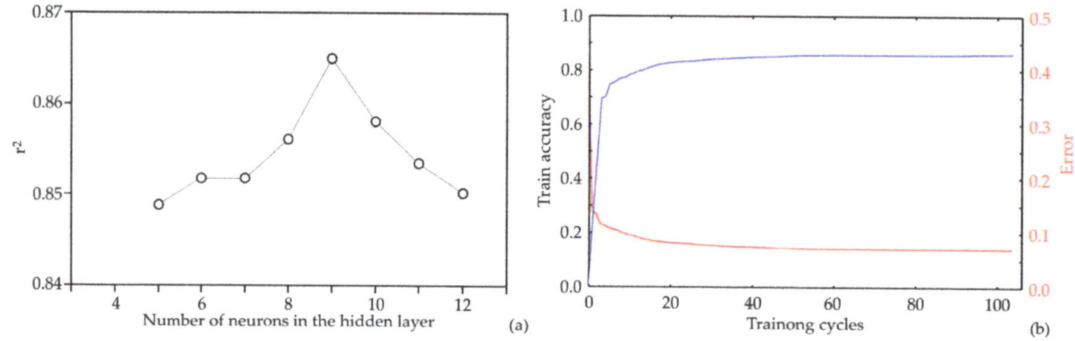

Figure 1. ANN calculation: (**a**) The dependence of the r^2 value of the number of neurons in the hidden layer in the ANN model, (**b**) Training results per epoch.

3. Discussion

3.1. Antimicrobial and Antibiofilm Activity

The antibacterial activity of mushroom-derived compounds or mushroom extracts has been extensively explored and reported for more than two decades. It was a step towards the search for naturally derived antibiotics due to the ever-more present threat of bacterial resistance. As stated by the World Health Organization (WHO) and CDC, microbial resistance presents a global health, development, and economic threat [31,32]. Alves proposed mushroom extracts as an alternative source of new antimicrobials [33]. The authors screened 13 wild mushroom species prepared as aqueous methanolic extracts against clinical isolates of multi-resistant bacteria. Several species turned out to be especially effective, with MIC in the range of 5–20 mg/mL (similar to this study, Table 1). Extracts were more effective against Gram-positive bacteria in which case microbicidal activity was reported, while in the case of Gram-negative species, extracts were bacteriostatic. The same was observed in this and several other studies [34–36]. Phenolic compounds and flavonoids have been marked as the molecules responsible for mushrooms' antimicrobial activity [37]. It has been reported that *Fomitopsis pinicola* possesses several compounds that strongly affect multidrug-resistant bacteria [36]. The same species tested here acted as an inhibitor of bacterial growth, and the alkali extract was more effective (MIC for both tested bacteria was 10 mg/mL). However, it was not the most potent among all 80 tested samples, probably due to the different solvents and bacterial strains used in this study. Concerning the method of extraction, it has been reported that methanol, ethyl acetate, and aqueous extracts accounted for 92.8% of the assays with antibacterial activity [35]. In the same study, aqueous extracts of *Clitocybe geotropa*, together with *Lentinula edodes*, had the highest antimicrobial activity against several tested pathogens. In this study, *C. geotropa* was among the least effective species (both types of extracts), which might be the consequence of the more aggressive extraction procedure applied here, which included high temperature and high pressure. In addition, alkali extraction is an efficient method for cell wall degradation, followed by the transformation of water-insoluble compounds [38]. Thus, the alkali samples were more water soluble and expressed higher antimicrobial activity. The type of solvent applied for mushroom extraction affects the type and concentration of polyphenols, and it has been recently reviewed [39]. For example, the concentration of polyphenols in turkey tail mushrooms extracted with water, ethanol, and methanol differed significantly, with the highest amount measured in the water extract. However, the highest amount of single polyphenol, p-hydroxybenzoic acid, has been confirmed in methanol extract. The overall antibacterial effect was not so strong, while almost all samples exhibited very strong (over 50%) antibiofilm activity. This is not unfounded because it has been proven that polysaccharides from bacteria such as *Escherichia coli* efficiently act as antibiofilm agents toward other pathogenic strains. They are defined as the key competition compounds and are even autoregulatory [40]. Because mushrooms live in a bacteria-loaded environment, such as soil and decaying plant material, it is possible that their compounds, including polysaccharides (which are dominant in the samples examined in this study), have a competitive function. In addition, the environment mushrooms populate is wet and, thus, encouraging biofilm formation [41]. Similarly, another group of researchers demonstrated that the ethanol extract of *Marasmius oreades* had a weak antimicrobial but a significant antibiofilm effect [42].

The problem of bacterial biofilms is well-known in the food industry and is usually treated by chemical and physical methods, which are expensive, hard to perform, vary in stability and thus efficiency, contribute to microbial resistance, and can even jeopardize consumer's health [43,44]. Especially challenging is mature biofilm eradication due to the increase in the structure's resistance; for example, fully formed biofilms are 10 to 1000 times more resistant to antibiotics than planktonic cells [45]. Among many food-borne pathogens, two species were selected, Gram-positive and Gram-negative, to cover principal differences connected with the bacterial structure. In addition, both species are often reported as the cause of food poisoning [7,46,47]. In this study, both adhesion and biofilm formation were prevented in the presence of various mushroom species extracts, and biofilm formation was almost completely stopped in several cases. Klančnik [16] tested crude and purified compounds from mushrooms as potential antibiofilm agents and found that crude extracts are more efficient. The percentage of efficiency, in this case, varied from 26.6 to 73.7, and the samples were stronger inhibitors of fungal biofilms. Here, the focus was on crude instead of more purified extracts because a synergistic effect was expected due to the wide palette of active compounds such as phenolic acids proven to be present in mushrooms [15,48]. The synergistic antibiofilm effect of mushroom extracts has also been reported and demonstrated by other authors [18]. However, it is not always the case, and the effect depends on the exact combination of phenolic acids and other compounds, as well as their concentrations. The same authors reported satisfactory inhibition of biofilm formation of different *L. edodes* extract samples, ranging from 20 to 30%, which is significantly lower than in the present study. They also established dose-dependent activity, although not in all cases. Lower doses when combined had additive outcomes, while higher doses acted antagonistically. The observed effect was attributed to the physicochemical interactions between the compounds in complex extracts. Kavita [49] discussed the antibiofilm activity of extracellular polymeric substances from *Oceanobacillus iheyensis*, noticing a dose-dependent relation up to a specific concentration of tested material. This was also observed in this study, and the cut-off value varied with different samples. In most cases, it was 0.312 or 0.625 mg/mL. Some of the species examined here have already been tested for their antibiofilm activity and reported by other authors, although the bacterial strains were not the same [50]. Their aqueous extract of *B. edulis* had high efficiency in removing the biofilms of *Staphylococcus aureus* and *E. coli* (78 and 94%, respectively), which is in agreement with the findings reported here for water extract of the same fungi species against *L. monocytogenes* and *S. enteritidis* (88 and 87%, respectively). In both studies, the antibiofilm effect of this popular edible mushroom was stronger against Gram-negative bacteria.

Several compounds might be responsible for the antibiofilm effect of mushrooms. Polysaccharides, proteins, peptides, and small water-soluble molecules, such as phenolic compounds, were identified as the responsible active agents [16]. Different authors pointed out that phenolic acids (gallic, ferulic, vanillic, malic, caffeic, and chlorogenic acid) are significant contributors to the antibiofilm activity of mushrooms [15,42]. Gallic, caffeic, and chlorogenic acids inhibit the metabolism of bacterial cells in a biofilm, leading to its disruption [44]. Another often-reported mechanism of the antibiofilm activity of mushrooms is the inhibition of quorum sensing [19,51,52]. Hereby, the focus was not on identifying the compounds responsible for the antibiofilm activity but to screen as many species as possible in order to set up and train a mathematical model capable of predicting the antibiofilm activity of mushrooms. However, previous studies showed that extracts prepared in the way described here mainly consisted of polysaccharides.

In addition, the mushroom extracts tested in this study mostly did not express bactericidal activity, while at the same time demonstrating an antibiofilm-forming effect. Thus, the prospect of building microbial resistance is non-existent or unlikely, which makes this material highly interesting for practical application. Moreover, mushroom polysaccharide extracts are water-soluble and mainly non-toxic, which is not the case with some other highly efficient antibiofilm polysaccharides, such as the ones isolated from non-pathogenic *E. coli* [20].

Although the predictive capabilities of the ANN modeling technique have been tested on different antimicrobial potential setups [26–28,53,54], this study enables the explication of the antiadhesion and antibiofilm-forming characteristics of mushroom extracts for the first time. The targeted physiological characteristics of bacterial cells relevant to the decreasing of food-borne infection have been observed by modest, routine, and repeatable assays. In addition, the mathematical methodology used in this study has been applied for the first time in the experimental investigation of water and alkali extracts of a high number of mushroom species.

3.2. ANN Model

The ANN model showed a good ability to generalize and predict experimental data. Based on its performance, the optimal number of neurons in the hidden layer for predicting the inhibition of adhesion and the inhibition of the biofilm-forming process was found to be 9 (MLP 25-9-2 network), resulting in high values of the coefficient of determination (r^2), with an overall value of 0.856 for the training period, and low values of the sum of squares (SOS), as seen in Table 2.

Table 2. ANN summary (performance and errors), for training, testing, and validation cycles.

Network Name	Performance			Error			Training Algorithm	Error Function	Hidden Activation	Output Activation
	Train.	Test.	Valid.	Train.	Test.	Valid.				
MLP 25-9-2	0.865	0.761	0.747	112.980	178.491	220.136	BFGS 54	SOS	Logistic	Identity

Performance term represent the coefficients of determination, while error terms indicate a lack of data for the ANN model; Train.—training process; Test.—testing process; Valid.—validation process.

Table S3 from supplementary materials presents the elements of matrix W_1 and vector B_1 (presented in the bias row), and Table S4 from supplementary materials presents the elements of matrix W_2 and vector B_2 (bias) for the hidden layer, for the ANN model, which were calculated using Equation (2). The performance of the ANN model was evaluated by comparing its calculated outputs to the experimental measurements, represented as the sum of the coefficient of determination (r^2) between measured and calculated values for the inhibition of adhesion and inhibition of the biofilm-forming process. The results showed that the goodness of fit was 0.894, 0.863, and 0.887 for the training, testing, and validation steps, respectively, for the inhibition of adhesion and 0.856, 0.796, and 0.781 for the inhibition of the biofilm-forming process. The ANN models were able to predict the experimental variables with good accuracy for a wide range of process variables, as seen in Figure 2, which shows the comparison between the experimentally measured and ANN model-predicted values.

The ANN models were highly successful in predicting values that were very close to the desired values, as indicated by the high r^2 value. This is in line with other studies in the literature that have reported similar results for the inhibition of adhesion and inhibition of biofilm-forming processes [55–57]. The ANN model used in this study was complex, with 254 weights and biases, due to the high nonlinearity of the system being investigated [55,58].

During the training period, the r^2 value between the experimental and ANN model outputs was 0.865 for the inhibition of adhesion and inhibition of biofilm-forming processes.

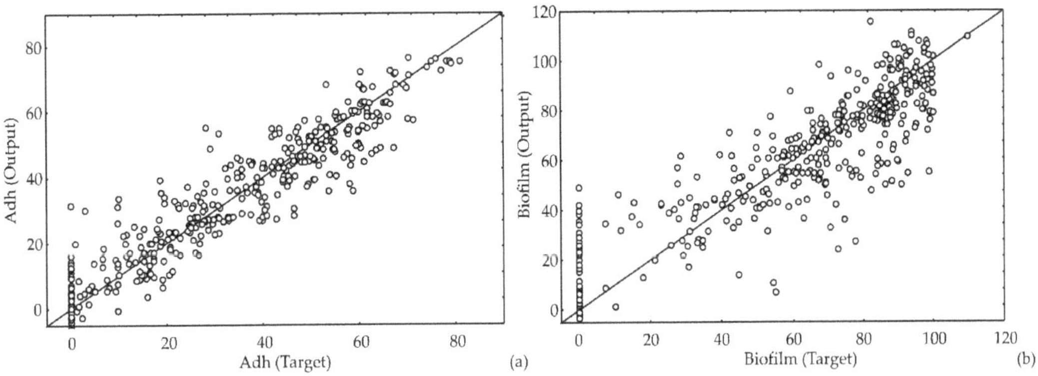

Figure 2. Experimental and predicted values obtained for (**a**) inhibition of adhesion and (**b**) inhibition of the biofilm-forming process.

The quality of the ANN model fit was assessed using χ^2, MBE, RMSE, and MPE values [59], which should be as low as possible. Additionally, a residual analysis was performed to further evaluate the model. Skewness measures the deviation from normal symmetry, and Kurtosis measures the peakedness of a distribution. If the skewness or kurtosis values are clearly different from zero, then the distribution is asymmetrical or more peaked than normal, respectively. A high r^2 value indicates that the variation was accounted for and that the data fit satisfactorily to the proposed model [60,61].

The predicted values were very close to the desired values in most cases, in terms of r^2 value [56].

The fit of the model was evaluated using Table 3, where the aim is to have a high coefficient of determination (r^2) value close to 1. Additionally, to achieve a good fit to the experimental values, it is desirable for the values of other tests, such as χ^2, MBE, RMSE, and MPE, to be as low as possible [60,61].

Table 3. The "goodness of fit" tests for the developed ANN models.

Output Variable	χ^2	RMSE	MBE	MPE	Skewness	Residual Analysis			
						Kurtoisis	Average	SD	Variance
Antiadhesion	59.777	7.722	−0.242	29.740	−0.454	1.373	−0.242	7.728	59.718
Antibiofilm forming	235.989	15.343	0.480	17.529	0.096	1.054	0.480	15.354	235.758

χ^2—reduced Chi-square, RMSE—root mean square error, MBE—mean bias error, SD—standard deviation of the residuals.

3.3. *Global Sensitivity Analysis-Yoon's Interpretation Method*

In this study, the relative influence of 25 input variables on the inhibition of adhesion and inhibition of the biofilm-forming process was analyzed. According to the results shown in Figure 3, the concentration of *L. monocytogenes* was found to have the greatest positive influence on the inhibition of adhesion, with a relative importance of approximately +8.72%. Conversely, the concentration of *S. enteritidis*, as well as the concentrations of extracts Fh and GI, were identified as the most negatively influential parameters on the inhibition of adhesion, with relative influences of −6.24%, −13.24%, and −10.81%, respectively.

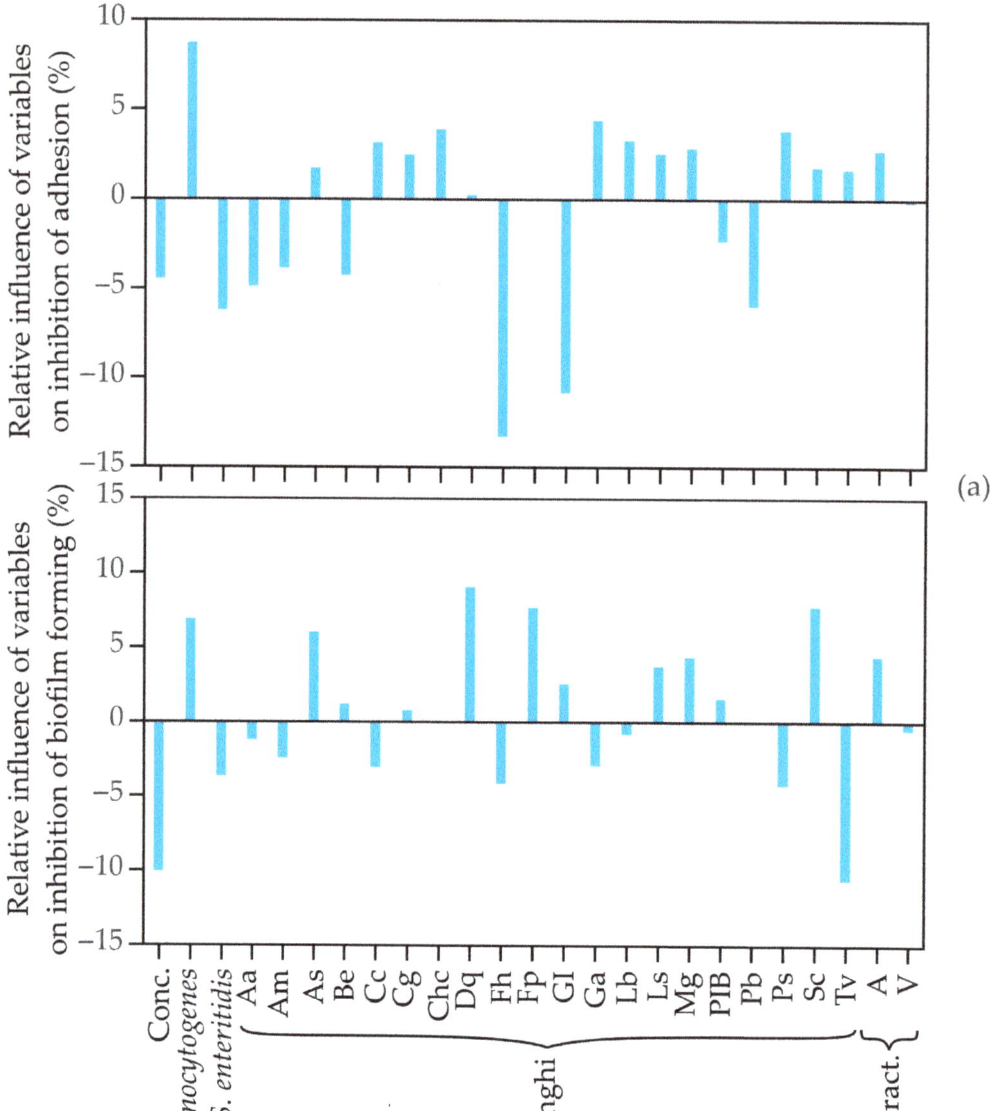

Figure 3. The relative importance of twenty-five input variables on (**a**) the inhibition of adhesion and (**b**) inhibition of the biofilm-forming process.

For the inhibition of the biofilm-forming process, a positive influence was observed for the concentration of *L. monocytogenes*, as well as extracts of mushrooms As, Dq, Fp, and Sc, with relative influences of +6.90%, +6.03%, +9.07%, +7.70%, and +7.76%, respectively. The most pronounced negative influence on the inhibition of the biofilm-forming process was observed for the Conc. and Tv mushroom extracts, with relative influences reaching −10.04% and −10.61%.

4. Materials and Methods

4.1. Reagents

Ethanol (96% w/v), tryptic soy broth, 2,3,5-triphenyltetrazoliumchloride (TTC), and crystal violet solution (1%) were all obtained from Sigma Aldrich (St. Louis, MO, USA).

4.2. Mushroom Samples Collection and Identification

Mushroom species, 20 of them, were collected in the period of spring 2019–autumn 2020 at different locations in the Republic of Serbia. The identification of carpophores was performed by the authors (K.A., V.J., and L.V.) according to the methods of classical herbarium taxonomy; the micro- and macromorphology of collected specimens were compared to standard descriptions in the taxonomic monographs. The representative voucher specimens, including their mycelial cultures, were deposited in the specimen collection of the Institute of Food Technology and Biochemistry, University of Belgrade—Faculty of Agriculture. To prepare them for extraction, mushroom samples were brush-cleaned and air-dried (40 °C) to constant mass. After being powdered in a Cyclotec mill (Tecator, Hoganas, Sweden), 40 mesh, the samples were stored in a cool and dark place prior to analysis.

4.3. Preparation of Mushroom Extracts

The dried powdered mushroom was soaked in ethanol (70% w/v) and mixed in a magnetic stirrer, filtered, mixed with water, and autoclaved for 1 h (120 °C, 1.2 bar). After being cooled, the material was filtered through cotton wool, and the liquid part was evaporated on a hot plate magnetic stirrer until 90% of the starting volume had been removed. The concentrated sample was next precipitated with a double amount of ethanol and centrifuged (Eppendorf 5804R, Hamburg, Germany) for 10 min at 9000 rpm. The supernatant was discarded, while the solid part was dried at 40 °C and powdered in a mortar. Thus, the water extract was obtained. A filter cake left after the liquid part was separated after autoclaving was mixed with sodium hydroxide (1 M) and again autoclaved under the same conditions. The material was then cooled to room temperature, filtered through cotton wool, neutralized, and centrifuged for 10 min at 9000 rpm. As with the water extract, the alkali sample was precipitated overnight with ethanol at 4°. The next day, it was centrifuged, and the solid part was collected and dried at 40 °C and powdered.

4.4. Bacterial Strains and Culture Conditions

The bacterial strains used in this study were Gram-positive *L. monocytogenes* ATTC 19111 and Gram-negative *S. enteritis* ATTC 13076. Both bacterial strains were obtained by aerobic subculturing in Tryptic Soy Broth (TSB), 24 h at 37 °C, before testing antimicrobial activity. The working concentration of the microbial suspension in the appropriate medium was 10^5 CFU/mL and was adjusted with a McFarland densitometer (Biosan, Latvia).

4.5. Determination of Minimum Inhibitory Concentrations (MIC)

The MIC was determined by the broth microdilution method [62]. The MIC was determined using serial dilutions in concentrations ranging from 0.156 to 20 mg/mL. An amount of 50 µL of sample dilutions and 50 µL of test microorganisms in a TSB were added to a sterile 96-well microtiter plate (Sarstedt, Germany). After aerobic incubation for 24 h at 37 °C, TTC, an indicator of cellular respiration, was added to the wells in a final concentration of 0.05%. After 1 h it was assessed whether a pink color has appeared. The MIC is taken as the first lowest concentration at which no color developed. From all wells where the color did not appear, the sample was sub-cultured on TSA plates for 24 h at 37 °C. The MBC represents the lowest concentration that prevents any growth of the organism after its subculturing. Every experiment was performed in triplicate.

4.6. Antiadhesion and Antibiofilm-Forming Assay

To determine the antiadhesion potential of mushroom extracts, the same bacteria as for the MIC assay were used. The antiadhesion ability was determined using a procedure established previously [19]. To adjust the final concentration of the overnight bacterial culture suspension to 10^5 CFU/mL, a McFarland densitometer (Biosan, Latvia) was used. The mushroom extract was dissolved in sterile Milli-Q (MQ) water in such a way as to obtain an initial concentration of 5 mg/mL, and then this solution was transferred to flatbottomed 96-well microtiter plates (Thermo Scientific™ Nunc™, Waltham, MA, USA). The bacterial culture (50 µL), previously prepared in sterile TSB, was added to the mushroom extracts. After 24 h of incubation, the plates were washed three times with sterile MQ water using a microplate washer (Rayto RT-3100, Rayto Life and Analytical Sciences Co. Ltd., Shenzhen, China). The samples were dried at 40 °C, and then a crystal violet solution (0.1 mL, 1%) was added to them. The dyeing lasted 15 min, so the dye was carefully washed off with tap water. To determine the inhibition of bacterial adhesion, a solution of acetic acid (33%) was added to the dried samples containing *L. monocytogenes*, while an ethanol solution (96%) was added to those with *S. enteritidis*, and absorbance was measured at a wavelength of 590 nm using a microplate reader (BioTek ELx 808, Winooski, VT, USA). The corresponding bacterial suspension in TSB was used as a control. The equation

$$\left(\frac{Ac - As}{Ac}\right) \cdot 100 \tag{1}$$

was used to determine the percentage of inhibition of bacterial adhesion (%IA) achieved in the presence of the appropriate concentration of mushroom extract. *Ac* is the absorbance of the control and *As* is the absorbance of the sample.

The antibiofilm potential of mushroom extracts was determined using the procedure already described, with the difference that samples in microtiter plates were incubated for 48 h instead of 24 h. In addition, Equation (1) was applied. In this case, the percentage of inhibition of biofilm formation (%IB) in the presence of the appropriate concentration of the mushroom extract was determined.

4.7. Artificial Neural Network (ANN)

The multi-layer perceptron (MLP) model was used, which is known for its accuracy in approximating non-linear functions [63], for modeling the anti-adhesion and anti-biofilm effects of the mushroom extracts. To optimize the model, the Broyden–Fletcher–Goldfarb–Shanno (BFGS) algorithm was used, with 100,000 repeating steps. The experimental data was divided into three parts: 60% for training, 20% for cross-validation, and 20%for testing. The weights and biases for the hidden and output layers were grouped into two matrices: W_1 and B_1 and W_2 and B_2, respectively:

$$Y = f_1(W_2 \cdot f_2(W_1 \cdot X + B_1) + B_2) \tag{2}$$

Weight coefficients were determined during the ANN learning cycle, with the intention to minimize the error between network results and experimental values [56,64].

Global Sensitivity Analysis

The relative impact of the input parameters on the output variables was calculated using Yoon's global sensitivity equation, which is based on the weight coefficients of the developed ANN models [65].

$$RI_{ij}(\%) = \frac{\sum_{k=0}^{n} (w_{ik} \cdot w_{kj})}{\sum_{i=0}^{m} \left| \sum_{k=0}^{n} (w_{ik} \cdot w_{kj}) \right|} \cdot 100\% \tag{3}$$

where w—weight coefficient in ANN model, i—input variable, j—output variable, k—hidden neuron, n—number of hidden neurons, m—number of inputs.

The numerical verification of the developed models was tested using reduced Chi-square (χ^2), root mean square error (RMSE), coefficient of determination (r^2), mean bias error (MBE), and mean percentage error (MPE) [59]:

$$\chi^2 = \frac{\sum_{i=1}^{N} (x_{\exp,i} - x_{pre,i})^2}{N - n} \tag{4}$$

$$\text{RMSE} = \left[\frac{1}{N} \cdot \sum_{i=1}^{N} (x_{pre,i} - x_{\exp,i})^2 \right]^{1/2} \tag{5}$$

$$\text{MBE} = \frac{1}{N} \cdot \sum_{i=1}^{N} (x_{pre,i} - x_{\exp,i}) \tag{6}$$

$$\text{MPE} = \frac{100}{N} \cdot \sum_{i=1}^{N} \left(\frac{|x_{pre,i} - x_{\exp,i}|}{x_{\exp,i}} \right) \tag{7}$$

where $x_{\exp,i}$ stands for the experimental values and $x_{pre,i}$ are the predicted values calculated by the model; N and n are the number of observations and constants, respectively.

4.8. Statistical Analyses

The data were processed statistically using the software package STATISTICA 10.0 (StatSoft Inc., Tulsa, OK, USA). The obtained results are expressed as the mean value with standard deviation (SD).

5. Conclusions

Discovering mushrooms as a source of novel antimicrobial agents in nature, this study offers the initial case study of their full potential in in vitro conditions against the bacterias *S. enteritidis* and *L. monocytogenes*. Namely, mushroom-derived extracts proved to be efficient food-borne pathogenic bacteria adhesion and biofilm-forming control agents, which is very important due to the unbefitting use of antibiotics and the unseemly control of human infections, which has led to the emergence of resistant bacterial species. Application of alternative sources of antimicrobials, which is proven in this study with 40 different water and alkali-based extracts of 20 different mushrooms, can lead to a decrease in the negative impact on public health and the global economy. For the first time, the ANN models were applied in the investigation of mushroom extracts as anti-biofilm and anti-adhesion agents, so these types of advanced mathematical tools were able to fit the experimental data well and successfully predict the output variables, with a good predictive capability. The overall coefficient of determination (r^2) for the inhibition of adhesion and inhibition of the biofilm-forming process was 0.865, which indicates the possibility of using this data analysis for cost- and time-consuming experiments such as this one with a high number of samples. Overall, the natural material tested in this study has several benefits of interest to the food industry, such as solubility, efficiency, and non-toxicity, and it has no bactericidal activity, while at the same time, the proposed ANN model can successfully predict its antibiofilm behavior. The features examined and validated in the presented paper provide a promising avenue for the industrial setting.

Supplementary Materials: The following supporting information can be downloaded at: https://www.mdpi.com/article/10.3390/antibiotics12030627/s1, Table S1: The list of mushroom species and their abbreviations; Table S2: Antiadhesion and antibiofilm-forming activity of water and alkali mushroom extracts against *L. monocytogenes* ATCC 19111 and *S. enteritidis* ATCC 13076; Table S3: Elements of matrix W_1 and vector B_1 (presented in the bias row), for the ANN model; Table S4: Elements of matrix W_2 and vector B_2 (presented in the bias column), for ANN model.

Author Contributions: Conceptualization J.V., L.P. and O.Š.; methodology, J.V., A.K. and L.P.; software, L.P.; validation, M.K. and D.R.; formal analysis, J.V., A.K. and V.L.; investigation, M.K. and V.L.; resources, A.K.; data curation, J.V., L.P. and O.Š.; writing—original draft preparation, J.V., A.K., D.R. and L.P.; writing—review and editing, J.V., A.K., M.K., D.R., O.Š. and L.P.; visualization, L.P.; supervision, J.V., A.K., O.Š. and L.P.; project administration, L.P. All authors have read and agreed to the published version of the manuscript.

Funding: The authors would like to thank the Serbian Ministry of Science, Technological Development and Innovation, agreement No. 451-03-47/2023-01/200051 and 451-03-47/2023-01-200116.

Institutional Review Board Statement: Not applicable.

Informed Consent Statement: Not applicable.

Data Availability Statement: Not applicable.

Conflicts of Interest: The authors declare no conflict of interest.

References

1. Food and Drug Administration, Outbreak Investigation of Listeria monocytogenes: Dole Packaged Salad (December 2021). Available online: https://www.fda.gov/food/outbreaks-foodborne-illness/outbreak-investigation-listeria-monocytogenes-dole-packaged-salad-december-2021 (accessed on 26 December 2022).
2. Food Safety News. Biofilms with Listeria Pose Persistent Threat in Food Production. Available online: https://www.foodsafetynews.com/2017/06/biofilms-with-listeria-pose-persistent-threat-in-food-production/#more-141170 (accessed on 26 December 2022).
3. Wagner, E.M.; Pracser, N.; Thalguter, S.; Fischel, K.; Rammer, N.; Pospíšilová, L.; Alispahic, M.; Wagner, M.; Rychli, K. Identification of biofilm hotspots in a meat processing environment: Detection of spoilage bacteria in multi-species biofilms. *Int. J. Food Microbiol.* **2020**, *328*, 108668. [CrossRef] [PubMed]
4. Highmore, C.J.; Melaugh, G.; Morris, R.J.; Parker, J.; Direito, S.O.L.; Romero, M.; Soukarieh, F.; Robertson, S.N.; Bamford, N.C. Translational challenges and opportunities in biofilm science: A BRIEF for the future. *NPJ Biofilms Microbiomes* **2022**, *8*, 68. [CrossRef] [PubMed]
5. Bai, X.; Nakatsu, C.H.; Bhunia, A.K. Bacterial Biofilms and Their Implications in Pathogenesis and Food Safety. *Foods* **2021**, *10*, 2117. [CrossRef] [PubMed]
6. Cámara, M.; Green, W.; MacPhee, C.E.; Rakowska, P.D.; Raval, R.; Richardson, M.C.; Slater-Jefferies, J.; Steventon, K.; Webb, J.S. Economic significance of biofilms: A multidisciplinary and cross-sectoral challenge. *NPJ Biofilms Microbiomes* **2022**, *8*, 42. [CrossRef] [PubMed]
7. Galié, S.; García-Gutiérrez, C.; Miguélez, E.M.; Villar, C.J.; Lombó, F. Biofilms in the Food Industry: Health Aspects and Control Methods. *Front Microbiol.* **2018**, *9*, 898. [CrossRef]
8. Toushik, S.H.; Mizan, F.R.; Hossain, I.; Ha, S.D. Fighting with old foes: The pledge of microbe-derived biological agents to defeat mono- and mixed-bacterial biofilms concerning food industries. *Trends Food Sci. Technol.* **2020**, *99*, 413–425. [CrossRef]
9. Kjelleberg, S.; McDougald, D.; Rasmussen, T.B.; Givskov, M. Quorum-sensing inhibition. In *Chemical Communication among Bacteria*; Winans, S.C., Bassler, B.L., Eds.; ASM Press: Washington, DC, USA, 2008; pp. 393–416.
10. Al-Dhabi, N.A.; Arasu, M.V.; Rejiniemon, T.S. In vitro antibacterial, antifungal, antibiofilm, antioxidant and anticancer properties of isosteviol isolated from endangered medicinal plant *Pittosporum tetrasoermum*. *Evid. Based Complement. Alternat. Med.* **2015**, *2015*, 164261.
11. Mishra, R.; Panda, A.K.; De Mandal, S.; Shakeel, M.; Bisht, S.S.; Khan, J. Natural Anti-biofilm Agents: Strategies to Control Biofilm-Forming Pathogens. *Front Microbiol.* **2020**, *11*, 566325. [CrossRef]
12. Golberg, K.; Markus, V.; Kagan, B.E.; Barzanizan, S.; Yaniv, K.; Teralı, K.; Kramarsky-Winter, E.; Marks, R.S.; Kushmaro, A. Anti-Virulence Activity of 3,3′-Diindolylmethane (DIM): A Bioactive Cruciferous Phytochemical with Accelerated Wound Healing Benefits. *Pharmaceutics* **2022**, *14*, 967. [CrossRef]
13. Balaban, M.; Koc, C.; Sar, T.; Akbas, M.Y. Antibiofilm effects of pomegranate peel extracts against *B. cereus*, *B. subtilis*, and *E. faecalis*. *Int. J. Food Sci. Technol.* **2021**, *56*, 4915–4924. [CrossRef]
14. Elisashvili, V.; Asatiani, M.D.; Khardziani, T.; Rai, M. Natural antimicrobials from Basidiomycota Mushrooms. In *Promising Antimicrobials from Natural Products*; Rai, M., Kosalec, I., Eds.; Springer: Cham, Switzerland, 2022; pp. 323–353.
15. Alves, M.J.; Ferreira, I.C.; Lourenço, I.; Costa, E.; Martins, A.; Pintado, M. Wild mushroom extracts as inhibitors of bacterial biofilm formation. *Pathogens* **2014**, *3*, 667–679. [CrossRef]
16. Klančnik, A.; Megušar, P.; Sterniša, M.; Jeršek, B.; Bucar, F.; SmoleMožina, S.; Kos, J.; Sabotič, J. Aqueous extracts of wild mushrooms show antimicrobial and antiadhesion activities against bacteria and fungi. *Phytother. Res.* **2017**, *31*, 1971–1976. [CrossRef]

17. Signoretto, C.; Marchi, A.; Bertoncelli, A.; Burlacchini, G.; Papetti, A.; Pruzzo, C.; Zaura, E.; Lingström, P.; Ofek, I.; Pratten, J.; et al. The anti-adhesive mode of action of purified mushroom (*Lentinus edodes*) extract with anticaries and antigingivitis properties in two oral bacterial pathogens. *Complement. Altern. Med.* **2014**, *14*, 75. [CrossRef] [PubMed]
18. Papetti, A.; Signoretto, C.; Spratt, D.A.; Pratten, J.; Lingström, P.; Zaura, E.; Ofek, I.; Wilson, M.; Pruzzo, C.; Gazzani, G. Components in *Lentinus edodes* mushroom with anti-biofilm activity directed against bacteria involved in caries and gingivitis. *Food Funct.* **2018**, *9*, 3489–3499. [CrossRef]
19. Vunduk, J.; Wan-Mohtar, W.A.A.Q.I.; Mohamad, S.A.; Halim, N.H.A.; Dzomir, A.Z.M.; Žižak, Ž.; Klaus, A. Polysaccharides of *Pleurotus flabellatus* strain Mynuk produced by submerged fermentation as a promising novel tool against adhesion and biofilm formation of foodborne pathogens. *LWT* **2019**, *112*, 108221. [CrossRef]
20. Song, X.; Gaascht, F.; Schmidt-Dannert, C.; Salomon, C.E. Discovery of antifungal and biofilm preventive compounds from mycelial cultures of a unique *North American Hericium* sp. fungus. *Molecules* **2020**, *25*, 963. [CrossRef]
21. Kim, Y.; Oh, S.; Kim, S.H. Released exopolysaccharide (r-ESP) produced from probiotic bacteria reduce biofilm formation of enterohemorrhagic *Escherichia coli* O157:H7. *Biochem. Biophys. Res. Commun.* **2009**, *379*, 324–329. [CrossRef] [PubMed]
22. U.S. National Library of Medicine. Available online: https://clinicaltrials.gov/ (accessed on 29 November 2022).
23. U.S. National Library of Medicine. Antibacterial and Anti-biofilm Activity of Frankincense Extract Against Porphyromonas Gingivalis. Available online: https://clinicaltrials.gov/ct2/show/NCT04705714?cond=antibiofilm&draw=2&rank=3 (accessed on 29 November 2022).
24. Shaban, T.F.; Alkawareek, M.Y. Prediction of qualitative activity of antibiotics using supervised machine learning techniques. *Comput. Biol. Med.* **2021**, *140*, 105065. [CrossRef]
25. Wawrzyniak, J. Application of Artificial Neural Networks to Assess the Mycological State of Bulk Stored Rapeseeds. *Agriculture* **2020**, *10*, 567. [CrossRef]
26. Tomić, A.; Šovljanski, O.; Nikolić, V.; Pezo, L.; Aćimović, M.; Cvetković, M.; Stanojev, J.; Kuzmanović, N.; Markov, S. Screening of Antifungal Activity of Essential Oils in Controlling Biocontamination of Historical Papers in Archives. *Antibiotics* **2023**, *12*, 103. [CrossRef]
27. Šovljanski, O.; Saveljić, A.; Aćimović, M.; Šeregelj, V.; Pezo, L.; Tomić, A.; Ćetković, G.; Tešević, V. Biological Profiling of Essential Oils and Hydrolates of *Ocimum basilicum* var. *Genovese* and var. *Minimum* Originated from Serbia. *Processes* **2022**, *10*, 1893. [CrossRef]
28. Aćimović, M.; Šovljanski, O.; Pezo, L.; Travičić, V.; Tomić, A.; Zheljazkov, V.D.; Ćetković, G.; Švarc-Gajić, J.; Brezo-Borjan, T.; Sofrenić, I. Variability in Biological Activities of *Satureja montana* Subsp. *montana* and Subsp. *variegata* Based on Different Extraction Methods. *Antibiotics* **2022**, *11*, 1235. [CrossRef]
29. Marks, B.P. Status of microbial modeling in food process models. *Compr. Rev. Food Sci. Food Saf* **2008**, *7*, 137–143. [CrossRef]
30. Rajković, D.; Marjanović Jeromela, D.; Pezo, L.; Lončar, B.; Zanetti, F.; Monti, A.; Kondić Špika, A. Yield and Quality Prediction of Winter Rapeseed—Artificial Neural Network and Random Forest Models. *Agronomy* **2022**, *12*, 58. [CrossRef]
31. World Health Organization. Antimicrobial Resistance. Available online: https://www.who.int/news-room/fact-sheets/detail/antimicrobial-resistance (accessed on 25 January 2023).
32. Center for Disease Control. Antibiotic Resistance: A Global Threat. Available online: https://www.cdc.gov/drugresistance/solutions-initiative/stories/ar-global-threat.html (accessed on 25 January 2023).
33. Alves, M.J.; Ferreira, I.C.F.R.; Martins, A.; Pintado, M. Antimicrobial activity of wild mushroom extracts against clinical isolates resistant to different antibiotics. *J. Appl. Microbiol.* **2012**, *113*, 466–475. [CrossRef] [PubMed]
34. Suay, I.; Arenal, A.; Asensio, F.J.; Basilio, A.; Cabello, M.A.; Diez, M.T.; Garcia, J.B.; González del Val, A.; Gorrochategui, J.; Hernández, P.; et al. Screening of basidiomycetes for antimicrobial activities. *Antonie Van Leeuwenhoek* **2000**, *78*, 129–139. [CrossRef] [PubMed]
35. Venturini, M.E.; Rivera, C.S.; Gonzalez, C.; Blanco, D. Antimicrobial activity of extracts of edible wild and cultivated mushrooms against foodborne bacterial strains. *J. Food Prot.* **2008**, *71*, 1701–1706. [CrossRef] [PubMed]
36. Huguet, C.; Bourjot, M.; Bellanger, J.M.; Prévost, G.; Urbain, A. Screening for antibacterial activity of French mushrooms against pathogenic and multidrug resistant bacteria. *Appl. Sci.* **2022**, *12*, 5229. [CrossRef]
37. Barros, L.; Calhelha, R.; Vaz, J.; Ferreira, I.C.F.R.; Baptista, P.; Estevinho, L.M. Antimicrobial activity and bioactive compounds of Portuguese wild edible mushrooms methanolic extracts. *Eur. Food Res. Technol.* **2007**, *225*, 151–156. [CrossRef]
38. Klaus, A.; Kozarski, M.; Niksic, M.; Jakovljevic, D.; Todorovic, N.; Van Griensven, L.J.L.D. Antioxidative activities and chemical characterization of polysaccharides extracted from the basidiomycete *Schizophyllum commune*. *LWT-Food Sci. Technol.* **2011**, *44*, 2005–2011. [CrossRef]
39. Kozarski, M.; Klaus, A.; van Griensven, L.; Jakovljevic, D.; Todorovic, N.; Wan-Mohtar, W.A.A.Q.I. Mushroom β-glucan and polyphenol formulations as natural immunity boosters and balancers: Nature of the application. *Food Sci. Hum. Wellness* **2023**, *12*, 378–396. [CrossRef]
40. Bernal, P.; Liamas, M.A. Promising biotechnological applications of antibiofilm exopolysaccharides. *Microb. Biotechnol.* **2012**, *5*, 670–673. [CrossRef]
41. Moussa, A.Y.; Fayez, S.; Xiao, H.; Xu, B. New insights into antimicrobial and antibiofilm effects of edible mushrooms. *Food Res. Int.* **2022**, *162*, 111982. [CrossRef]

42. Shomali, N.; Onar, O.; Cihan, A.C.; Akata, I.; Yildirim, O. Antioxidant, anticancer, antimicrobial, and antibiofilm properties of the culinary-medicinal fairy ring mushroom, *Marasmius oreades* (Agaricomycetes). *Int. J. Med. Mushrooms* **2019**, *21*, 571–582. [CrossRef] [PubMed]
43. Deng, Q.; Pu, Y.; Sun, L.; Wang, Y.; Liu, Y.; Wang, R.; Liao, J.; Xu, D.; Liu, Y.; Yr, R.; et al. Antimicrobial peptide AMPNT-6 from bacillus subtilis inhibits biofilm formation by *Shewanella putrefaciens* and disrupts its preformed biofilms on both abiotic and shrimp shell surfaces. *Food Res. Int.* **2017**, *102*, 8–13. [CrossRef] [PubMed]
44. Bai, J.R.; Zhong, K.; Wu, Y.P.; Elena, G.; Gao, H. Antibiofilm activity of shikimic acid against *Staphylococcus aureus*. *Food Control* **2019**, *95*, 327–333. [CrossRef]
45. Ye, J.; Shao, C.; Zhang, X.; Guo, X.; Gao, P.; Cen, Y.; Ma, S.; Liu, Y. Effects of DNase I coating of titanium on bacterial adhesion and biofilm formation. *Mater. Sci. Eng. C* **2017**, *78*, 738–747. [CrossRef] [PubMed]
46. Younus, M.; Wilkins, M.J.; Arshad, M.M.; Rahbar, M.H.; Saeed, A.M. Demographic risk factors and incidence of Salmonella enteritidis infection in Michigan. *Foodborne Pathog. Dis.* **2006**, *3*, 266–273. [CrossRef]
47. Shamloo, E.; Hosseini, H.; Abdi Moghadam, Z.; Halberg, L.M.; Haslberger, A.; Alebouyeh, M. Importance of *Listeria monocytogenes* in food safety: A review of its prevalence, detection, and antibiotic resistance. *Iran. J. Vet. Res.* **2019**, *20*, 241–254.
48. Al-Bakri, A.G.; Othman, G.; Afifi, F.U. Determination of the antibiofilm, antiadhesive, and anti-MRSA activities of seven Salvia species. *Pharmacogn. Mag.* **2010**, *6*, 264–270. [CrossRef]
49. Kavita, K.; Singh, V.K.; Mishra, A.; Jha, B. Characterization and anti-biofilm activity of extracellular polymeric substances from *Oceanobacillus iheyensis*. *Carbohydr. Polym.* **2014**, *101*, 29–35. [CrossRef] [PubMed]
50. Garcia, J.; Rodrigues, F.; Castro, F.; Aires, A.; Marques, G.; Saavedra, M.J. Antimicrobial, antibiofilm, and antioxidant properties of *Boletus edulis* and *Neoboletus luridiformis* against multidrug-resistant ESKAPE pathogens. *Front. Nutr.* **2022**, *8*, 1093. [CrossRef]
51. Soković, M.; Ćirić, A.; Glamočlija, J.; Nikolić, M.; van Griensven, L.J.L.D. *Agaricus blazei* hot water extract shows anti quorum sensing activity in the nosocomial human pathogen *Pseudomonas aeruginosa*. *Molecules* **2014**, *19*, 4189–4199. [CrossRef] [PubMed]
52. De Carvalho, M.P.; Gulotta, G.; do Amaral, M.W.; Lünsdorf, H.; Sasse, F.; Abraham, W.R.A. Coprinuslactone protects the edible mushroom Coprinus comatus against biofilm infections by blocking both quorum-sensing and MurA. *Environ. Microbiol.* **2016**, *18*, 4254–4264. [CrossRef] [PubMed]
53. Šeregelj, V.; Šovljanski, O.; TumbasŠaponjac, V.; Vulić, J.; Ćetković, G.; Markov, S.; Čanadanović-Brunet, J. Horned Melon (*Cucumis metuliferus* E. Meyer Ex. Naudin)—Current Knowledge on Its Phytochemicals, Biological Benefits, and Potential Applications. *Processes* **2022**, *10*, 94. [CrossRef]
54. Aćimović, M.; Šovljanski, O.; Šeregelj, V.; Pezo, L.; Zheljazkov, V.D.; Ljujić, J.; Tomić, A.; Ćetković, G.; Čanadanović-Brunet, J.; Miljković, A.; et al. Chemical Composition, Antioxidant, and Antimicrobial Activity of *Dracocephalum moldavica* L. Essential Oil and Hydrolate. *Plants* **2022**, *11*, 941. [CrossRef]
55. Pezo, L.; Curcic, B.; Filipovic, V.; Nicetin, M.; Koprivica, G.; Misljenovic, N.; Levic, L. Artificial neural network model of pork meat cubes osmotic dehydration. *Hem. Ind.* **2013**, *67*, 465–475. [CrossRef]
56. Basheer, I.A.; Hajmeer, M. Artificial neural networks: Fundamentals, computing, design, and application. *J. Microbiol. Methods* **2000**, *43*, 3–31. [CrossRef]
57. Montaño, J.J.; Palmer, A. Numeric sensitivity analysis applied to feedforward neural networks. *Neural Comput. Appl.* **2003**, *12*, 119–125. [CrossRef]
58. Chattopadhyay, P.B.; Rangarajan, R. Application of ANN in sketching spatial nonlinearity of unconfined aquifer in agricultural basin. *Agric. Water Manag.* **2014**, *113*, 81–91. [CrossRef]
59. Arsenovic, M.; Pezo, L.; Stankovic, S.; Radojevic, Z. Factor space differentiation of brick clays according to mineral content: Prediction of final brick product quality. *Appl. Clay Sci.* **2015**, *115*, 108–114. [CrossRef]
60. Montgomery, D.C. *Design and Analysis of Experiments*; John Wiley and Sons Ltd.: Hoboken, NJ, USA, 1984.
61. Madamba, P.S. The Response Surface Methodology: An Application to Optimize Dehydration Operations of Selected Agricultural Crops. *LWT* **2002**, *35*, 584–592. [CrossRef]
62. Klaus, A.; Kozarski, M.; Vunduk, J.; Todorovic, N.; Jakovljevic, D.; Zizak, Z.; Pavlovic, V.; Levic, S.; Niksic, M.; Van Griensven, L.J.L.D. Biological potential of extracts of the wild edible Basidiomycete mushroom *Grifola frondosa*. *Food Res. Int.* **2015**, *67*, 272–283. [CrossRef]
63. Momenzadeh, L.; Zomorodian, A.; Mowla, D. Experimental and theoretical investigation of shelled corn drying in a microwave assisted fluidized bed dryer using Artificial Neural Network. *Food Bioprod. Process.* **2011**, *89*, 15–21. [CrossRef]
64. Trelea, I.C.; Raoult-Wack, A.L.; Trystram, G. Note: Application of neural network modelling for the control of dewatering and impregnation soaking process (osmotic dehydration). *Food Sci. Technol. Int.* **1997**, *3*, 459–465. [CrossRef]
65. Yoon, Y.; Swales, G.; Margavio, T.M. A comparison of discriminant analysis versus artificial neural networks. *J. Oper. Res. Soc.* **2017**, *44*, 51–60. [CrossRef]

antibiotics

MDPI

Article

Antibacterial Activity of Selected Essential Oils against Foodborne Pathogens and Their Application in Fresh Turkey Sausages

Branislav Šojić [1], Predrag Ikonić [2], Sunčica Kocić-Tanackov [1], Tatjana Peulić [2], Nemanja Teslić [2], Miloš Županjac [2], Ivana Lončarević [1], Zoran Zeković [1], Milica Popović [2], Stefan Vidaković [1] and Branimir Pavlić [1,*]

1 Faculty of Technology Novi Sad, University of Novi Sad, Bulevar cara Lazara 1, 21000 Novi Sad, Serbia
2 Institute of Food Technology in Novi Sad, University of Novi Sad, Bulevar cara Lazara 1, 21000 Novi Sad, Serbia
* Correspondence: bpavlic@uns.ac.rs

Abstract: Essential oils (EOs) isolated from different plant materials, namely *Origanum majorana* L., *Satureja hortensis* L., and *Satureja montana* L. (OMEO, SHEO, and SMEO, respectively), were used in fresh turkey sausage processing. The chemical composition and in vitro antimicrobial potential of selected EOs and their mixture were determined. The minimum inhibitory concentration (MIC) and minimum bactericidal concentration (MBC) against foodborne pathogens (*Escherichia coli*, *Salmonella* Enteritidis, and *Listeria monocytogenes*) ranged in the interval of 0.44–7.1 μL/mL. Fresh turkey sausages were produced with EOs addition and marked as follows: TOMEO—0.150 μL/g OMEO; TSHEO—0.150 μL/g SHEO; TSMEO—0.150 μL/g SMEO; TEOM—0.050 μL/g OMEO, 0.050 μL/g SHEO and 0.050 μL/g SMEO, and control (C) (without EOs). Microbiological profile and biogenic amines content in fresh turkey sausages were recorded during storage. The selected EOs and their mixture efficiently reduced bacterial growth and biogenic amines formation and accumulation. The lowest *Enterobacteriaceae* count and total biogenic amine (BA) concentration were determined through treatment TSHEO. The results of this study show that selected EOs could be useful in fresh turkey sausage processing in order to improve safety and shelf-life.

Keywords: biogenic amines; essential oils; fresh sausages; shelf-life; turkey meat

1. Introduction

In the past two decades, poultry meat production has gradually increased worldwide [1]. According to FAO predictions, in 2030, poultry meat production will reach an amount of nearly 151 million tons [2]. The increase in demand for poultry meat among consumers is related to its low cost of production, absence of cultural and religious restrictions, and relatively high nutritive potential [1]. The demand for turkey meat is also constantly increasing, and presently this type of poultry meat accounts close to 30% of total poultry meat production [2]. Turkey meat is marked as an essential part of healthy nutrition due to its high level of vital minerals (iron, zinc, phosphorus, potassium, and magnesium), which helps to maintain the normal functioning of the human immune and nervous system [3,4]. Additionally, turkey meat is characterized by high levels of easily digestible proteins ($\leq$28%) and relatively low levels of fat ($\leq$5%) and cholesterol [4]. Turkey meat also possesses high-quality sensory attributes (color, flavor, and texture) [4,5]. Concerning high nutritive and sensory quality, turkey meat is widely used in processing different types of meat products, including fresh sausages [5].

Fresh sausages are widely consumed processed meat products worldwide [6]. According to Serbian legislation [7], these products are manufactured by grinding and mixing meat (pork, beef, or poultry) with different components: table salt, spice mixtures, carbohydrates, and water. Fresh sausages are manufactured without food preservatives (nitrites and nitrates) and thermal treatments. Hence, these products are usually characterized by relatively high numbers of microorganisms, and they undergo spoilage even during refrigerated storage, resulting in a relatively short shelf-life [6]. Along with the microbial growth, proteolysis occurs, leading to a generation of polypeptides, peptides, free amino acids, aldehydes, organic acids, etc. [8–10]. Following this process, biogenic amines (BA) are formed and accumulated due to the metabolic activity of present decarboxylating bacteria. BA are the anti-nutritional organic bases of low molecular weight, which are regularly found in a range of food products (meat and meat products, fish, dairy products, fermented vegetables, beer, wine, etc.), and might have a toxicological influence on human health. Their content in meat products is affected by several factors, including the quality of raw material (meat hygienic status and composition, pH, water activity, etc.), ingredients (food additives, starter cultures, etc.), manufacturing practices, processing operations and conditions, and storage conditions (time, temperature, packaging methods, etc.) [10–12]. Thus, the assessment of BA in different types of meat products is essential as an indicator of food hygiene and freshness, as well as from toxicological viewpoint [12–15].

One of the critical approaches to decrease microbiological growth and prolong the meat products shelf-life is the usage of food additives, including nitrites and nitrates. However, these food additives are considered unhealthy [16].

Therefore, scientists in the field of meat technology are oriented towards various natural substitutes to synthetic additives, concentrating on plant extracts, including essential oils (EOs) [17]. EOs are remarkable since they are noticeable as GRAS (generally recognized as safe) and enjoy wide acceptance by consumers [18]. Several authors have already determined the strong antimicrobial potential of different essential oils in the processing of fresh sausages [14,19–23]. Hence, this study aimed to assess the antimicrobial and antioxidative potential of selected Eos, namely *Origanum majorana* essential oil (OMEO), *Satureja hortensis* essential oil (SHEO), *Satureja montana* essential oil (SMEO) and their mixtures (EOM), against foodborne pathogens in vitro and on the quality and shelf-life of fresh turkey sausages.

2. Results and Discussion

2.1. Chemical Composition of Applied Essential Oils

The chemical profile of three EOs obtained from the *Lamiaceae* species is given in Table 1 and chromatograms are given in Figure S1 (Supplementary Materials). GC-MS analysis showed that EOs consist of several groups of components, i.e., monoterpene hydrocarbons, oxygenated monoterpenes, sesquiterpene hydrocarbons, and oxygenated sesquiterpenes. The EOs of all samples showed a predominant presence of oxygenated monoterpenes, which is clearly visible in terms of the contents of major compounds in each sample: terpinen-4-ol (OMEO), thymol (SHEO), and carvacrol (SMEO).

Table 1. Chemical profile of selected essential oils.

Name	RT [min]	OMEO		SHEO		SMEO	
		RP [%]	SD	RP [%]	SD	RP [%]	SD
α-Thujene	3.767	1.67^{iA}	0.06	1.67^{hA}	0.07	1.44^{ghB}	0.01
α-Pinene	3.883	0.70^{noC}	0.02	1.49^{hiA}	0.08	1.16^{iB}	0.03
Camphene	4.169	nd	n/a	1.06^{jkA}	0.08	0.46^{lB}	0.04
Sabinene	4.672	3.54^{e}	0.04	nd	n/a	nd	n/a
β-Pinene	4.768	1.29^{kA}	0.04	0.13^{nB}	0.02	0.11^{oB}	0.01
1-Octen-3-ol	4.815	nd	n/a	1.59^{hiA}	0.61	1.36^{ghA}	0.10
β-Myrcene	5.064	1.11^{lA}	0.02	1.53^{hiA}	0.98	1.79^{fA}	0.10
α-Phellandrene	5.408	0.58^{noA}	0.01	0.38^{lmnB}	0.03	0.28^{mnC}	0.01
δ-3-Carene	5.567	nd	n/a	0.12^{n}	0.01	nd	n/a

Table 1. *Cont.*

Name	RT [min]	OMEO		SHEO		SMEO	
		RP [%]	SD	RP [%]	SD	RP [%]	SD
α-Terpinene	5.79	9.57 ^{cA}	0.14	2.89 ^{efB}	0.08	2.24 ^{eC}	0.03
p-Cymene	5.954	3.49 ^{eC}	0.01	10.20 ^{bB}	0.25	12.12 ^{cA}	0.15
o-Cymene+Limonene	6.065	2.39 ^{g}	0.01	nd	n/a	nd	n/a
Eucalyptol (1,8-Cineole)	6.15	nd	n/a	nd	n/a	0.78 ^{jk}	0.02
o-Cymene+β-Phellandrene	6.15	nd	n/a	2.13 ^{g}	0.00	nd	n/a
β-Phellandrene	6.139	1.39 ^{jk}	0.13	nd	n/a	nd	n/a
γ-Terpinene	6.928	14.33 ^{bA}	0.13	9.77 ^{cB}	0.05	14.39 ^{bA}	0.05
cis-Sabinene hydrate	7.203	2.08 ^{hA}	0.01	0.41 ^{lmnB}	0.01	nd	n/a
Terpinolene	7.855	3.05 ^{fA}	0.01	0.26 ^{mnB}	0.02	0.14 ^{noC}	0.01
trans-Sabinene hydrate	8.188	4.40 ^{d}	0.16	nd	n/a	nd	n/a
Linalool	8.31	3.09 ^{fA}	0.17	0.77 ^{klC}	0.05	1.33 ^{hB}	0.05
cis-Menth-2-en-1-ol	8.983	2.05 ^{h}	0.04	nd	n/a	nd	n/a
trans-Menth-2-en-1-ol	9.643	1.30 ^{jk}	0.01	nd	n/a	nd	n/a
Borneol	10.582	nd	n/a	2.52 ^{fA}	0.01	1.48 ^{gB}	0.02
Terpinen-4-ol	10.984	27.69 ^{aA}	0.46	1.43 ^{hijB}	0.01	0.86 ^{jkC}	0.02
α-Terpineol	11.572	4.41 ^{dA}	0.02	0.40 ^{lmnB}	0.01	0.21 ^{mnoC}	0.03
cis-Piperitol	11.768	0.67 ^{no}	0.01	nd	n/a	nd	n/a
Estragole	11.89	0.89 ^{m}	0.07	nd	n/a	nd	n/a
trans-Piperitol	12.255	0.72 ^{no}	0.11	nd	n/a	nd	n/a
Thymol methyl ether	13.293	nd	n/a	0.33 ^{mn}	0.02	nd	n/a
Carvone	13.616	0.64 ^{no}	0.01	nd	n/a	nd	n/a
Carvacrol methyl ether	13.648	nd	n/a	0.66 ^{lm}	0.01	nd	n/a
Linalool acetate	14.162	1.28 ^{k}	0.04	nd	n/a	nd	n/a
Terpinen-4-ol acetate	15.872	1.47 ^{j}	0.02	nd	n/a	nd	n/a
Thymol	16.02	0.69 ^{noB}	0.06	41.10 ^{aA}	0.39	0.17 ^{noC}	0.01
Carvacrol	16.359	0.55 ^{oC}	0.05	9.99 ^{bcB}	0.16	53.58 ^{aA}	0.31
δ-Elemene	17.286	0.22 ^{p}	0.03	nd	n/a	nd	n/a
Neryl acetate	18.604	0.09 ^{p}	0.00	nd	n/a	nd	n/a
Thymol acetate	18.837	nd	n/a	1.24 ^{ijA}	0.02	0.88 ^{jB}	0.04
Geranyl acetate	19.388	0.11 ^{p}	0.00	nd	n/a	nd	n/a
trans-Caryophyllene	20.479	2.20 ^{hC}	0.04	3.25 ^{deA}	0.03	2.91 ^{dB}	0.05
β-Gurjunene	20.908	nd	n/a	nd	n/a	0.13 ^{o}	0.01
Aromadendrene	21.289	0.17 ^{pA}	0.00	0.14 ^{nB}	0.00	nd	n/a
α-Humulene (α-Caryophyllene)	21.845	0.12 ^{pA}	0.00	0.11 ^{nB}	0.00	0.10 ^{oC}	0.01
γ-Muurolene	22.867	nd	n/a	nd	n/a	0.17 ^{no}	0.01
Germacrene D	22.989	nd	n/a	nd	n/a	0.45 ^{l}	0.01
Viridiflorene (Ledene)	23.540	nd	n/a	0.18 ^{n}	0.00	nd	n/a
Bicyclogermacrene	23.543	0.77 ^{mn}	0.02	nd	n/a	nd	n/a
β-Bisabolene	24.175	nd	n/a	3.45 ^{dA}	0.03	0.74 ^{kB}	0.05
γ-Cadinene	24.366	nd	n/a	nd	n/a	0.18 ^{mno}	0.03
δ-Cadinene	24.651	0.07 ^{pC}	0.00	0.21 ^{nB}	0.01	0.31 ^{mA}	0.01
n.i.	25.536	nd	n/a	0.08 ^{n}	0.00	nd	n/a
Spathulenol	26.685	0.58 ^{no}	0.04	nd	n/a	nd	n/a
Caryophyllene oxide	26.833	0.61 ^{noA}	0.06	0.19 ^{nC}	0.01	0.24 ^{mnoB}	0.01

RT—retention time [min]; RP—relative percentage [%]; SD—standard deviation; nd—not detected; n/a—not applicable; n.i.—not identified. Means ± SD with different letters $^{(A–C)}$ in the same row are significantly different ($p < 0.05$); values with different letters $^{(a–p)}$ in the same column are significantly different ($p < 0.05$).

OMEO samples obtained from *O. majorana* showed the most diverse terpenoid profile among exanimated EOs. Two major compounds identified in this sample were γ-terpinene and terpinen-4-ol, with relative percentages of 14.33 and 27.69%, respectively. Results are in accordance with the literature data, since it has been reported that the content of these two compounds in OMEO were 9.5 and 32.1% [24]. According to Ghazal et al. [25], *trans*-sabinene hydrate (25.18%) and terpinen-4-ol (24.92%) were the most abundant compounds in the Hungarian variety of the *O. majorana* essential oil, while the content of γ-terpinene (6.48%) was lower compared to the OMEO obtained in this work. The OMEO samples also showed a very balanced content of less abundant compounds. It was observed that 18 compounds exhibited relative percentages from 1 to 10% (Table 1). This could be particularly interesting since these compounds could contribute to the synergistic effects and improve the bioactive potential of the sample.

On the other hand, fewer compounds were identified in SHEO and SMEO essential oils obtained from *S. hortensis* and *S. montana*. It was observed that both samples had a similar content of oxygenated monoterpene phenols (Table 1). In SHEO, thymol and carvacrol comprised 41.10 and 9.99% relative percentages, while carvacrol (53.58%) was the most abundant in SMEO, while the content of thymol was negligible. This was expected since both plant species are from the genus *Satureja*, and the same observation was reported in a systematic review that evaluated the chemical profile of all *Satureja* species [26]. The content of major compounds was followed by *p*-cymene and γ-terpinene, which were similar in SHEO (10.20 and 9.77%) and (12.12 and 14.39%). Minor compounds that were identified in both samples with a relative percentage higher than 1% were α-thujene, α-pinene, 1-octen-3-ol, β-myrcene, α-terpinene, borneol, and *trans*-caryophyllene.

2.2. Minimal Inhibitory Concentration and Minimal Bactericidal Concentration of the Selected Essential Oils

The antibacterial potential of selected EOs (OMEO, SHEO, SMEO, and EOM) was expressed by the microdilution method (Table 2). Minimal inhibitory concentration (MIC) and minimal bactericidal concentration (MBC) are determined for the most common pathogens in meat processing: *Escherichia coli*, *Salmonella* Enteritidis, and *Listeria monocytogenes*.

Table 2. Minimal inhibitory concentration (MIC) and minimal bactericidal concentration (MBC) of the selected essential oils.

Essential Oils	Test Microorganism					
	Escherichia Coli		*Salmonella* Enteritidis		*Listeria Monocytogenes*	
	MIC (μL/mL)	MBC (μL/mL)	MIC (μL/mL)	MBC (μL/mL)	MIC (μL/mL)	MBC (μL/mL)
OMEO	0.89	1.78	3.55	7.1	1.78	7.1
SHEO	0.89	1.78	0.44	0.89	0.44	0.89
SMEO	3.55	7.1	1.78	3.55	0.89	1.78
EOM	0.44	0.89	0.44	0.89	0.44	1.78

O. majorana essential oil (OMEO); *S. hortensis* essential oil (SHEO); *S. montana* essential oil (SMEO); Essential oils mixture (EOM).

The MICs of EOs against all tested pathogen bacteria were low and ranged in the interval 0.44–3.55 μL/mL. There is no agreement on the acceptable inhibition level for plant extracts and EOs when compared with standards. However, Duarte et al. [27] recommended a classification of plant extracts based on MIC results (strong inhibitors: MIC up to 500 μg/mL; moderate inhibitors: MIC between 500 and 1500 μg/mL; weak inhibitors: MIC above 1500 μg/mL). According to this recommendation, it was observed that all selected EOs and their mixture could be marked as strong inhibitors against pathogenic bacteria: *E. coli, S.* Enteritidis, *and L. monocytogenes*. In the case of bactericidal potential, the MBC of SHEO was lower than those determined for OMEO and SMEO against all three pathogenic bacteria. The strong antimicrobial effect of SHEO is probably related to its chemical profile and high content of terpenoids: thymol—41.10%; carvacrol—9.99% [28]. Additionally, Burt [29] suggested that essential oil that contains a high percentage of these terpenoids possesses strong antimicrobial potential. These terpenoids stimulate the weakening of the lipid cell membrane, initiating the leakage of cellular contents and, finally, bacterial death [30]. Additionally, it should be noted that the lowest MIC/MBC against *E.*

coli was determined in the mixture of EOs. This could be the result of the synergistic effect of bioactive terpenoids contained in EOs [30].

2.3. Physicochemical Characteristics of Fresh Turkey Sausages

The pH and water activity (a_w) values of fresh turkey sausages ranged from 6.15 to 6.37 and from 0.949 to 0.960, respectively (Table 3). The pH of all the treatments decreased ($p < 0.05$) during the initial 24 h of storage. This could be attributed to the formation of organic acids, primarily lactic acid, due to the metabolic activity of lactic acid bacteria (LAB) [16]. Additionally, a significant ($p < 0.05$) increase in the pH values in all the treatments was recorded on 2nd day of storage. This was most likely related to the accumulation of alkaline compounds, including peptides, amines, and amino acids [31]. At the end of storage, the difference between treatments was approximately 0.05 pH units. Therefore, it was concluded that the addition of selected EOs did not affect ($p > 0.05$) the pH values of fresh turkey sausages.

Table 3. pH and water activity (a_w) values of fresh turkey sausages.

	pH Values				
Storage Day	**Treatments**				
	C	**TOMEO**	**TSHEO**	**TSMEO**	**TEOM**
0	6.35 ± 0.03 ^{aA}	6.37 ± 0.03 ^{aA}	6.37 ± 0.03 ^{aA}	6.36 ± 0.03 ^{aA}	6.37 ± 0.03 ^{aA}
1	6.15 ± 0.02 ^{dA}	6.17 ± 0.04 ^{dA}	6.17 ± 0.02 ^{dA}	6.18 ± 0.00 ^{cA}	6.17 ± 0.02 ^{cA}
2	6.26 ± 0.02 ^{bA}	6.28 ± 0.01 ^{bcA}	6.33 ± 0.02 ^{bB}	6.35 ± 0.02 ^{aBC}	6.36 ± 0.01 ^{aC}
3	6.32 ± 0.01 ^{aA}	6.31 ± 0.02 ^{bA}	6.37 ± 0.02 ^{aC}	6.34 ± 0.01 ^{aA}	6.28 ± 0.02 ^{bB}
4	6.22 ± 0.04 ^{cA}	6.26 ± 0.04 ^{cA}	6.24 ± 0.06 ^{cA}	6.27 ± 0.05 ^{bA}	6.24 ± 0.01 ^{bA}
	a_w Values				
Storage Day	Treatments				
	C	TOMEO	TSHEO	TSMEO	TEOM
0	0.960 ± 0.010 ^{cB}	0.951 ± 0.002 ^{cA}	0.954 ± 0.001 ^{cAB}	0.958 ± 0.001 ^{cAB}	0.951 ± 0.002 ^{cA}
1	0.971 ± 0.002 ^{dC}	0.959 ± 0.002 ^{dA}	0.959 ± 0.002 ^{dA}	0.954 ± 0.001 ^{dB}	0.958 ± 0.001 ^{dA}
2	0.958 ± 0.003 ^{bcA}	0.956 ± 0.001 ^{bcA}	0.951 ± 0.001 ^{bcB}	0.952 ± 0.000 ^{bcB}	0.956 ± 0.001 ^{bcA}
3	0.948 ± 0.002 ^{aA}	0.949 ± 0.001 ^{aA}	0.956 ± 0.001 ^{aC}	0.959 ± 0.002 ^{aB}	0.959 ± 0.001 ^{aB}
4	0.949 ± 0.002 ^{abA}	0.950 ± 0.001 ^{abAB}	0.951 ± 0.001 ^{abAB}	0.954 ± 0.001 ^{abC}	0.952 ± 0.001 ^{abB}

TOMEO—0.150 μL/g *O. majorana* essential oil; TSHEO—0.150 μL/g *S. hortensis* essential oil; TSMEO—0.150 μL/g *S. montana* essential oil; TEOM—0.050 μL/g *O. majorana* essential oil; 0.050 μL/g *S. hortensis* essential oil; and 0.050 μL/g *S. montana* essential oil. Control (C). Means ± SD with different letters $^{(A–E)}$ in the same row are significantly different ($p < 0.05$); values with different letters $^{(a–d)}$ in the same column are significantly different ($p < 0.05$).

The antioxidant potential of fresh turkey sausages is displayed in Figure 1. The induction period is an interval (min) until oxygen pressure drops by 10% from the recorded maximum pressure. The registered values of this indicator ranged in the interval from 511 min (C) to 717 min (TEOM). The differences among the treatments were set as follows: TEOM ≥ TSMEO > TSHEO > TOMEO > C. Thus, the addition of selected EOs and their mixture slowed down the consumption of oxygen, i.e., provided the better oxidative stability of fresh turkey sausages. This finding could be the consequence of the antioxidant potential of terpenoids: terpinen-4-ol (OMEO), thymol (SHEO), and carvacrol (SMEO). The strong antioxidant potential of terpinen-4-ol was previously observed by Li et al. [32]. Moreover, de Oliveira et al. [33] suggested that thymol and carvacrol efficiently reduced lipid oxidation in meat products by scavenging free radicals. Due to the strong antioxidant capacity of these terpenoids, SMEO influenced the efficient reduction of lipid oxidation in fresh pork sausages during cold storage [34].

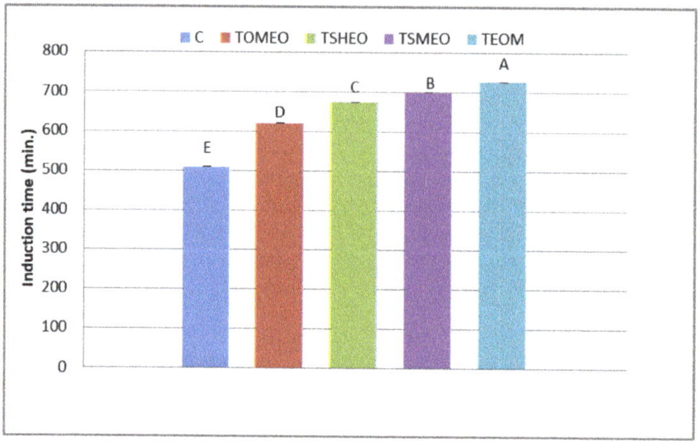

Figure 1. Oxidative stability of fresh turkey sausages. TOMEO—0.150 μL/g *O. majorana* essential oil; TSHEO—0.150 μL/g *S. hortensis* essential oil; TSMEO—0.150 μL/g *S. montana* essential oil; TEOM—0.050 μL/g *O. majorana* essential oil; 0.050 μL/g *S. hortensis* essential oil; and 0.050 μL/g *S. montana* essential oil. Control (C). Different upper cases in superscripts (A–E) indicate difference ($p < 0.05$) between treatments.

2.4. Microbiological Profile of Fresh Turkey Sausages

The microbiological profile of fresh turkey sausages is listed in Table 4. On the 1st day of storage, the total plate count (TPC) fluctuated from 4.33 log cfu/g (TEOM) to 5.44 log cfu/g (C). During the storage, TPC significantly ($p < 0.05$) increased for all five treatments. On 3rd day of storage, acceptable TPC was determined in TOMEO and TSHEO. According to the European Commission [35], the adequate microbiological quality of ground meat is reached when the TPC is lower than 6 log cfu/g. At the end of storage, the following differences in TPC were determined: C > TSHEO ≥ TSMEO > TEOM ≥ TOMEO. Generally, the addition of EOs significantly ($p < 0.05$) reduced TPC [29]. These outcomes established the strong antibacterial potential of selected EOs, particularly OMEO. The antimicrobial effect of *Origanum* species positively correlates with terpinen-4-ol content as the most dominant compound of OMEO [28]. Moreover, Cox et al. [36] observed that terpinene, as one of the main compounds of OMEO, inhibits the oxidative respiration of bacterial strains, causing damage to cytoplasmic membranes. According to this study, Yasar et al. [37] determined that OMEO possess a strong antimicrobial capacity regarding TPC in fresh beef meat.

Enterobacteriaceae count (TEC) and LAB counts generally increased during storage (Table 4). All three EOs and their mixture efficiently reduced TEC and LAB counts compared to C. The differences for both TEC and LAB counts were determined as follows: C > TSMEO > TOMEO > TEOM > TSHEO, at the end of storage. Generally, these bacteria possess very similar sensitivity against selected EOs. SHEO possesses the highest antimicrobial potential against the aforementioned microorganisms. This could be the consequence of the antimicrobial potential of thymol and carvacrol [29]. Carvacrol is marked as the terpenoid phenol with the highest antimicrobial potential. The high content of carvacrol causes the increased permeability of cell membranes. It simultaneously affects a reduction in pH gradient across the cytoplasm membrane, as well as the inhibition of ATP synthesis and, finally, the death of bacterial cells [28]. In this study, the highest antimicrobial potential against TEC and LAB was determined in the TSHEO. Although SHEO contains a lower percentage of carvacrol than SMEO, the most pronounced antimicrobial potential of SHEO could be the consequence of the synergistic effect of thymol and carvacrol with minor terpenoids, including *trans*-caryophyllene (3.25%) and β-bisabolene (3.45%). Carneiro et al. [38] and Ghavam et al. [39] determined the strong antibacterial potential of β-bisabolene and *trans*-caryophyllene.

Table 4. Microbiological profile of fresh turkey sausages.

Storage Day	Total Plate Count—TPC (log cfu/g)				
	Treatments				
	C	TOMEO	TSHEO	TSMEO	TEOM
1	5.44 ± 0.16^{aD}	4.87 ± 0.02^{aA}	4.67 ± 0.03^{aC}	4.95 ± 0.01^{aA}	4.33 ± 0.03^{aB}
2	6.08 ± 0.07^{bB}	5.76 ± 0.02^{bA}	4.98 ± 0.02^{bC}	6.07 ± 0.11^{bB}	5.67 ± 0.03^{bA}
3	6.50 ± 0.03^{cC}	5.99 ± 0.01^{cA}	6.00 ± 0.11^{cA}	6.19 ± 0.02^{cB}	6.09 ± 0.08 c^{AB}
4	7.00 ± 0.05^{dC}	6.12 ± 0.06^{dA}	6.28 ± 0.00^{dB}	6.26 ± 0.05^{dB}	6.14 ± 0.06^{dA}
	Total *Enterobacteriaceae* Count—TEC (log cfu/g)				
Storage Day	Treatments				
	C	TOMEO	TSHEO	TSMEO	TEOM
1	2.66 ± 0.18^{aC}	2.04 ± 0.04^{aAB}	2.12 ± 0.12^{aAB}	2.22 ± 0.06^{aB}	1.96 ± 0.00^{aA}
2	3.50 ± 0.02^{bD}	3.02 ± 0.02^{bC}	2.00 ± 0.00^{bB}	2.80 ± 0.10^{bA}	2.85 ± 0.05^{bA}
3	3.93 ± 0.03^{cE}	3.74 ± 0.04^{cD}	3.39 ± 0.09^{cC}	3.00 ± 0.00^{cA}	3.15 ± 0.15^{cB}
4	4.50 ± 0.02^{dE}	3.52 ± 0.01^{dC}	3.06 ± 0.02^{dA}	4.09 ± 0.01^{dD}	3.31 ± 0.01^{dB}
	Lactic acid Bacteria—LAB Count (log cfu/g)				
Storage Day	Treatments				
	C	TOMEO	TSHEO	TSMEO	TEOM
1	2.98 ± 0.02^{aD}	2.50 ± 0.03^{aA}	2.42 ± 0.12^{aA}	2.79 ± 0.09^{aC}	1.85 ± 0.00^{aB}
2	3.61 ± 0.00^{bD}	2.69 ± 0.09^{bA}	2.15 ± 0.15^{B}	2.93 ± 0.03^{C}	2.74 ± 0.04^{A}
3	3.26 ± 0.26^{cC}	2.97 ± 0.07^{cAB}	2.78 ± 0.0^{cA}	3.65 ± 0.12^{cD}	3.20 ± 0.05^{cBC}
4	3.97 ± 0.07^{dD}	3.06 ± 0.06^{dA}	2.71 ± 0.11^{dB}	3.40 ± 0.10^{dC}	2.95 ± 0.17^{dA}

TOMEO—0.150 µL/g *O. majorana* essential oil; TSHEO—0.150 µL/g *S. hortensis* essential oil; TSMEO—0.150 µL/g *S. montana* essential oil; TEOM—0.050 µL/g *O. majorana* essential oil, 0.050 µL/g *S. hortensis* essential oil; and 0.050 µL/g *S. montana* essential oil. Control (C). Means ± SD with different letters $^{(A–E)}$ in the same row are significantly different ($p < 0.05$); values with different letters $^{(a–d)}$ in the same column are significantly different ($p < 0.05$).

The strong antimicrobial potential of SHEO in minced poultry meat was determined by Azimi et al. [40]. Moreover, SHEO efficiently reduced the growth of *Staphylococcus aureus* and *E. coli* in minced beef meat [41]. Previously, the antimicrobial potential of SMEO was confirmed, as it reduced the growth of TEC in fresh pork sausage when applied in similar concentrations (0.075–0.150 µL/g) [34].

Foodborne pathogens (*E. coli*, *L. monocytogenes* and S. spp.) were not detected in any treatment of fresh turkey sausages analyzed in this study. This finding could be an indicator of good hygienic practices applied during manufacturing in the meat processing pilot plant.

2.5. Biogenic Amines Contents in Fresh Turkey Sausages

Six BA were analyzed in samples of fresh turkey sausages using the HPLC method, and the determined BA profile is presented in Figure 2. Tryptamine (TRY), phenylethylamine (PHE), and histamine (HIS) were not detected in any sausage sample during four days of storage, while tyramine (TIR) was the dominant amine found in all samples starting from the first day until the end of storage, except in treatments TSHEO and TEOM after one day.

Values of TIR ranged from 19.3 mg/kg (TSMEO, 1st day) to 184 mg/kg (C, 4th day). The storage time significantly influenced ($p < 0.05$) this BA content in all treatments, except in TEOM, where it remained almost the same between the second and third day ($p > 0.05$). Additionally, treatment significantly influenced ($p < 0.05$) TIR formation, i.e., addition of EOs significantly ($p < 0.05$) reduced TIR concentration during the whole storage period. TIR level was higher than 100 mg/kg in C samples after only two days, in TOMEO and TSMEO after 3 days, and in TSHEO after 4 days. Thus it exceeded the previously reported threshold value for potential poisoning due to TIR [11,14,22]. On the other hand, the concentration of this BA in TEOM remained below this level throughout the storage period. This finding is in accordance with previously published results by several authors [9,12,15] regarding the positive correlation between the LAB counts and the concentration of TIR in sausages.

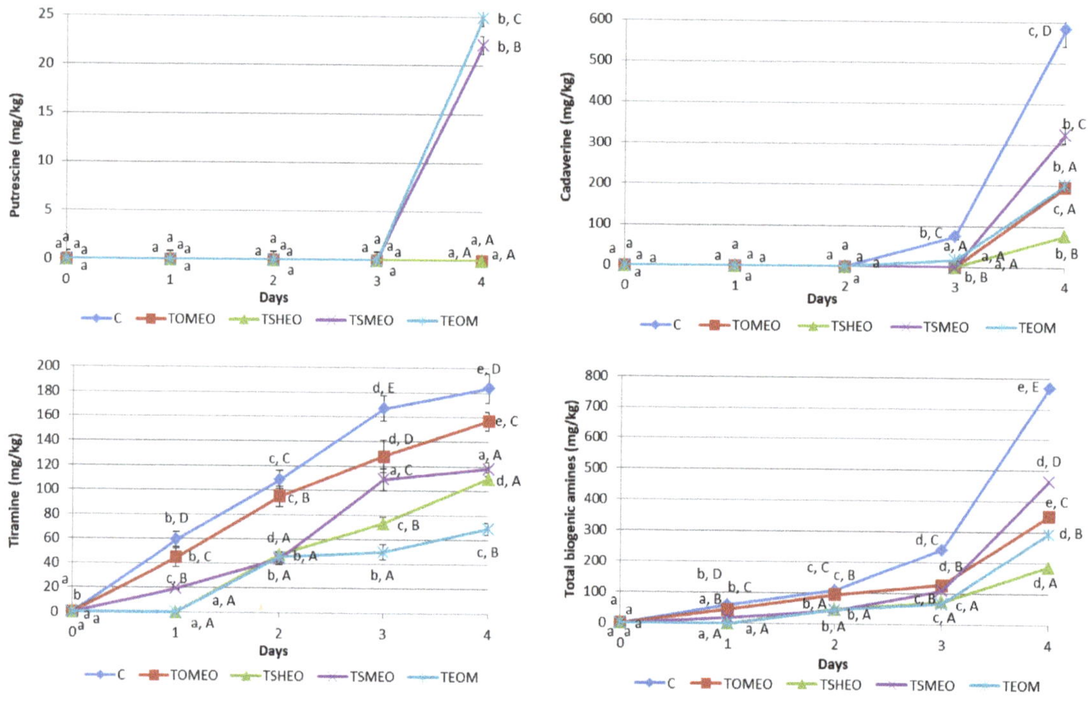

Figure 2. Evolution of biogenic amines (mg/kg) in fresh turkey sausages during storage. TOMEO—0.150 μL/g *O. majorana* essential oil; TSHEO—0.150 μL/g *S. hortensis* essential oil; TSMEO—0.150 μL/g *S. montana* essential oil; TEOM—0.050 μL/g *O. majorana* essential oil; 0.050 μL/g *S. hortensis* essential oil; and 0.050 μL/g *S. montana* essential oil; Control (C). Different upper cases (A–E) indicate difference ($p < 0.05$) between treatments at the same storage day. Different lower cases (a–e) indicate difference ($p < 0.05$) between different storage day, for each treatment.

Putrescine (PUT) was found just in sausages from TSMEO (22.1 mg/kg) and TEOM (24.9 mg/kg), after four days of refrigerated storage. Cadaverine (CAD) was determined for the first time after 3 days in C (75.2 mg/kg) and TEOM (17.5 mg/kg) sausages. The highest value of CAD was found at the end of the storage period in C sample, being 582 mg/kg. On the contrary, the sausages made with the addition of EOs were characterized by a much lower level of CAD at the end of the storage period, varying in a relatively wide range, from 77 mg/kg (TSHEO) to 324 mg/kg (TSMEO). Thus, most of the obtained values for this BA were significantly different ($p < 0.05$), except the ones registered for TOMEO and TEOM. High levels of PUT and CAD can contribute to food poisoning even though they do not have a direct negative health effect. However, it is known that these BA can potentiate the toxicity of HIS [13,14]. Considering the fact that HIS was not registered in all tested sausages during the storage period, it can be concluded that the risk level of poisoning due to their consumption is very low. Nevertheless, the accumulation of PUT and CAD in meat products could be correlated with the growth and metabolic activity of contaminant bacteria, i.e., *Enterobacteriaceae*, indicating lower quality (freshness) of raw materials and processing hygiene [11,14,15].

Regarding the total BA concentration, the following order was registered: C > TSMEO > TOMEO > TEOM > TSHEO. It can be seen that the levels of total BA were in complete accordance with the previously shown results concerning TEC and LAB counts (Table 4), confirming these microorganisms' significant influence on BA generation. The storage time had a significant influence ($p < 0.05$) on total BA content both in C and treated sausages (TOMEO, TSHEO, TSMEO, and TEOM). Additionally, the influence of added EOs on total BA concentration was significant ($p < 0.05$), being especially noticeable after 4 days of storage. According to the results obtained in this study, it could be concluded that adding selected EOs into basic sausage formulation significantly reduced ($p < 0.05$) the formation and accumulation of BA in fresh turkey sausage. This finding is consistent with the previously published results obtained by a number of authors investigating the effects of different plant EOs on BA levels in meat products [14,22,31].

3. Materials and Methods

3.1. Plant Material and Essential Oils

O. majorana L. (OM), grown in Serbia, was produced by the Geneza d.o.o., Kanjiža, Serbia. OMEO was obtained according to the official Ph. Eur. VII procedure [42]. *S. hortensis* L. (SH) and *S. montana* L. (SM) were produced by Herba d.o.o (Serbia). The procedure was repeated in order to collect the proper level of obtained EOs (OMEO, SHEO, and SMEO) for further application in fresh turkey sausage processing.

3.2. GC-MS Analysis of Essential Oils

The terpenoids profile of EOs was determined by GC system (7890A, Agilent Technologies, Santa Clara, CA, USA) coupled with MS detector (5975C, Agilent Technologies, USA) and capillary column (30 m × 0.25 mm, 0.25 μm; 19091S-433UI HP-5MSUI, Agilent Technologies, USA). The samples were dissolved and properly diluted in methylene chloride prior to GC analysis. Injection volume was set at 1 μL and prepared samples were injected into the GC system via autosampler (7683B, Agilent Technologies, USA). The mobile phase was helium (>99.9997%), which was set at a constant flow rate of 2 mL/min. The temperature regime of GC oven was set as follows: starting temperature was 60 °C; 0–30 min temperature was increasing up to 150 °C at a rate of 3 °C/min; 30–35 min temperature was increasing up to 250 °C at a of rate 20 °C/min; and 35–40 min temperature was constant at 250 °C for 5 min. The injection temperature was set at a 250 °C. The terpenoids were identified using the NIST database of MS spectra and the database in the literature [43]. For the additional confirmation of terpenoids, the linear retention indices (LRI) were calculated for all identified compounds and compared with LRI reported in the literature [43]. The final results were expressed as a relative percentage (%) ± standard deviation.

3.3. Antimicrobial Activity of Essential Oils

The antimicrobial activity of selected EOs and their mixture was performed using the microdilution method. The MIC and MBC of the EOs were determined using the broth microdilution method according to Kocić-Tanackov et al. [44]. The antimicrobial activity of selected EOs was evaluated on *Escherichia coli* ATCC 8739; *Salmonella enterica* subsp. *enterica* serovar Enteritidis (group D) ATCC 14028; and *Listeria monocytogenes*, ATCC 13932, obtained from the American Type Culture Collection.

The MIC was determined as the lowest EOs concentration that inhibited the growth in the well (clear broth suspension) but still showed slightly visible growth on the plate. MBC was determined at the EOs concentration that inhibited growth in the well and showed no visible growth on the plate (the presence of ≤2 cfu per plate is acceptable). All tests were performed in duplicates for each EO.

3.4. Preparation of Fresh Sausage

Fresh turkey sausages were manufactured in a meat processing pilot plant (Institute of Food Technology, Novi Sad, Serbia) according to principles of good manufacturing practice (GMP) and good hygienic practice (GHP). Firstly, fresh turkey shoulders were deboned and trimmed to remove visible fat and connective tissues. The prepared meat at 3 ± 1 °C was minced using a stainless steel electric meat grinder (Titan 70 mm, Slovenia) until 8 mm meat particles were obtained. Further, ground meat was manually mixed with the seasonings for approximately 5 min. The basic formulation of fresh turkey sausages involved 98% lean turkey meat and 2% salt. Formerly, the following treatments (5) were processed with the supplementation of EOs: TOMEO—0.150 μL/g OMEO; TSHEO—0.150 μL/g SHEO; TSMEO—0.150 μL/g SMEO; TEOM—0.050 μL/g OMEO; 0.050 μL/g SHEO; 0.050 μL/g SMEO; and control (C) (without EOs). The sample sausages were stuffed in natural casings (pig small intestines; Ø ≈ 32 mm) using stainless steel piston filler SC-13 STAR (Talleres Ramon SL, Spain). The all sample sausages were processed under the same hygienic conditions, which implied low ambient temperature (10 °C) and the usage of sanitized accessories and equipment. Subsequently, sausages (approximately 0.1 kg each) were stored in the refrigerator at 3 ± 1 °C for 4 days. Samples were taken at different periods, after 0, 1, 2, 3, and 4 days of refrigerated storage, consisting of three randomly selected fresh turkey sausages from each treatment.

3.5. Physicochemical Analysis of Fresh Turkey Sausages

The oxidative stability of fresh turkey sausages was analyzed by RapidOxy 100 (Anton Paar, Blankenfelde-Mahlow, Germany). The method was described in detail by Jovanović et al. [45]. The samples were subjected to analysis immediately after the stuffing.

The pH was measured using a digital pH meter Testo 205 (Testo SE & Co. KGaA, Titisee-Neustadt, Germany), which was calibrated using standard buffers (pH = 4.00 ± 0.05 and pH = 7.00 ± 0.01 at 20 ± 2 °C) before measurements. Water activity (a_w) was measured using a LabSwift-a_w measuring instrument (NovasinaAG, Lachen, Switzerland).

3.6. Microbiological Analysis of Fresh Turkey Sausages

The following microbiological analyses were performed: TPC—total plate count [46], TEC—*Enterobacteriaceae* count [47]; LAB—lactic acid bacteria count [48]; *E. coli* [49]; *L. monocytogenes* [50]; *Salmonella* spp. [51]; and sulfite-reducing clostridia count [52]. Results were expressed as a log cfu/g.

3.7. Biogenic Amines Determination in Fresh Turkey Sausages

BA were analyzed using high-performance liquid chromatography—HPLC (Agilent 1200 series, Agilent Technologies, Inc., Santa Clara, CA, USA). Tryptamine (TRY), phenylethylamine (PHE), putrescine (PUT), cadaverine (CAD), histamine (HIS), and tyramine (TIR) were determined as their dansyl derivatives, after homogenization (T18 Basic Ultra Turrax; IKA-Werke GmbH & Co. KG) and extraction with 0.4 M perchloric acid solution [15]. The single analysis lasted for 12 min, and the system was equilibrated for 6 min before the next analysis.

3.8. Statistical Analysis

Statistical analysis was conducted using STATISTICA 14.0 (TIBCO Software Inc., Palo Alto, CA, USA). All data were shown as mean values with their standard deviation indicated (mean value ± SD). Differences among treatments were assessed using Duncan's post hoc test and were considered significant at $p < 0.05$.

4. Conclusions

The most dominant compounds in selected EOs were: terpinen-4-ol (27.69%)—OMEO; thymol (41.10%)—SHEO; and carvacrol (53.58%)—SMEO. The SHEO and the mixture of selected EOs possess the highest antimicrobial potential against pathogen bacteria (*E. coli*, *S.* Enteritidis, and *L. monocytogenes*) in vitro. The highest antioxidant potential in sausage samples was determined in the mixture of EOs. Moreover, all three EOs and their mixtures influenced the reduction of TPC, TEC, and LAB counts in sausage samples during refrigerated storage. The supplementation of selected EOs into sausage formulation affected a significant reduction ($p < 0.05$) in the formation and accumulation of BA in fresh turkey sausages. TRY, PHE, and HIS were not detected in any sausage sample during four days of storage, while TIR was the predominant amine found in almost all samples starting from the 1st day. The highest concentration of a particular BA was registered for CAD at the end of the storage period in the C sample. At the same time, the sausages made with the addition of EOs were characterized by much lower levels of CAD. These data strongly suggest that all selected EOs and their mixture could be used as natural antimicrobials in fresh turkey sausages. Thus, meat processors could be strongly encouraged to use these EOs as natural additives in meat processing.

Supplementary Materials: The following supporting information can be downloaded at: https://www.mdpi.com/article/10.3390/antibiotics12010182/s1, Figure S1: GC-MS Total ion chromatograms of (a) *Origanum majorana*; (b) *Satureja hortensis*; (c) *Satureja montana* essential oils.

Author Contributions: Conceptualization, B.Š., B.P. and P.I.; methodology, B.Š., B.P. and S.K.-T.; software, M.Ž. and T.P.; validation, Z.Z., S.K.-T. and T.P.; formal analysis, T.P., N.T., I.L., M.P. and M.Ž.; investigation, B.Š., P.I., N.T., I.L. and T.P.; resources, B.P., P.I. and S.K.-T.; data curation, M.Ž., M.P., S.V. and I.L.; writing—original draft preparation, B.Š., B.P., P.I., I.L.,T.P. and S.K.-T.; writing—review and editing, B.Š., Z.Z., N.T. and P.I.; visualization, T.P., M.P., M.Ž. and S.V.; supervision, B.Š, B.P. and Z.Z.; project administration, B.P.; funding acquisition, B.P., S.V., I.L., T.P., S.K.-T. and P.I. All authors have read and agreed to the published version of the manuscript.

Funding: The research in this paper was financed by the Science Fund of Republic Serbia: "Novel extracts and bioactive compounds from under-utilized resources for high-value applications"—BioUtilize, No: 7750168, as well as by the Ministry of Education, Science and Technological Development of the Republic of Serbia (Agreement No: 451-03-68/2022-14/200222).

Institutional Review Board Statement: Not applicable.

Informed Consent Statement: Not applicable.

Data Availability Statement: The data presented in this study are available in article and Supplementary Material.

Conflicts of Interest: The authors declare no conflict of interest.

References

1. Biogenic, D.; Biesek, J.; Banaszak, M.; Adamski, M.; Wójcik, W.; Łukasiewicz-Mierzejewska, M.; Damaziak, K.; Bié, D. Biogenic Amines in Poultry Meat and Poultry Products: Formation, Appearance, and Methods of Reduction. *Animals* **2022**, *12*, 1577. [CrossRef]
2. FAO. *World Food and Agriculture—Statistical Yearbook 2020*; FAO: Rome, Italy, 2020.
3. Amirkhanov, K.; Igenbayev, A.; Nurgazezova, A.; Okuskhanova, E.; Kassymov, S.; Muslimova, N.; Yessimbekov, Z. Comparative analysis of red and white Turkey meat quality. *Pakistan J. Nutr.* **2017**, *16*, 412–416. [CrossRef]
4. Askerov, P.F.; Rabadanovich, A.; Kibirov, K.G.; Tolparov, E.B.; Bondarenko, O.V.; Khairbekov, A.U. Role and Importance of Turkey Meat Production in Poultry Farming in Russia: Prospects for Further Development. *Entomol. Appl. Sci. Lett.* **2021**, *8*, 15–20. [CrossRef]
5. Igenbayev, A.; Okuskhanova, E.; Nurgazezova, A.; Ya, R.; Kassymov, S.; Nurymkhan, G.; Tazeddinova, D.; Mironova, I.; Rebezov, M. Fatty acid composition of female turkey muscles in Kazakhstan. *J. World's Poult. Res.* **2019**, *9*, 78–81. [CrossRef]
6. Georgantelis, D.; Ambrosiadis, I.; Katikou, P.; Blekas, G.; Georgakis, S.A. Effect of rosemary extract, chitosan and α-tocopherol on microbiological parameters and lipid oxidation of fresh pork sausages stored at 4 °C. *Meat Sci.* **2007**, *76*, 172–181. [CrossRef]

7. Regulation on the Quality of Ground Meat, Meat Preparations and Meat Products. UNEP Law and Environment Assistance Platform. Available online: https://leap.unep.org/countries/rs/national-legislation/regulation-quality-ground-meat-meat-preparations-and-meat (accessed on 21 December 2022).
8. Ikonić, P.; Jokanović, M.; Petrović, L.; Tasić, T.; Škaljac, S.; Šojić, B.; Džinić, N.; Tomović, V.; Tomić, J.; Danilović, B.; et al. Effect of Starter Culture Addition and Processing Method on Proteolysis and Texture Profile of Traditional Dry-Fermented Sausage Petrovská klobása. *Int. J. Food Prop.* **2016**, *19*, 1924–1937. [CrossRef]
9. Domínguez, R.; Munekata, P.E.; Agregán, R.; Lorenzo, J.M. Effect of commercial starter cultures on free amino acid, biogenic amine and free fatty acid contents in dry-cured foal sausage. *LWT—Food Sci. Technol.* **2016**, *71*, 47–53. [CrossRef]
10. Triki, M.; Herrero, A.M.; Jiménez-Colmenero, F.; Ruiz-Capillas, C. Quality Assessment of Fresh Meat from Several Species Based on Free Amino Acid and Biogenic Amine Contents during Chilled Storage. *Foods* **2018**, *7*, 132. [CrossRef]
11. Fraqueza, M.J.; Alfaia, C.M.; Barreto, A.S. Biogenic amine formation in turkey meat under modified atmosphere packaging with extended shelf life: Index of freshness. *Poult. Sci.* **2012**, *91*, 1465–1472. [CrossRef]
12. Latorre-Moratalla, M.L.; Bover-Cid, S.; Bosch-Fusté, J.; Veciana-Nogués, M.T.; Vidal-Carou, M.C. Amino acid availability as an influential factor on the biogenic amine formation in dry fermented sausages. *Food Control* **2014**, *36*, 76–81. [CrossRef]
13. Rabie, M.A.; Siliha, H.; El-Saidy, S.; El-Badawy, A.A.; Malcata, F.X. Effects of γ-irradiation upon biogenic amine formation in Egyptian ripened sausages during storage. *Innov. Food Sci. Emerg. Technol.* **2010**, *11*, 661–665. [CrossRef]
14. Zhang, X.; Wang, H.; Li, X.; Sun, Y.; Pan, D.; Wang, Y.; Cao, J. Effect of cinnamon essential oil on the microbiological and physiochemical characters of fresh Italian style sausage during storage. *Anim. Sci. J.* **2019**, *90*, 435–444. [CrossRef] [PubMed]
15. Ikonić, P.; Jokanović, M.; Ćućević, N.; Peulić, T.; Šarić, L.; Tomičić, Z.; Škaljac, S.; Delić, J.; Lakićević, B.; Tomašević, I. Effect of different ripening conditions on amino acids and biogenic amines evolution in Sjenički sudžuk. *J. Food Compos. Anal.* **2023**, *115*, 105009. [CrossRef]
16. Sharma, H.; Mendiratta, S.K.; Agrawal, R.K.; Gurunathan, K.; Kumar, S.; Singh, T.P. Use of various essential oils as bio preservatives and their effect on the quality of vacuum packaged fresh chicken sausages under frozen conditions. *LWT—Food Sci. Technol.* **2017**, *81*, 118–127. [CrossRef]
17. Tomović, V.; Jokanović, M.; Šojić, B.; Škaljac, S.; Ivić, M. Plants as natural antioxidants for meat products. *IOP Conf. Ser. Earth Environ. Sci.* **2017**, *85*, 012030. [CrossRef]
18. Putnik, P.; Lorenzo, J.M.; Barba, F.J.; Roohinejad, S.; Jambrak, A.R.; Granato, D.; Montesano, D.; Kovačević, D.B. Novel Food Processing and Extraction Technologies of High-Added Value Compounds from Plant Materials. *Foods* **2018**, *7*, 106. [CrossRef] [PubMed]
19. Da Silveira, S.M.; Luciano, F.B.; Fronza, N.; Cunha, A.; Scheuermann, G.N.; Vieira, C.R.W. Chemical composition and antibacterial activity of *Laurus nobilis* essential oil towards foodborne pathogens and its application in fresh Tuscan sausage stored at 7 °C. *LWT—Food Sci. Technol.* **2014**, *59*, 86–93. [CrossRef]
20. Araújo, M.K.; Gumiela, A.M.; Bordin, K.; Luciano, F.B.; de Macedo, R.E.F. Combination of garlic essential oil, allyl isothiocyanate, and nisin Z as bio-preservatives in fresh sausage. *Meat Sci.* **2018**, *143*, 177–183. [CrossRef]
21. Šojić, B.; Pavlić, B.; Zeković, Z.; Tomović, V.; Ikonić, P.; Kocić-Tanackov, S.; Džinić, N. The effect of essential oil and extract from sage (*Salvia officinalis* L.) herbal dust (food industry by-product) on the oxidative and microbiological stability of fresh pork sausages. *LWT—Food Sci. Technol.* **2018**, *89*, 749–755. [CrossRef]
22. Carballo, D.E.; Mateo, J.; Andrés, S.; Giráldez, F.J.; Quinto, E.J.; Khanjari, A.; Operta, S.; Caro, I. Microbial Growth and Biogenic Amine Production in a Balkan-Style Fresh Sausage during Refrigerated Storage under a CO2-Containing Anaerobic Atmosphere: Effect of the Addition of *Zataria multiflora* Essential Oil and Hops Extract. *Antibiotics* **2019**, *8*, 227. [CrossRef]
23. Šojić, B.; Pavlić, B.; Ikonić, P.; Tomović, V.; Ikonić, B.; Zeković, Z.; Kocić-Tanackov, S.; Jokanović, M.; Škaljac, S.; Ivić, M. Coriander essential oil as natural food additive improves quality and safety of cooked pork sausages with different nitrite levels. *Meat Sci.* **2019**, *157*, 107879. [CrossRef] [PubMed]
24. Paudel, P.N.; Satyal, P.; Satyal, R.; Setzer, W.N.; Gyawali, R. Chemical Composition, Enantiomeric Distribution, Antimicrobial and Antioxidant Activities of *Origanum majorana* L. Essential Oil from Nepal. *Molecular* **2022**, *27*, 6136. [CrossRef] [PubMed]
25. Ghazal, T.S.A.; Schelz, Z.; Vidács, L.; Szemerédi, N.; Veres, K.; Spengler, G.; Hohmann, J. Antimicrobial, Multidrug Resistance Reversal and Biofilm Formation Inhibitory Effect of *Origanum majorana* Extracts, Essential Oil and Monoterpenes. *Plants* **2022**, *11*, 1432. [CrossRef] [PubMed]
26. Tepe, B.; Cilkiz, M. A pharmacological and phytochemical overview on *Satureja*. *Pharm. Biol.* **2015**, *54*, 375–412. [CrossRef] [PubMed]
27. Duarte, M.C.T.; Leme, E.E.; Delarmelina, C.; Soares, A.A.; Figueira, G.M.; Sartoratto, A. Activity of essential oils from Brazilian medicinal plants on *Escherichia coli*. *J. Ethnopharmacol.* **2007**, *111*, 197–201. [CrossRef]
28. Marques, J.D.L.; Volcão, L.M.; Funck, G.D.; Kroning, I.S.; da Silva, W.P.; Fiorentini, Â.M.; Ribeiro, G.A. Antimicrobial activity of essential oils of *Origanum vulgare* L. and *Origanum majorana* L. against *Staphylococcus aureus* isolated from poultry meat. *Ind. Crops Prod.* **2015**, *77*, 444–450. [CrossRef]
29. Burt, S. Essential oils: Their antibacterial properties and potential applications in foods—A review. *Int. J. Food Microbiol.* **2004**, *94*, 223–253. [CrossRef]

30. Lages, L.Z.; Radünz, M.; Gonçalves, B.T.; Silva da Rosa, R.; Fouchy, M.V.; de Cássia dos Santos da Conceição, R.; Gularte, M.A.; Barboza Mendonça, C.R.; Gandra, E.A. Microbiological and sensory evaluation of meat sausage using thyme (*Thymus vulgaris*, L.) essential oil and powdered beet juice (*Beta vulgaris* L., Early Wonder cultivar). *LWT* **2021**, *148*, 111794. [CrossRef]
31. Huang, L.; Wang, Y.; Li, R.; Wang, Q.; Dong, J.; Wang, J.; Lu, S. Thyme essential oil and sausage diameter effects on biogenic amine formation and microbiological load in smoked horse meat sausage. *Food Biosci.* **2021**, *40*, 100885. [CrossRef]
32. Li, Z.; Wei, Y.; Xu, Y.; Han, P.; Jiang, S.; Xu, F.; Wang, H.; Tao, N.; Shao, X. Terpinen-4-ol treatment maintains quality of strawberry fruit during storage by regulating sucrose-induced anthocyanin accumulation. *Postharvest Biol. Technol.* **2021**, *174*, 111461. [CrossRef]
33. Coutinho de Oliveira, T.L.; Malfitano de Carvalho, S.; de Araújo Soares, R.; Andrade, M.A.; Cardoso, M.D.G.; Ramos, E.M.; Piccoli, R.H. Antioxidant effects of *Satureja montana* L. essential oil on TBARS and color of mortadella-type sausages formulated with different levels of sodium nitrite. *LWT—Food Sci. Technol.* **2012**, *45*, 204–212. [CrossRef]
34. Šojić, B.; Pavlić, B.; Tomović, V.; Ikonić, P.; Zeković, Z.; Kocić-Tanackov, S.; Đurović, S.; Škaljac, S.; Jokanović, M.; Ivić, M. Essential oil versus supercritical fluid extracts of winter savory (*Satureja montana* L.)—Assessment of the oxidative, microbiological and sensory quality of fresh pork sausages. *Food Chem.* **2019**, *287*, 280–286. [CrossRef] [PubMed]
35. EUR-Lex-L:2005:338:TOC-EN-EUR-Lex. Available online: https://eur-lex.europa.eu/legal-content/EN/TXT/?uri=OJ:L:2005:338:TOC (accessed on 22 December 2022).
36. Cox, S.D.; Mann, C.M.; Markham, J.L.; Bell, H.C.; Gustafson, J.E.; Warmington, J.R.; Wyllie, S.G. The mode of antimicrobial action of the essential oil of *Melaleuca alternifolia* (tea tree oil). *J. Appl. Microbiol.* **2000**, *88*, 170–175. [CrossRef] [PubMed]
37. Yasar, S.; Nizamlloğlu, N.M.; Gücüş, M.O.; Bildik Dal, A.E.; Akgül, K. *Origanum majorana* L. Essential Oil-Coated Paper Acts as an Antimicrobial and Antioxidant Agent against Meat Spoilage. *ACS Omega* **2022**, *7*, 9033–9043. [CrossRef]
38. Carneiro, N.S.; Alves, C.C.F.; Alves, J.M.; Egea, M.B.; Martins, C.H.G.; Silva, T.S.; Bretanha, L.C.; Balleste, M.P.; Micke, G.A.; Silveira, E.V.; et al. Chemical composition, antioxidant and antibacterial activities of essential oils from leaves and flowers of *Eugenia klotzschiana* Berg (Myrtaceae). *An. Acad. Bras. De Ciênc.* **2017**, *89*, 1907–1915. [CrossRef] [PubMed]
39. Ghavam, M.; Bacchetta, G.; Castangia, I.; Manca, M.L. Evaluation of the composition and antimicrobial activities of essential oils from four species of *Lamiaceae* Martinov native to Iran. *Sci. Rep.* **2022**, *12*, 17044. [CrossRef]
40. Azimi, M.; Naghadehi, M.N.; Moulodi, F.; Mehdi, S.; Rohani, R.; Khaledabad, M.A. The Effects of *Satureja hortensis* L. Essential Oil on the Growth and Survival of *Salmonella typhimorium* in Minced Poultry Meat During Refrigerated Storage. *J. Kermanshah Univ. Med. Sci.* **2018**, *22*, 69640. [CrossRef]
41. Djenane, D.; Yangüela, J.; Amrouche, T.; Boubrit, S.; Boussad, N.; Roncalés, P. Chemical composition and antimicrobial effects of essential oils of *Eucalyptus globulus*, *Myrtus communis* and *Satureja hortensis* against *Escherichia coli* O157:H7 and Staphylococcus aureus in minced beef. *Food Sci. Technol. Int.* **2011**, *17*, 505–515. [CrossRef]
42. Council of, Europe. 2.9.18 Preparations for Inhalation: Aerodynamic Assessment of Fine Particles. In *European Pharmacopoeia 7.0.*; Council of Europe: Strasbourg, France, 2010; pp. 274–285.
43. Adams, R.P. *Identification of Essential Oil Components by Gas Chromatography/Quadrupole Mass Spectroscopy*, 4th ed.; Allured Publishing Corporation: Carol Stream, IL, USA, 2017, ISBN 9781932633214.
44. Kocić-Tanackov, S.; Blagojev, N.; Suturović, I.; Dimić, G.; Pejin, J.; Tomović, V.; Sojić, B.; Savanović, J.; Kravić, S.; Karabasil, N. Antibacterial activity of essential oils against *Escherichia coil*, *Salmonella enterica* and *Listeria monocytogenes*. *J. Food Saf. Food Qual. Fur Leb.* **2017**, *68*, 88–95.
45. Jovanović, P.; Pajin, B.; Lončarić, A.; Jozinović, A.; Petrović, J.; Fišteš, A.; Zarić, D.; Tumbas Šaponjac, V.; Ačkar, Đ.; Lončarević, I. Whey as a Carrier Material for Blueberry Bioactive Components: Incorporation in White Chocolate. *Sustainability* **2022**, *14*, 14172. [CrossRef]
46. *ISO 4833-1:2003*; Microbiology of the Food Chain—Horizontal Method for the Enumeration of Microorganisms—Part 1: Colony Count at 30 °C by the Pour Plate Technique. International Organization for Standardization: Geneva, Switzerland, 2003.
47. *ISO 21528-2:2017*; Microbiology of the Food Chain—Horizontal Method for the Detection and Enumeration of Enterobacteriaceae—Part 2: Colony-Count Technique. International Organization for Standardization: Geneva, Switzerland, 2017.
48. *ISO 15214:1998*; Microbiology of Food and Animal Feeding Stuffs—Horizontal Method for the Enumeration of Mesophilic Lactic Acid Bacteria—Colony-Count Technique at 30 °C. International Organization for Standardization: Geneva, Switzerland, 1998.
49. *ISO 16649-2:2005*; Microbiology of Food and Animal Feeding Stuffs—Horizontal Method for the Enumeration of Beta-Glucuronidase-Positive Escherichia coli—Part 2: Colony-Count Technique at 44 °C Using 5-bromo-4-chloro-3-indolyl beta-D-glucuronide. International Organization for Standardization: Geneva, Switzerland, 2005.
50. *ISO 11290-2:2017*; Microbiology of the Food Chain—Horizontal Method for the Detection and Enumeration of Listeria Monocytogenes and of Listeria spp.—Part 2: Enumeration Method. International Organization for Standardization: Geneva, Switzerland, 2017.

51. *ISO 6579-1:2017*; Microbiology of the Food Chain—Horizontal Method for the Detection, Enumeration and Serotyping of Salmonella—Part 1: Detection of Salmonella spp. International Organization for Standardization: Geneva, Switzerland, 2017.
52. *ISO 15213:2003*; Microbiology of Food and Animal Feeding Stuffs—Horizontal Method for the Enumeration of Sulfite-Reducing Bacteria Growing Under Anaerobic Conditions. International Organization for Standardization: Geneva, Switzerland, 2003.

antibiotics

MDPI

Article

Screening of Antifungal Activity of Essential Oils in Controlling Biocontamination of Historical Papers in Archives

Ana Tomić [1,*], Olja Šovljanski [1,*], Višnja Nikolić [2], Lato Pezo [3], Milica Aćimović [4], Mirjana Cvetković [5], Jovana Stanojev [6], Nebojša Kuzmanović [2] and Siniša Markov [1]

1 Faculty of Technology Novi Sad, University of Novi Sad, Bulevar Cara Lazara 1, 21000 Novi Sad, Serbia
2 The Archives of Vojvodina, Žarka Vasiljevića 2A, 21000 Novi Sad, Serbia
3 Instutute of General and Physical Chemistry, Studenski trg 10-12, 11000 Belgrade, Serbia
4 Institute of Field and Vegetable Crops Novi Sad, University of Novi Sad, Maksima Gorkog 30, 21000 Novi Sad, Serbia
5 Institute of Chemistry, Technology and Metallurgy, University of Belgrade, Njegoševa 12, 11000 Belgrade, Serbia
6 Biosense Institute, University of Novi Sad, Dr Zorana Đinđića 1, 21000 Novi Sad, Serbia
* Correspondence: anav@uns.ac.rs (A.T.); oljasovljanski@uns.ac.rs (O.Š.)

Abstract: The main challenge in controlling the microbiological contamination of historical paper is finding an adequate method that includes the use of cost-effective, harmless, and non-toxic biocides whose effectiveness is maintained over time and without adverse effects on cultural heritage and human health. Therefore, this study demonstrated the possibility of using a non-invasive method of historical paper conservation based on plant essential oils (EOs) application. Evaluation of antimicrobial effects of different EOs (lemongrass, oregano, rosemary, peppermint, and eucalyptus) was conducted against *Cladosporium cladosporoides*, *Aspergillus fumigatus*, and *Penicillium chrysogenum*, which are commonly found on archive papers. Using a mixture of oregano, lemongrass and peppermint in ratio 1:1:1, the lower minimal inhibition concentration (0.78%) and better efficiency during a vapour test at the highest tested distance (5.5 cm) compared with individual EOs was proven. At the final step, this EOs mixture was used in the in situ conservation of historical paper samples obtained from the Archives of Vojvodina. According to the SEM imaging, the applied EOs mixture demonstrates complete efficiency in the inhibition of fungi colonization of archive papers, since fungal growth was not observed on samples, unlike the control samples.

Keywords: paper conservation; paper biodegradation; fungal contamination; essential oil application; fungicide effect

1. Introduction

Nowadays, a great interest in the investigation of using essential oils (EOs) in diverse applications has emerged. This came about as a consequence of the high antimicrobial and antioxidant potential of EOs, so they could be used as a possible replacement for antibiotics and fungicides. EOs are commonly used in cosmetics and perfumes, and the food industry, but also have medicinal applications due to their therapeutic properties [1]. Taking into account the power of EOs, the newest research works are based on their alternative applications, such as part of smart packaging systems or as agents for controlling biocontamination in archives and libraries [2,3].

The prevention and treatment of biological degradation of paper is one of the biggest concerns in the field of preservation of paper materials of archival, library and museum collections. The combination of a high degree of biodegradation of paper with inappropriate microclimate conditions of storage and preservation make this material very sensitive to mould development [4]. In recent decades, much attention in the scientific research community has been focused on the evaluation of antimicrobial substances and testing methods of different materials depending on the characteristics of the material, the type and method of application, and the method of disposal/use [5–8]. The main challenges in the control of microbiological contamination of paper are reflected in finding methods and procedures that include the application of economically profitable biocides that contain harmless and non-toxic active compounds, and whose effectiveness is maintained over time and without harmful effects on cultural heritage and human health [7,8]. Due to their antimicrobial properties, well known since ancient times, natural molecules in plant essential oils are applied to suppress biological colonization. Essential oils contain a spectrum of plant secondary metabolites that can inhibit mould growth [9,10]. They act directly on the microbial cell by inhibiting its growth, causing ruptures of the cytoplasmic membrane, regulating intermediate metabolism, inhibiting enzymatic reactions, etc. [9]. On the other hand, their relationship to paper material is characterized by a high degree of inertness. Due to their highly effective antimicrobial activity against moulds, essential oils represent a potential ecological and economically viable solution for the biodegradation of archival paper materials [4,6,7].

Throughout history, several methods have been developed to prevent and stop the deterioration of paper-based archival materials that represent a significant cultural heritage of a country (e.g., birth records, death records, original historical records, unique and church records, clerical records, etc.) [11]. Most chemical and chemical–physical conservation procedures for the primary prevention of microbiological colonization are based on highly toxic compounds such as benzalkonium chloride, ethylene oxide, permethrin, sodium fluoride, etc. [5,11,12]. These compounds are also characterized by potential carcinogenicity, low degree of degradability, the possibility of uncontrolled pollution in the application environment, but also a minimal conservation effect in cases of already microbiologically contaminated samples of paper materials, which represents a big problem both for operators/conservators and for the treated material [12]. Additionally, most of these compounds are associated with shortcomings in application resulting from insufficient testing of their antimicrobial effect [5,13]. Moreover, there is increasing concern about the environmental and health issues of the use of toxic chemical agents in current conservation treatments. All the above-mentioned facts have led to the necessity of antimicrobial alternatives with lower toxicity as a long-term solution to improve the conservation and protection of historically important papers. Several scientific papers deal with using essential oils as alternative substances for antimicrobial treatment of historical papers [3,4,14–16], indicating the potential of these natural oils in the prevention and inhibition of fungal colonization of paper-based cultural heritage samples.

Based on the above facts, the aim of this paper is to investigate the possibility of using different EOs to control fungal contamination of historical paper. In order to improve further conservation and protection steps of archival materials, a comprehensive approach of selection and application of alternative biocides such as essential oils against archive-originated fungi was involved in this paper. To our knowledge, this is the first study that combines mathematical modelling with microbiological and chemical analysis to obtain the most efficient application method of EOs in historical paper treatment.

2. Results

2.1. Screening of the EOs' Antifungal Activity

The antifungal activity of five EOs against three representative fungi commonly found on archive papers was evaluated by diameters of the inhibition zone by using disc diffusion method. As shown in Table 1, the highest antifungal activity against all tested strains was observed for oregano, lemongrass and peppermint EOs. The activity of these EOs was significantly higher than the activity of actidion, which was used as a positive control. On the other hand, rosemary and eucalyptus EOs exhibit moderate activity against *C. cladosporoides* (5/1), while no antifungal activity was observed against *A. fumigatus* (6/1) and *P. chrysogenum* (7/1). In this step, the inactivity of 5% DMSO against the tested fungi was confirmed, so it can be used for the preparation of lower concentrations of EOs.

Table 1. Inhibition zones (mean value diameter (mm) ± standard deviation) observed on Sabouraud Dextrose Agar.

Essential Oil	Fungal Strain		
	C. cladosporoides (5/1)	*A. fumigatus* (6/1)	*P. chrysogenum* (7/1)
Lemongrass	39.33 ± 1.15	39.00 ± 1.00	38.33 ± 1.53
Oregano	40.00 ± 0.00	40.00 ± 0.00	40.00 ± 0.00
Rosemary	21.33 ± 3.46	nd *	nd
Peppermint	40.00 ± 0.00	39.33 ± 1.15	40.00 ± 0.00
Eucalyptus	14.67 ± 3.21	nd	nd
Actidion	26.67 ± 0.58	25.67 ± 0.58	22.20 ± 2.00
Sterile distilled water	nd	nd	nd
DMSO 5%	nd	nd	nd

* nd—not detected.

2.2. Minimal Inhibitory Concentration Determination

Further testing of the antimicrobial effect against selected fungal representatives included a determination of minimal inhibitory concentrations (MICs) of EOs which have previously showed antifungal activity. According to the obtained results for individual essential oils (Table 2), MICs ranged between 0.78 and 6.75% of the initial concentration of EOs. Additionally, a mixture of efficient EOs (MIX) was tested and the obtained values of MIC of each EO was lower (0.78% for each EO) compared with individual MICs of tested EOs, which indicates a synergistic antifungal effect of tested EOs.

Table 2. The results of minimal inhibitory concentration (%) * ± standard deviation.

Essential Oil	Fungal Strain		
	C. cladosporoides (5/1)	*A. fumigatus* (6/1)	*P. chrysogenum* (7/1)
Lemongrass	1.56 ± 0.00 *	6.75 ± 0.00	6.75 ± 0.00
Oregano	0.78 ± 0.00	1.56 ± 0.00	1.56 ± 0.00
Peppermint	1.56 ± 0.00	6.75 ± 0.00	1.56 ± 0.00
MIX	0.78 ± 0.00	0.78 ± 0.00	0.78 ± 0.00

* the initial concentration of EO was determined as 100% and all lower concentration was obtained using the dilution method.

2.3. Time-Kill Kinetics Study

The time-kill kinetics profile of essential oils was determined against selected fungi using MICs of individual essential oil as well as the mixture of all three together in its MIC values (marked as MIX). Figure 1 shows kinetic models for control samples (non-treated fungal suspensions) and time-kill kinetics models for treated suspensions.

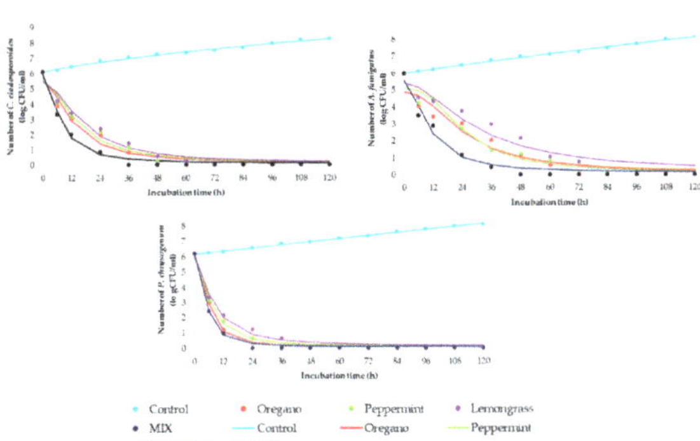

Figure 1. Time-kill kinetics study between MIC values of essential oils (markers signify the experimental data; lines indicate predictive results.

Additionally, Table 3 summarizes the regression coefficients of the observed control and time-kill kinetics models to clarify the speed and intensity of the used concentration of essential oils.

Table 3. Regression coefficients (a, b, c and d) for time-kill kinetics models (directed to Equation (2)).

Sample	Control	Oregano	Peppermint	Lemongrass	MIX
Fungal isolate			*C. cladosporoides* (5/1)		
d	16.261	0.100	0.100	0.100	0.100
a	6.081	5.642	5.592	5.493	5.925
c	549.710	12.062	13.871	16.368	7.337
b	0.862	1.811	1.852	1.890	1.838
			A. fumigatus (6/1)		
d	18.448	0.100	0.100	0.100	0.100
a	6.022	4.893	5.118	5.429	5.578
c	549.684	24.337	24.366	29.861	10.142
b	1.055	2.155	2.484	1.811	1.854
			P. chrysogenum (7/1)		
d	18.654	0.100	0.100	0.100	0.100
a	6.178	6.079	6.081	6.072	6.159
c	549.680	5.685	6.396	7.452	4.739
b	1.092	2.128	1.830	1.596	2.047

The goodness of fit between experimental quantities and model planned results are presented in Table 4. The gained kinetics models can be described as accurate since the coefficient of determination is high (r^2 > 0.938). According to the time-kill kinetic models (Figure 1, Table 4), statistically calculated parameters fitted in well with obtained experimental data, with coefficients of determination between 0.938 and 0.998.

Table 4. The goodness of fit between experimental quantities and model planned results.

Fungi Isolate	Sample	Mathematical Model Quality Parameters									
		χ^2	RMSE	MBE	MPE	r^2	Skew	Kurt	Mean	StDev	Var
C. cladosporoides (5/1)	Control	0.006	0.076	0.002	0.927	0.988	−0.018	−1.33	0.0023	0.0795	0.006
	Oregano	0.148	0.369	−0.117	5.071	0.972	0.976	0.233	−0.117	0.365	0.133
	Peppermint	0.150	0.371	−0.113	20.223	0.972	1.074	0.008	−0.113	0.369	0.136
	Lemongrass	0.152	0.373	−0.103	20.307	0.971	1.06	−0.011	−0.103	0.374	0.140
	MIX	0.051	0.217	−0.109	3.268	0.992	0.754	−0.403	−0.11	0.195	0.038
A. fumigatus (6/1)	Control	0.003	0.057	0.001	0.642	0.993	−0.180	−0.566	0.001	0.059	0.003
	Oregano	0.287	0.513	−0.09	10.769	0.938	1.197	0.938	−0.09	0.528	0.279
	Peppermint	0.17	0.396	−0.061	7.400	0.965	0.86	1.821	−0.061	0.409	0.167
	Lemongrass	0.304	0.528	−0.146	11.658	0.949	0.459	−1.533	−0.1456	0.53	0.280
	MIX	0.109	0.317	−0.112	7.373	0.979	0.880	0.409	−0.112	0.309	0.096
P. chrysogenum (7/1)	Control	0.001	0.037	0.000	0.450	0.997	0.064	−1.202	−0.0003	0.038	0.001
	Oregano	0.029	0.163	−0.103	0.683	0.998	0.048	0.926	−0.103	0.132	0.017
	Peppermint	0.037	0.185	−0.108	2.001	0.995	0.881	0.407	−0.108	0.157	0.024
	Lemongrass	0.062	0.238	−0.109	4.752	0.989	0.741	−0.761	−0.109	0.221	0.049
	MIX	0.023	0.144	−0.103	0.754	0.998	0.0704	0.725	−0.103	0.105	0.011

Legend: χ^2—reduced chi-square; RMSE—root mean square error; MBE—mean bias error; MPE—mean percentage error; r^2—coefficient of determination; Skew—skewedness; Kurt—kurtosis; StDev—standard deviation; Var—variance.

2.4. Chemical Composition of Selected EOs

The main compounds detected in three effective essential oils are presented in Table 5, while complete chemical compositions were shown in Supplementary Table S1. According to the gained results, the most abundant compounds in oregano essential oil (66 compounds, comprising 99.9%) were γ-terpinene (19.6%), carvacrol (15.6%), p-cymene (11.0%), and sabinene (8.8%). Menthol (30.3%), menthone (23.8%), menthouran (7.5%), and menthyl acetate (5.6%) were dominant in the chemical composition of peppermint essential oil (50 compounds, comprising 100%). In lemongrass essential oil (23 compounds, comprising 99.8%), geranial (51.5%) and neral (36.9%) were dominant followed by myrcene (4.8%) and geraniol (2.9%).

Table 5. The dominant compounds in selected essential oil (complete chemical composition was given in Supplementary Table S1).

Essential Oil					
Oregano (*Origanum vulgare*)		**Peppermint (*Mentha piperita*)**		**Lemongrass (*Cymbopogon citratus*)**	
Compounds	%	**Compounds**	%	**Compounds**	%
γ-terpinene	19.6	Menthol	30.3	Geranial	51.5
Carvacrol	15.6	Menthone	23.8	Neral	36.9
p-cymene	11.0	Menthouran	7.5	Myrcene	4.8
Sabinene	8.8	Menthyl acetate	5.6	Geraniol	2.9

2.5. EOs Efficiency in Vapour Phase

After validation of high antifungal activity of the chosen three EOs in direct contact with fungal isolates, the efficiency of the EOs' vapour phase on the fungal growth was evaluated using predictive mathematical analysis based on the surface area of fungal growth on Petri plates. Different distances between EO samples and inoculated Petri plates (1–5.5 cm) were analysed. The obtained images of Petri plates were presented in Supplementary Figures S1–S3. The obtained data were subjected to computer determination of the contaminated area, and the obtained surface area values were presented in Table 6. The complete absent of fungal growth was defined as 0% (negative result), while the fungal growth on the entire plate surface was determined as 100% (positive result). All presented results are quantified between these two values.

Table 6. Interpretation of data * for EOs efficiency in vapour phase based on contaminated surface area.

		Contaminated Area (%) *											
Microorganism		***C. cladosporoides* (5/1)**				***A. fumigatus* (6/1)**				***P. chrysogenum* (7/1)**			
Essential Oil		**Oregano**	**Peppermint**	**Lemongrass**	**MIX**	**Oregano**	**Peppermint**	**Lemongrass**	**MIX**	**Oregano**	**Peppermint**	**Lemongrass**	**MIX**
Distance (cm)	1	0	0	0	0	0	0	0	0	0	0	0	0
	2.5	0	0	0	0	0	0	0	0	0	0	0	0
	3.5	0	0	0	0	0	0	0	0	0	0	0	0
	4.5	0	0	0	0	0	32	43	0	0	15	54	0
	5.5	0	0	0	0	32	53	61	0	11	91	92	0

* The complete absent of fungal growth was defined as zero (0)—negative result, while the fungal growth on the entire plate surface was determined as one (1)—positive result.

The obtained results of fungal growth on Petri plates were evaluated through regression coefficients, as presented in Table 7. The calculation was carried out using exponential model analysis based on Equation (3). Due to the absence of growth in the case of *C. cladosporoides* (5/1) for all essential oils and the mix, a regression coefficient cannot be determined (Table 8). The same situation was observed for *P. chrysogenum* (7/1) in the case of using a mixture of essential oils.

Table 7. Regression coefficients (a and b) for evaluation of EOs' efficiency in vapour phase.

Regression Coefficients	Microorganisms											
	C. cladosporoides (5/1)				*A. fumigatus* (6/1)				*P. chrysogenum* (7/1)			
Essential Oil	Oregano	Peppermint	Lemongrass	MIX	Oregano	Peppermint	Lemongrass	MIX	Oregano	Peppermint	Lemongrass	MIX
a	-	-	-	-	0.676	0.897	0.821	0	0.496	1.233	0.912	-
b	-	-	-	-	0.003	0.004	0.007	0	0.004	0.001	0.006	-

As the next step in the evaluation of EOs, efficiency in vapour phase, the predictive modelling was conducted. The goodness of fit between experimental quantities and model planned results are presented in Table 8. The gained kinetics models can be described as accurate since the coefficient of determination is high ($r^2 > 0.721$). According to the gained models, statistically calculated parameters fitted in well with obtained experimental data, with coefficients of determination between 0.721 and 0.985.

Table 8. The "goodness of fit" between experimental quantities and model planned results.

Fungi Isolate	Sample	Mathematical Model Quality Parameters									
		χ^2	RMSE	MBE	MPE	r^2	Skew	Kurt	Mean	StDev	Var
C. cladosporoides (5/1)	Oregano	-	-	-	-	-	-	-	-	-	-
	Peppermint	-	-	-	-	-	-	-	-	-	-
	Lemongrass	-	-	-	-	-	-	-	-	-	-
	MIX	-	-	-	-	-	-	-	-	-	-
A. fumigatus (6/1)	Oregano	0.011	0.096	0.018	12.646	0.794	2.019	4.300	0.018	0.105	0.011
	Peppermint	0.005	0.062	−0.013	6.746	0.925	1.003	2.183	−0.013	0.068	0.005
	Lemongrass	0.010	0.091	−0.017	7.942	0.887	1.256	2.555	−0.017	0.100	0.010
	MIX	-	-	-	-	-	-	-	-	-	-
P. chrysogenum (7/1)	Oregano	0.001	0.030	−0.005	9.264	0.721	1.623	3.118	−0.005	0.033	0.001
	Peppermint	0.005	0.061	−0.035	14.865	0.985	−0.280	−1.523	−0.035	0.055	0.003
	Lemongrass	0.013	0.103	−0.022	6.539	0.931	0.952	2.119	−0.022	0.113	0.013
	MIX	-	-	-	-	-	-	-	-	-	-

Legend: χ^2—reduced chi-square; RMSE—root mean square error; MBE—mean bias error; MPE—mean percentage error; r^2—coefficient of determination; Skew—skewedness; Kurt—kurtosis; StDev—standard deviation; Var—variance.

2.6. EOs In Situ Application onto Historical Paper Samples

In order to verify decent results provided in previous experiments, the efficacy of an EOs mixture in vapour phase was tested in situ on the historical paper samples. SEM analysis of the samples was carried out in order to detect the difference in microstructure of the historical paper samples artificially contaminated with fungi after the treatment with vapour of EOs mixture, and the same artificially contaminated samples that were not treated with vapour of EOs. In Figure 2a–f, the SEM micrographs for artificially contaminated historical paper substrates non-treated and treated with the vapour of EOs mixture are shown, while in Figure 2g the SEM micrograph of the paper which was used as a blank sample is presented. All of the micrographs were carried out at the magnification ×500.

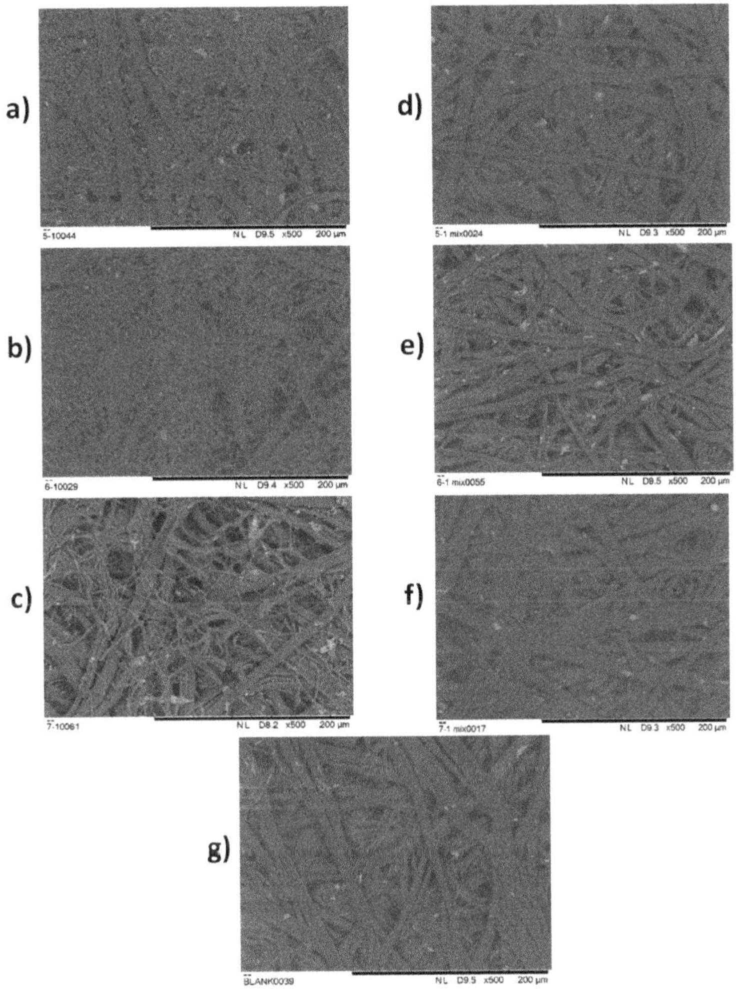

Figure 2. SEM micrographs for: (**a–c**) non treated samples *C. cladosporoides* (5/1), *A. fumigatus* (6/1), and *P. chrysogenum* (7/1), respectively; (**d–f**) treated samples *C. cladosporoides* (5/1) mix, *A. fumigatus* (6/1) mix and *P. chrysogenum* (7/1) mix, respectively; (**g**) blank historical paper sample.

3. Discussion

In recent decades, natural molecules in plant essential oils have been utilized for the suppression of biological colonization in/on different materials. The antimicrobial potential of essential oils is based on their wide range of secondary metabolites that can inhibit mould growth but also possess inert relationships to materials [9,10]. Therefore, the in vitro antimicrobial activity was verified through comprehensive testing, which included several steps: the screening of antifungal activity (Table 1) for five essential oils (lemongrass, oregano, rosemary, peppermint, and eucalyptus), the determination of MIC concentrations (Table 2) for EOs which have fungicide effect, as well as time-kill kinetics for gained MICs against all fungal representatives (Figure 1, Tables 3 and 4).

According to the gained results of the disc-diffusion method, the EOs of oregano, lemongrass and peppermint showed significant antifungal activity against all three tested fungi representatives. The wide inhibition zones with values greater than 38 mm for all tested fungi imply the possibility of using these EOs as fungicide agents. These results are in correlation with the results obtained by other researchers for peppermint [17–20], lemongrass [21–24] and oregano EOs [25–27]. The EOs of the mentioned plants had relatively high antimicrobial activities against many microorganisms, but especially against eukaryotic microorganisms such as the test organisms in this study. The average antimicrobial effect was detected in the case of rosemary and eucalyptus EOs against *C. cladosporoides* (inhibition zones were 21.33 and 14.67 mm, respectively), while the antimicrobial activity against *A. fumigatus* and *P. chrysogenum* were not detected. Based on these results, in can be concluded that *Cladosporium* representative is the most sensitive tested microorganism, while *Aspergillus* and *Penicillium* have similar resistant potential. Considering the gained results, oregano, lemongrass and peppermint EOs were chosen as the most potent EOs for further experiments. In the following test, the MIC values for selected EOs were determined. The obtained results have confirmed that the most sensitive fungus was *C. cladosporoides*, since the concentration of 1.56% was sufficient for the fungicide effect in the case of lemongrass and peppermint EOs, and 0.78% when Oregano EO was applied. For a fungicide effect against *A. fumigatus* and *P. chrysogenum*, the same MICs of 6.75% and 1.56% were determined for lemongrass and oregano, respectively. Only in the case of peppermint EO were the MIC values different, implying a four times higher concentration against *A. fumigatus* (Table 2). Additionally, a fungicide effect against all three fungal representatives can be achieved with lower values of the mentioned EOs (0.78%), using the MIX where the synergistic effect of EOs was accomplished.

In addition to antimicrobial profiling of the selected essential oil, the time-kill kinetics study was conducted. Sim et al. [28] emphasized that monitoring the in vitro pharmacodynamics potential of plant based-substances through a time-kill kinetics study can be a basis for understanding the biocide effect of MIC concentration during contact time. Therefore, the gained results are presented in Figure 1 and Tables 3 and 4. Briefly, the time-kill kinetics profiles for *C. cladosporoides* indicated the relatively rapid fungicide effect of the tested oils, showing the greatest results in the case of using a mixture of essential oils (MIX). A total reduction in fungal viability was observed after the first 36 h in the case of the MIX, while the same effect for the individual effect of essential oil was determined after 60 h. Time-kill kinetics profiles for A. *fumigatus* suggest a slight prolongation of time required for the fungicide effect of individual oils, as well as MIX. Briefly, the mentioned effect was achieved for 72 h in the case of individual oils, videlicet 48 h for the MIX. Comparing the obtained results for *C. cladosporoides* and *A. fumigatus*, it can be observed for *P. chrysogenum* during contact time with different oils and their MIX that the killing rates were higher and inactivation profile was more prompt in all tested cases. The fungicide effect was observed 12 h and 24 h earlier compared with the same effect in the case of contact of MIX and *C. cladosporoides* or *A. fumigatus*, respectively. The individual effect of essential oil on the total reduction of viability of *P. chrysogenum* can be observed in the first 48 h. It can be concluded that the MIX of essential oils accelerates the fungicide effect for all tested fungal isolates, so its use can be economically and time acceptable.

Based on a review of the scientifically relevant literature, different spectra of plant metabolites can be involved in a high antimicrobial response during contact with EOs. In this study, selected EOs were conducted to GC-MS analysis in order to determine chemical profiles and compositions. Comparing the referenced data from the literature about chemical composition with the obtained chemical compositions of EOs in this study (Table 5, Supplementary Table S1), it could be assumed that the largest number of *O. vulgare* essential oil do not have the same chemical composition compared with the presented oil in this study [29–37]. Briefly, the most abundant compound in this oil, γ-terpinene, was not defined in other studies as the most dominant compound. The most usual chemotypes are carvacrol, germacrene D, sabinene, β-ocimene, and β-caryophyllene chemotype. The reason for this variety in chemical composition can be based on different geographical origins, since the mentioned research was conducted in more than 20 different countries across the world. On the other hand, the essential oils *Mentha piperita* and *Cymbopogon citratus* have the usual chemical composition, less dependent on the geographical area of plant growth [20–24,38–43]. In summary, antifungal activity of the dominant compounds in all three tested essential oils was observed, especially γ-terpinene [25–27] and menthol [17–19]. As two dominant compounds which together represent citral, geranial (trans-citral) and neral (cis-citral) in *C. citratus* essential oil have also been studied as effective agents against different fungi in vitro [44]. It is known that many extrinsic and intrinsic factors greatly influence the composition of the EO and the concentration of major and minor components in its chemical profile. Additionally, there is limited information about the influence of individual compounds on antimicrobial properties. For example, it is proven that carvacrol damages the cell membrane of fungi by inhibiting the ergosterol synthesis, which constitutes the backbone of the fungal cell membrane [45]. On the other hand, in one experiment, the vapour of peppermint oil and two its main compounds (menthol and menthone) were tested toward antifungal efficiency against *Sclerotinia sclerotiorum* and *Mucor* spp. The result of this experiment indicates that menthol alone was found to be the compound that carries the antifungal properties of peppermint oil, whereas menthone alone did not show any action [46]. When it comes to geraniol and citral as main compounds in essential oils, it is found that they show signs of apoptosis mediated by DNA fragmentation in yeasts cells [47].

The efficiency of EOs' vapour phase on the fungal growth was evaluated using EOs with the highest antifungal activity in preceding experimental steps. The natural vapouring capacity of EOs at ambient temperature was involved in this step, while distance between inoculated Petri plates and EOs source was varied between 1.0 and 5.5 cm. Monitoring of samples was carried out for 21 days and imaged using a digital camera (Supplementary Figures S1–S3). The fungal growth, i.e., contaminated areas at Petri plates, served for the determination of surface area using a computer quantification method. According to Table 6, distances between 1 and 3.5 cm were designated efficiency for all tested essential oils and the mixture in the case of all three fungi representatives. The first differences at fungal strain as well as distance level were observed at a distance of 4.5 cm between inoculated Petri plates and EO samples. Briefly, *C. cladosporoides* (5/1) did not grow regardless of applied essential oil sample. On the other hand, complete growth inhibition of *A. fumigatus* (6/1) was observed in the case of using oregano EO or EOs mixture (MIX), while contaminated areas of 32 and 43% were observed in the case of peppermint and lemongrass essential oils, respectively. A similar situation can be noticed for *P. chrysogenum* (7/1), since the contamination area of 15 and 54% was obtained for the same two mentioned essential oils as for *A. fumigatus* (6/1). A further increase of the distance to a value of 5.5 cm reduced the efficiency of oregano EO in the case of *A. fumigatus* (6/1) and *P. chrysogenum* (7/1), since contamination areas of 32 and 11% were observed, respectively. In summary, only the mixture of essential oils was completely efficient at all tested distances. These results were evaluated using mathematical modelling (Tables 7 and 8), where the obtained predictive quality parameters point out that statistically calculated parameters fitted in well with obtained experimental data. The gained coefficients of determination are very high, and predictive capacity of the models can be used for following application of EOs mixture during in situ treatments.

The absent of fungal growth indicates the strong potential of a mixture of oregano, peppermint, and lemongrass EOs for the inhibition of fungal growth of *C. cladosporoides* (5/1), *A. fumigatus* (6/1) and *P. chrysogenum* (7/1) at a distance greater that 5 cm (Tables 6–8). In order to demonstrate the potential of the in situ application of the created EOs mixture, historical paper samples were treated with the EOs mixture and SEM imaging was conducted. In Figure 2a, the micrograph of *C. cladosporoides* (5/1) is presented. Analysing the microstructure, apart from the cellulose fibres, hyphae and spores originating from fungi are clearly distinguished. Spores are the roundish structures and hyphae are thinner threads, connected to the round spores. In Figure 2b, spores and hyphae of *A. fumigatus* (6/1) on the cellulose fibre matrix are clearly observed, as well as in Figure 2c for *P. chrysogenum* (7/1). In comparison to Figure 2a–c, in Figure 2d–f there are no observed spores nor hyphae structures. In addition, Figure 2d–f is very similar to Figure 2g, which represents the blank historical paper sample. In these figures, only the cellulose fibres and irregular residues left after the manual paper production can be observed. This confirms that the treatment with EOs mix in vapour phase was lethal for the *C. cladosporoides* (5/1), *A. fumigatus* (6/1) and *P. chrysogenum* inoculated on archive paper substrates.

4. Materials and Methods

4.1. Tested Fungi

In this study, the following three fungi are used: *Cladosporium cladosporoides*, *Aspergillus fumigatus* and *Penicillium chrysogenum*. Throughout the manuscript they are labelled as 5/1, 6/1 and 7/1, respectively (Figure 3). These strains belong to the private collection of the Laboratory of Microbiology, Faculty of Technology Novi Sad, University of Novi Sad. All three strains have been earlier reported as paper biodeteriogens [48]. The chosen fungi were maintained and cultured onto Potato Dextrose Agar (HiMedia, Mumbai, India). During culturing the inoculated medium was incubated at 25 °C for 7 days. Sterile Petri dishes, without venting, were used in all further experiments.

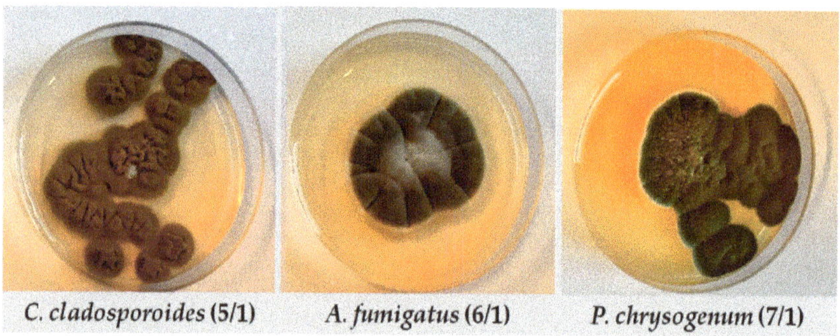

Figure 3. Tested fungal strains.

4.2. EOs

Five different commercial essential oils (lemongrass, oregano, rosemary, peppermint and eucalyptus) purchased from AlekPharm (Belgrade, Serbia), were utilized in the preliminary screening of antifungal activity. Information about product INCI and CAS numbers are given in Table 9, while detail chemical composition (GC-MS) is given in Supplementary Table S1.

Table 9. Product specification of essential oils.

Essential Oil	Lemongrass	Oregano	Rosemary	Peppermint	Eucalyptus
Product INCI	*Cymbopogon citratus* leaf oil	*Origanum vulgare* oil	*Rosmarinus officinalis* leaf oil	*Mentha piperita* oil	*Eucalyptus globulus* leaf oil
CAS Number	8007-02-1	84012-24-8	8000-25-7	84082-70-2	84625-32-1

4.3. Screening of the EOs Antifungal Activity

Five selected essential oils were utilized in the preliminary screening of antifungal activity by disc-diffusion method, which was completely performed according to Aćimović et al. [49]. Some important steps of this method imply the use of freshly prepared fungal culture (obtained as described in Section 4.1) for the inoculation of Sabouraud Dextrose Agar (HiMedia, Mumbai, India) and application of the EOs (15 µL) onto sterile discs in triplicate for each culture onto solidified media. As a positive control actidione (30 µg/mL) was used, while as a negative control sterile distilled water and 5% DMSO were chosen. After 7 days at 25 ± 2 °C, the halo zones around discs were measured using HiAntibiotic Zone Scale^{TM} (HiMedia, Mumbai, India). The obtained results of the antifungal activity of EOs were interpreted as follows: resistant—halo zone lower than 22 mm, intermediary effect—range of halo zone is 22–26 mm, and sensitive—halo zone above 26 mm.

4.4. MIC Determination

Minimal inhibitory concentration (*v/v*) was assessed for EOs that achieved the biggest halo zone in screening of their antifungal activity evaluated by disc-diffusion method. The decreasing concentrations of EOs (100−0.78%) were tested while determining the *MIC* value, following the procedure explained in detail by Micić et al. [50]. The dissolution of essential oils was performed by using 5% DMSO solution. The final *MIC* value was determined using Equation (1), in which the number of microorganisms in the positive control is labelled as N_c, while N_t stands for the number of microorganisms in the treated sample.

$$MIC = \left(\frac{N_C \quad N_t}{N_c}\right) \cdot 100(\%) \tag{1}$$

4.5. Time-Kill Kinetics Study

For monitoring microbial behaviour during contact with MIC concentration of selected essential oils and fungi, the time-kinetics study was carried out using the procedure described by Aćimović et al. [51]. In brief, the contact time of the MIC concentration of EOs with fungal spore suspension (prepared in the nutrient medium using McFarland standard, spore suspension approx. 6 log CFU/mL) was conducted at 25 °C for 120 h, while the sampling time was in 0, 6, 12, 24, 36, 48, 60, 72, 84, 96, 108 and 120 h. The number of survival cells was determined after streaking of the sample aliquot onto SMA plates and incubation at 25 °C for 5 days. As well as tracking the effect of individual EOs, the mix of equal portion of three tested EOs was also monitored regarding the number of cells. The time-kill kinetics modelling was conducted to obtain the four-parameter sigmoidal numerical model which is suitable for biological systems [49], and which can be represented as an S-shaped model. The formula for modelling the mentioned system was presented as Equation (2), where ($y(t)$) is the number of viable/survival cells during the contact time between the MIC concentration of essential oil and cells, while *a*,*b*,*c* and d represent a minimum of the experimentally obtained values (t = 0), the Hill's slope, the inflection point and the maximally obtained value ($t - \infty$), respectively.

$$y(t) = d + \frac{a - d}{1 + \left(\frac{t}{c}\right)^b} \tag{2}$$

4.6. Chemical Composition of Selected EOs

The selected essential oils used were exposed to GC-MS analysis with an Agilent 7890A apparatus equipped with a 5975 C MSD, FID, and an HP-5MS fused-silica capillary column (30 m × 0.25 mm, film thickness 0.25 μm). The carrier gas was helium, and its inlet pressure was 19.6 psi and linear velocity of 1 mL min^{-1} at 210 °C. The injector temperature was 250 °C, the injection volume was 1 μL, split ratio was 10:1. The components were identified based on their linear retention index relative to C8-C32 n-alkanes, in comparison with data reported in the literature (Adams4 and NIST17 databases). The relative percentage of the oil constituents were expressed as percentages by FID peak area normalization.

4.7. EOs Efficiency in Vapour Phase

For dominant fungal strains isolated from archive paper, the antifungal efficiency of the vapour phase of EOs which showed the highest antifungal activity in previous experimental steps was evaluated. For this purpose, standard disc-diffusion method as described in Section 4.2. was employed, with some modifications. Namely, sterile discs were not applied onto inoculated and solidified media, rather the disc was laid on the inside surface of the upper lid and 15 μL of individual 100% EO or their mix (5 μL of each EO) was placed onto the disc. The distance between the inoculated media and the upper lid was varied as follows: 1, 2.5, 3.5, 4.5 and 5.5 cm by setting the additional Petri dish circuit onto a previous one (Figure 4). As the negative control 15 μL of sterile distilled water instead of EOs was applied onto sterile disc, while actidione (30 μg/mL) was used as a positive control. The prepared Petri dishes were inverted on top of the lid and sealed with parafilm to prevent leakage of the vapour. The experiment was performed in triplicate.

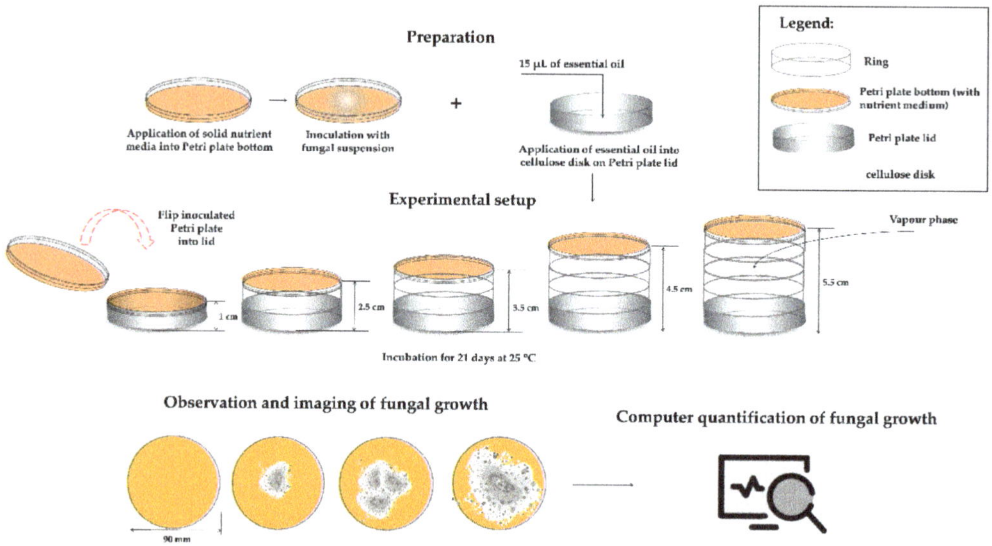

Figure 4. Schematic presentation of method for determination of EOs efficiency in vapour phase.

The prepared groups of the samples were monitored at 25 °C for 21 days' storage period. Each sample image was recorded with a common digital camera, which captured a region of roughly Ø90 mm (the macro function was used, for a more clear photograph). The obtained pictures were used to determine the contaminated area of the sample using ImageJ 1.53 r (used for masking the contaminated area) and Inkscape 1.0 (applied to measure the distances in pictures). The values of the recorded images' surface area were assigned to the values between 0 and 1 (negative control images surface gained value 0, while positive control images surface was assumed to be 1).

The data are presented as an exponential model (Equation (3)).

$$SE(t) = a \cdot \exp(b \cdot t) \tag{3}$$

The surface area $SE(t)$ at time t was the targeted output, while a and b were the regression coefficients. The suitability of the gained mathematical models was tested using the mathematical quality parameters through numerical verification of the obtained models according to Equations (4)–(7) [52,53].

$$\chi^2 = \frac{\sum_{i=1}^{N} \left(x_{exp,i} - x_{pre,i}\right)^2}{N-n}, \tag{4}$$

$$RMSE = \left[\frac{1}{N} \cdot \sum_{i=1}^{N} \left(x_{pre,i} - x_{exp,i}\right)^2\right]^{1/2}, \tag{5}$$

$$MBE = \frac{1}{N} \cdot \sum_{i=1}^{N} \left(x_{pre,i} - x_{exp,i}\right), \tag{6}$$

$$MPE = \frac{100}{N} \cdot \sum_{i=1}^{N} \left(\frac{|x_{pre,i} - x_{exp,i}|}{x_{exp,i}} \right) \quad (7)$$

The $x_{exp,i}$ represents experimental values, while $x_{pre,i}$ are the predicted values calculated from the model. N and n are the numbers of observations and constants, respectively. In order to compare samples means, analysis of variance (ANOVA) was conducted.

4.8. EOs In Situ Application onto Historical Paper Samples

The samples for the in situ experiment were taken from a fragment of the handmade paper; it was impossible to determine to which document it belonged to while lacking text, seals and other insignia, and it is assumed to be a part of the fond F.2 Bačka-Bodrog County—Baja, Sombor, Serbia (1699–1849), 1688–1849. The date when this type of the paper was made is believed to be the end of the 18th and the beginning of the 19th century, at a time when the manufacturing of paper included the use of quality materials—fibre of more pure or less pure cellulose obtained from old cotton, linen and hemp rags, which had a certain amount of glue added. It is a strong, elastic and durable type of paper. Under optimal conditions for preservation, the properties of this type of paper do not experience significant changes over time, unlike the paper created by wooden materials. The paper is without visible damage, while a lesser discoloration (yellowing) is a consequence of the natural process of aging. The preparation of the samples included the cutting of the paper in equal parts with 1 × 1 cm dimensions.

Onto prepared historical paper samples 100 μL of prepared fungal suspensions (approx. spore concentration 6 log CFU/mL) was applied and placed in the bottom of the Petri dish, while the sterile disc with 15 μL of EOs mix (5 μL of each EO) or equal amount of distilled water for control samples was laid onto the inside of the upper lid. The distance between the artificially contaminated historical paper sample and soaked disc with mix of EOs was 3.5 cm. The experiment was carried out at 25 °C for 21 days. After three weeks, the state of the artificially contaminated and treated historical paper surface was evaluated by scanning electron microscopy (SEM Hitachi TM3030) under a high vacuum (acceleration voltage 15 kV, beam current 20 nA, spot size 1 mm).

5. Conclusions

The antifungal efficiency of three EOs (lemongrass, oregano and peppermint) against *Cladosporium cladosporoides*, *Aspergillus fumigatus* and *Penicillium chrysogenum* was demonstrated in liquid and vapour phase. Furthermore, through obtaining MIC values and time-kill kinetic study, the high antifungal potential of the tested EOs individually and in mixture have been shown. For the first time, mathematical modelling has been employed in order to track the efficacy of the EOs in vapour phase, where it was concluded that only a mixture of essential oils was completely efficient at all tested distances. Following the obtained results, the equal proportion of the tested oils was applied in situ onto small fragments of historical papers that had previously been artificially contaminated, and the same high efficiency of the EOs mixtures in vapour phase was confirmed by scanning electron microscopy.

After such promising results presented in this manuscript, the future plan of the authors is to accomplish a suitable protocol for the treatment of archival documents with EOs as well as to conducting experiments with the complete fonds of documents.

Supplementary Materials: The following supporting information can be downloaded at: https://www.mdpi.com/article/10.3390/antibiotics12010103/s1, Table S1: Chemical composition of essential oils; Figure S1: EOs efficiency in vapour phase against *C. cladosporoides*; Figure S2: EOs efficiency in vapour phase against *A. fumigatus*; Figure S3: EOs efficiency in vapour phase against *P. chrysogenum*.

Author Contributions: Conceptualization, A.T., V.N. and O.Š.; methodology, A.T. and O.Š.; validation, L.P.; formal analysis, A.T., J.S., M.C. and M.A.; investigation, A.T. and O.Š.; resources, A.T.; data curation, O.Š. and L.P.; writing—original draft preparation, A.T. and O.Š; writing—review and editing, A.T. and O.Š.; visualization, L.P. and J.S.; supervision, S.M. and N.K. All authors have read and agreed to the published version of the manuscript.

Funding: This research was funded by the Ministry of Education, Science, and Technological Development of the Republic of Serbia (grant no. 451-03-68/2023-14/200134).

Institutional Review Board Statement: Not applicable.

Informed Consent Statement: Not applicable.

Data Availability Statement: Not applicable.

Acknowledgments: The authors would like to express their gratitude to the Ministry of Education, Science, and Technological Development of the Republic of Serbia for financial support. Special gratitude is directed to the Archives of Vojvodina for cooperation, and BioSense Institute, University of Novi Sad, Serbia, for the use of measurement equipment.

Conflicts of Interest: The authors declare no conflict of interest.

References

1. Kozics, K.; Buckova, M.; Puskarova, A.; Kalaszova, V.; Cabicarova, T.; Pangallo, D. The effect of ten essential oils on several cutaneous drug-resistant microorganisms and their cyto/genotoxic and antioxidant properties. *Molecules* **2019**, *24*, 4570. [CrossRef] [PubMed]
2. Borrego, S.; Guiamet, P.; Vivar, I.; Battiston, P. Fungal involved in biodeterioration of documents in paper and effect on substrate. *Acta Microsc.* **2018**, *27*, 37–44.
3. Díaz-Alonso, J.; Bernardos, A.; Regidor-Ros, J.L.; Martínez-Manez, R.; Bosch-Roig, P. Innovative use of essential oil cold diffusion system for improving air quality on indoor cultural heritage spaces. *Int. Biodet. Biodeg.* **2021**, *162*, 105–125. [CrossRef]
4. Bosco, F.; Mollea, C.; Demichela, M.; Fissore, D. Application of Essential Oils to Control the Biodeteriogenic Microorganisms in Archives and Libraries. *Heritage* **2022**, *5*, 2181–2195. [CrossRef]
5. Michaelsen, A.; Pinzari, F.; Barbabietola, N.; Piñar, G. Monitoring the effects of different conservation treatments on paper-infecting fungi. *Int. Biodeterior. Biodegrad.* **2013**, *84*, 333–341. [CrossRef]
6. Kwasna, H.; Karbowska-Berent, J.; Behnke-Borowczyk, J. Effect of Fungi on the Destruction of Historical Parchment and Paper Documents. *Pol. J. Environ. Stud.* **2020**, *29*, 2679–2695. [CrossRef]
7. Rakotonirainy, M.S.; Lavédrine, B. Screening for antifungal activity of essential oils and related compounds to control the biocontamination in libraries and archives storage areas. *Int. Biodeterior. Biodegrad.* **2005**, *55*, 141–147. [CrossRef]
8. Verticchio, E.; Frasca, F.; Bertolin, C.; Siana, A.M. Climate-induced risk for the preservation of paper collections: Comparative study among three historic libraries in Italy. *Build Environ.* **2021**, *206*, 108394. [CrossRef]
9. Prakash, B.; Kedia, A.; Mishra, P.K.; Dubey, N.K. Plant essential oils as food preservatives to control moulds, mycotoxin contamination and oxidative deterioration of agri-food commodities—Potentials and challenges. *Food Control* **2015**, *47*, 381–391. [CrossRef]
10. Perczak, A.; Gwiazdowska, D.; Marchwińska, K.; Juś, K.; Gwiazdowski, R.; Waśkiewicz, A. (Antifungal activity of selected essential oils against *Fusarium culmorum* and *F. graminearum* and their secondary metabolites in wheat seeds. *Arch. Microbiol.* **2019**, *20*, 1085–1097. [CrossRef]
11. Alexopoulou, I.; Zervos, S. Paper conservation methods: An international survey. *J. Cult. Herit.* **2016**, *21*, 922–930. [CrossRef]
12. Zervos, S.; Alexopoulou, I. Paper conservation methods: A literature review. *Cellulose* **2015**, *22*, 2859–2897. [CrossRef]
13. Sequeira, S.; Cabrita, E.J.; Macedo, M.F. Antifungals on paper conservation: An overview. *Int. Biodeterior. Biodegrad.* **2012**, *74*, 67–86. [CrossRef]
14. Palla, F.; Bruno, M.; Mercurio, F.; Tantillo, A.; Rotolo, V. Essential Oils as Natural Biocides in Conservation of Cultural Heritage. *Molecules* **2020**, *25*, 730. [CrossRef] [PubMed]
15. Borrego, S.; Lavin, P.; Perdomo, I.; Gómez de Saravia, S.; Guiamet, P. Determination of Indoor Air Quality in Archives and Biodeterioration of the Documentary Heritage. *Int. Schol. Res. Not.* **2012**, *2012*, 680598. [CrossRef] [PubMed]
16. Casiglia, S.; Bruno, M.; Scandolera, E.; Senatore, F.; Senatore, F. Influence of harvesting time on composition of the essential oil of Thymus capitatus (L.) Hoffmanns. & Link. growing wild in northern Sicily and its activity on microorganisms affecting historical art crafts. *Arab. J. Chem.* **2019**, *12*, 2704–2712.
17. Moghtader, M. In vitro antifungal effects of the essential oil of *Mentha piperita* L. and its comparison with synthetic menthol on *Aspergillus niger*. *Afr. J. Plant Sci.* **2013**, *7*, 521–527. [CrossRef]
18. Moghaddam, M.; Pourbaige, M.; Tabar, H.K.; Farhadi, N.; Hosseini, S.M.A. Composition and Antifungal Activity of Peppermint (*Mentha piperita*) Essential Oil from Iran. *J. Essent. Oil-Bear. Plants* **2013**, *16*, 506–512. [CrossRef]

19. İşcan, G.; Kirimer, N.; Kürkcüoğlu, M.; Can Başer, H.; Demirci, F. Antimicrobial Screening of *Mentha piperita* Essential Oils. *J. Agric. Food Chem.* **2002**, *50*, 3943–3946. [CrossRef] [PubMed]
20. Hussain, A.I.; Anwar, F.; Nigam, P.S.; Ashraf, M.; Gilani, A.H. Seasonal variation in content, chemical composition and antimicrobial and cytotoxic activities of essential oils from four Mentha species. *J. Sci. Food Agric.* **2010**, *90*, 1827–1836. [CrossRef] [PubMed]
21. Ali, M.M.; Yusuf, M.A.; Abdalaziz, M.N. GC-MS analysis and antimicrobial screening of essential oil from lemongrass (*Cymbopogon citratus*). *Int. J. Pharm. Chem.* **2017**, *3*, 72–76.
22. Gao, S.; Liu, G.; Li, J.; Chen, J.; Li, L.; Zhang, X.; Zhang, S.; Thorne, R.F.; Zhang, S. Antimicrobial Activity of Lemongrass Essential Oil (*Cymbopogon flexuosus*) and Its Active Component Citral Against Dual-Species Biofilms of *Staphylococcus aureus* and *Candida* Species. *Front. Cell. Infect.* **2020**, *10*, 603858. [CrossRef]
23. Shaaban, H.A.; Ramadan, M.M.; Amer, M.M.; El-Sideek, L.; Osman, F. Chemical composition of *Cymbopogon citratus* essential oil and antifungal activity against some species of mycotoxigenic *Aspergillus fungi*. *Res. J. Appl. Sci.* **2013**, *9*, 5770–5779.
24. Degnon, R.G.; Allagbe, A.C.; Adjou, E.S.; Dahouenon-Ahoussi, E. Antifungal activities of *Cymbopogon citratus* essential oil against *Aspergillus* species isolated from fermented fish products of Southern Benin. *J. Food Qual. Hazards Control* **2019**, *6*, 53–57. [CrossRef]
25. Ličina, B.Z.; Stefanović, O.D.; Vasić, S.M.; Radojević, I.D.; Dekić, M.S.; Čomić, L.R. Biological activities of the extracts from wild growing *Origanum vulgare* L. *Food Control* **2013**, *33*, 498–504. [CrossRef]
26. Bendahou, M.; Muselli, A.; Grignon-Dubois, M.; Benyoucef, M.; Desjobert, J.-M.; Bernardini, A.-F.; Costa, J. Antimicrobial activity and chemical composition of *Origanum glandulosum* Desf. essential oil and extract obtained by microwave extraction: Comparison with hydrodistillation. *Food Chem.* **2008**, *106*, 132–139. [CrossRef]
27. Couto, C.; Raposo, N.; Rozental, S.; Borba-Santos, L.; Bezerra, L.; De Almeida, P.; Brandão, M. Chemical Composition and Antifungal Properties of Essential Oil of *Origanum vulgare* Linnaeus (Lamiaceae) against *Sporothrix schenckii* and *Sporothrix brasiliensis*. *Trop. J. Pharm. Res.* **2015**, *14*, 1207. [CrossRef]
28. Sim, J.H.; Jamaludin, N.S.; Khoo, C.H.; Cheah, Y.K.; Halim, S.N.B.A.; Seng, H.L.; Tiekink, E.R.T. In vitro antibacterial and time-kill evaluation of phosphanegold(I) dithiocarbamates, R3PAu[$S_2CN(iPr)CH_2CH_2OH$] for R = Ph, Cy and Et, against a broad range of Gram-positive and Gram-negative bacteria. *Gold Bulletin.* **2014**, *47*, 225–236. [CrossRef]
29. Stešević, D.; Jaćimović, Ž.; Šatović, Z.; Šapčanin, A.; Jančan, G.; Kosović, M.; Damjanović-Vratnica, B. Chemical characterization of wild growing *Origanum vulgare* populations in Montenegro. *Nat. Prod. Commun.* **2018**, *13*, 1357–1362. [CrossRef]
30. Gonceariuc, M.; Balamus, Z.; Sandu, T.; Romanciuc, G.; Gonceariuc, N. Essential oil of *Origanum vulgare* ssp. *vulgare* L. and *Origanum vulgare* ssp. hirtum (Link) Ietswaart from Moldova: Content and chemical composition. *Int. J. Agric. Innov. Res.* **2014**, *3*, 659–663.
31. Lukas, B.; Schmiderer, C.; Novak, J. Essential oil diversity of European *Origanum vulgare* L. (Lamiaceae). *Phytochemistry* **2015**, *119*, 32–40. [CrossRef] [PubMed]
32. Mockute, D.; Bernotiene, G.; Judzentiene, A. The essential oil of *Origanum vulgare* L. ssp. vulgare growing wild in Vilnius district (Lithuania). *Phytochemistry* **2001**, *57*, 65–69. [CrossRef]
33. Gong, H.Y.; Liu, W.H.; LV, G.Y.; Zhou, X. Analysis of essential oils of *Origanum vulgare* from six production areas of China and Pakistan. *Rev. Bras. Farmacogn.* **2014**, *24*, 25–32. [CrossRef]
34. Vazirian, M.; Mohammadi, M.; Faraei, M.H.; Amin, G.; Amanzadeh, Y. Chemical composition and antioxidant activity of *Origanum vulgare* subsp. *vulgare* essential oil from Iran. *Res. J. Pharmacogn* **2015**, *2*, 41–46.
35. Kosakowska, O.; Czupa, W. Morphological and Chemical variability of common origanum (*Origanum vulgare* L. subsp. *vulgare*) occurring in eastern Poland. *Herba Pol.* **2018**, *64*, 11–21. [CrossRef]
36. Moghadam, A.R.L. Chemical composition of the essential oils of *Origanum vulgare*. *Bull. Environ. Pharmacol. Life Sci.* **2015**, *4*, 150–152.
37. Chrishti, S.; Kaloo, Z.; Sultan, P.; Nisa, H.T.; Nisa, N.T. Quantitative analysis of the essential oil of *Origanum vulgare* (L) growing in the Kashmir valley. *Int. J. Appl. Res.* **2016**, *2*, 552–557.
38. McKay, D.L.; Blumberg, J.B. A review of the bioactivity and potential health benefits of peppermint tea (*Mentha piperita* L.). *Phytother. Res.* **2006**, *20*, 619–633. [CrossRef]
39. Salim, R. Carvone content and chemical composition in spearmint (*Mentha spicata* var. *Viridis* l.) as affected by herb storage under ambient temperature. *J. Food Nutr. Popul. Health* **2016**, *1*, 5.
40. Buleandra, M.; Oprea, E.; Popa, D.E.; David, I.G.; Moldovan, Z.; Mihai, I.; Badea, I.A. Comparative chemical analysis of mentha piperita and m. spicata and a fast assessment of commercial peppermint teas. *Nat. Prod. Commun.* **2016**, *11*, 551–555.
41. Do, D.N.; Nguyen, D.P.; Phung, V.D.; Le, X.T.; Le, T.M.; Do, V.M.; Minh, B.Q.; Luu, X.C. Fractionating of Lemongrass (*Cymbopogon citratus*) Essential Oil by Vacuum Fractional Distillation. *Processes* **2021**, *9*, 593. [CrossRef]
42. Bossou, A.D.; Ahoussi, E.; Ruysbergh, E.; Adams, A.; Smagghe, G.; Kimpe, N.D.; Avlessi, F.; Sohounhloue, D.C.K.; Mangelinckx, S. Characterization of volatile compounds from three *Cymbopogon* species and *Eucalyptus citrodora* from Benin and their insecticidal activities against *Tribolium castaneum*. *Ind. Crops Prod.* **2015**, *76*, 306–317. [CrossRef]
43. Hannaa, A.R.M.; Sallam, Y.I.; El-Leithy, A.S.; Aly, S.E. Lemongrass (*Cymbopogon citratus*) essential oil as affected by drying methods. *Ann. Agric. Sci.* **2012**, *57*, 113–116.

44. Zheng, Y.; Shang, Y.; Li, M.; Li, Y.; Ouyang, W. Antifungal Activities of cis-trans Citral Isomers against Trichophyton rubrum with ERG6 as a Potential Target. *Molecules* **2021**, *26*, 4263. [CrossRef] [PubMed]
45. Karadayi, M.; Yildim, V.; Güllüce, M. Antimicrobial Activity and Other Biological Properties of Oregano Essential Oil and Carvacrol. *Anatol. J. Biol.* **2020**, *2*, 52–68.
46. Kamatou, G.P.P.; Vermaak, I.; Viljoen, A.M.; Lawrence, B.M. Menthol: A Simple monoterpene with remarkable biological properties. *Phytochemistry* **2013**, *96*, 15–25. [CrossRef]
47. Gaonkar, R.; Avti, P.K.; Hegde, G. Differential Antifungal Efficiency of Geraniol and Citral. *NPC Nat. Product Commun.* **2018**, *13*, 1609–1614. [CrossRef]
48. Skóra, J.; Gutarowska, B.; Pielech-Przybylska, K.; Stępień, L.; Pietrzak, K.; Piotrowska, M.; Pietrowski, P. Assessment of microbiological contamination in the work environments of museums, archives and libraries. *Aerobiologia* **2015**, *31*, 389–401. [CrossRef]
49. Aćimović, M.; Šovljanski, O.; Pezo, L.; Travičić, V.; Tomić, A.; Zheljazkov, V.D.; Ćetković, G.; Švarc-Gajić, J.; Brezo-Borjan, T.; Sofrenić, I. Variability in biological activities of *Satureja montana* Subsp. *montana* and Subsp. *variegate* based on different extraction methods. *Antibiotics* **2022**, *11*, 1235. [CrossRef] [PubMed]
50. Micić, D.; Đurović, S.; Riabov, P.; Tomić, A.; Šovljanski, O.; Filip, S.; Tosti, T.; Dojčinović, B.; Božović, R.; Jovanović, D.; et al. Rosemary essential oils as a promising source of bioactive compounds: Chemical composition, thermal properties, biological activity and gastronomical perspectives. *Foods* **2021**, *10*, 2734. [CrossRef]
51. Aćimović, M.; Šovljanski, O.; Šeregelj, V.; Pezo, L.; Zheljazkov, V.D.; Ljujić, J.; Tomić, A.; Ćetković, G.; Čanadanović-Brunet, J.; Miljković, A.; et al. Chemical Composition, Antioxidant, and Antimicrobial Activity of *Dracocephalum moldavica* L. Essential Oil and Hydrolate. *Plants* **2022**, *11*, 941. [CrossRef]
52. Šovljanski, O.; Tomić, A.; Pezo, L.; Ranitović, A.; Markov, S. Prediction of denitrification capacity of alkalotolerant bacterial isolates from soil—An artificial neural network model. *J. Serb. Chem. Soc.* **2020**, *85*, 1417–1427. [CrossRef]
53. Šovljanski, O.; Saveljić, A.; Aćimović, M.; Šeregelj, V.; Pezo, L.; Tomić, A.; Cetković, G.; Tešević, V. Biological Profiling of Essential Oils and Hydrolates of *Ocimum basilicum* var. *Genovese* and var. *Minimum* Originated from Serbia. *Processes* **2022**, *10*, 1893. [CrossRef]

antibiotics

MDPI

Article

Agar Plate Methods for Assessing the Antibacterial Activity of Thyme and Oregano Essential Oils against *S. epidermidis* and *E. coli*

Chiara Mollea, Francesca Bosco * and Davide Fissore

Department of Applied Science and Technology, Politecnico di Torino, 10129 Turin, Italy
* Correspondence: francesca.bosco@polito.it

Abstract: The resistance to antimicrobials (AMR), especially antibiotics, represents a serious problem and, at the same time, a challenge. In the last decade, a growing interest in the use of essential oils (EOs) as antimicrobial substances was observed. Commercial thyme and oregano EOs are reported to be the main responsible of the oil antimicrobial efficacy against both Gram-positive and Gram-negative pathogenic bacteria. The aim of the present work was to study the efficacy of EOs against *Staphylococcus epidermidis* and *Escherichia coli* in long-time treatments. In a preliminary microdilution test, a MIC value was obtained for thyme EO against *S. epidermidis* and *E. coli*. After that, disk diffusion and disk volatilization tests were set up to study the influence of main cultural parameters on EO activity in liquid or vapor phase. Both bacteria were inhibited by thyme and oregano EOs when applied pure (100% v/v) or diluted (75% and 50% v/v): a higher inhibition was observed in a disk diffusion test in which the antimicrobial effect was due to both liquid and vapor phase components. Finally, a comparison with literature data was carried out even if it was not so easy because standard methods are usually modified and adapted to specific case study. For this reason, the results have to be interpreted in relation to the analytical method applied.

Keywords: *Thymus vulgaris* EO; *Origanum vulgaris* EO; *S. epidermidis*; *E. coli*; agar disk diffusion test; disk volatilization test

1. Introduction

The problem of resistance to antimicrobials (AMR) necessitates the identification of new, safe, and effective substances. In recent years, particular attention was paid to products of natural origin due to their low toxicity, biodegradability, and their broad spectrum of action compared to synthetic antimicrobial substances [1]. In this regard, a growing interest in the use of essential oils (OE) was observed since they have two interesting properties: the synergy of action with antibiotics and the absence of acquisition of microbial resistance to their constituents [1].

Essential oils (EOs), secondary metabolites of vegetable origin, are known to be blends of various polar and non-polar chemical molecules such as terpenes, terpenoids, and phenolics [2]. Thanks to this chemical composition, EOs have been studied for many years for their peculiar antimicrobial, antiviral, and antioxidant properties. On the other hand, they also possess some characteristics that can pose some concerns when used: in fact, EOs are volatile, scarcely water soluble (they can be dissolved only in alcohols or organic solvents), and often are characterized by a distinguishing aroma due to volatile components [3]. Nevertheless, thanks to their predominant biological activities, EOs can be utilized in very different fields, from healthcare to the field of food preservation but also in cosmetic product formulations or as repellents in the agricultural environment [4]. EOs can be divided into two main chemical groups: the one of terpenes and that of the aromatic and aliphatic molecules, which includes alcohols, aldehydes, phenols, heterocycles, and methoxy derivatives [5]. Among this last, carvacrol and thymol are reported to be the main ones responsible for the oils' antimicrobial efficacy. Thyme and oregano, containing these two phenolic compounds, are reported in the scientific literature for their antimicrobial activity against both Gram-positive and Gram-negative pathogenic bacteria such as *Escherichia coli*, *Staphylococcus aureus*, and *Staphylococcus epidermidis* and are mainly tested with agar diffusion assays [6,7]. As an example, in [6], 10 μL of thyme EO obtained similar results against both *E. coli* and *S. aureus* (inhibition halo greater than 20 mm); in [7], *S. aureus* and *S. epidermidis* proved to be resistant to the same volume of thyme EO.

Thyme EO was described as a natural preservative with antimicrobial properties more evident against Gram-positive bacteria probably due to the absence of the external membrane and a cell wall less resistant to the activity of EOs and their components [8]. It contains both thymol and carvacrol in different quantities depending on the plant origin: the antimicrobial activity is mainly ascribed to thymol, but both compounds can have antagonistic or synergistic effects depending on the temperature, the oxygen content, and the pH values [9]. Thanks to its broad spectrum of action, thyme EO was studied for the potential antibacterial activity against food pathogens: in fact, it was added to the formulation of meat, fish, and sea-food in the range 0.1–1%. Moreover, numerous medical applications consider the utilization of thyme EO for its anti-inflammatory, antitussive, analgesic, sedative, and anti-broncholitic properties [8,10].

As regards the antimicrobial efficacy of oregano EO, it mainly depends on the presence of carvacrol, which can interact with the other oregano constituents to enhance efficacy [11]. As for the Thyme EO, its applications are numerous, with oregano being utilized as a food preservative (e.g., in food packaging) or for the treatment of numerous diseases and infections [12].

In a recent review of [13], methods for in vitro evaluation of antimicrobial activity were reported and compared. The authors clearly identified the most important factors that influence the minimum inhibitory concentration (MIC): incubation conditions, culture media, and the use of emulsifiers or solvents. Other factors, such as inoculum size and end-points determination, were mentioned by [14]. In the work of [15], the influence of the most common media used for MIC determination of oregano EO by broth dilution method were reported.

Agar methods for the in vitro evaluation of the EO antimicrobial activity are reported in [14]; among them, the most known is the disk-diffusion assay, based on the Kirby–Bauer standard method, which allows to evaluate antimicrobial activity of the non-volatile components of the EOs [16]. A typical method to test the efficacy of the volatile components of EOs is the inverted lid test that is based on the generation of EO vapor and the creation of an atmosphere at the selected temperature. This is not a standard assay although it is often recommended to evaluate the microbial inactivation by the volatile components of the EOs [17].

Based on the previously reported papers, it appears clear that it is very difficult to reliably compare data from the literature because many parameters have an influence on the results due to the strong variance of the used antimicrobial susceptibility testing methods, as reported by [18].

In the present work, in order to overcome safety risk during test execution, two Biosafety Level 1 bacteria, *S. epidermidis* and *E. coli*, were used. MIC values were first investigated for commercial thyme and oregano EOs against both bacteria by applying a microdilution test. After that, specific antimicrobial tests were set up to study the influence of main parameters (i.e., EO concentrations and absolute quantity, temperature of incubation, EO treatment duration considering time intervals larger than in previous studies) on EO efficacy in liquid and vapor phases; the obtained values were compared with MIC results. The results obtained with the selected bacteria were compared with available literature data on pathogenic strains to possibly validate them as surrogate microorganisms.

2. Results

2.1. Preliminary Test—Microdilution in Broth

The microdilution test was carried out diluting commercial thyme and oregano EOs with 1.5% TEGO; the EO concentrations were in the range 7.5–0.03 µg/mL. At the tested cultural conditions, only thyme EO inhibited the growth of *Staphylococcus epidermidis* and *Escherichia coli*, and the obtained MIC value was 7.5 µg/mL for both bacteria. On the contrary, for oregano EO, a MIC value was not obtained.

2.2. Agar Disk Diffusion Tests

In order to distinguish the activity of the EOs in the liquid and in the vapor phase, specific antimicrobial tests were set up against the chosen *S. epidermidis* and *E. coli* strains. As regard the liquid phase, the agar disk diffusion test was used to examine, at the same time, the EO effect in the liquid and vapor phase. As reported by [19], the inhibition zone caused by EOs depends on both the uniform diffusion of the substance into the agarized medium and the release of vapors above the tested bacteria. Generally, the antimicrobial efficacy of the EOs is evaluated at 24 h [20,21]; in the present work, in order to check the EO influence on the bacterial growth over time, inhibition was evaluated and compared at both 24 and 48 h.

2.2.1. Test with a Gram-Positive Bacterium: *S. epidermidis*

The antimicrobial effect of 100%, 75%, and 50% EOs diluted with 1.5% TEGO on *S. epidermidis* grown at 37 °C is described. The measures of the inhibition halo diameter, checked after 24 and 48 h from the EO addition, are reported in Figure 1.

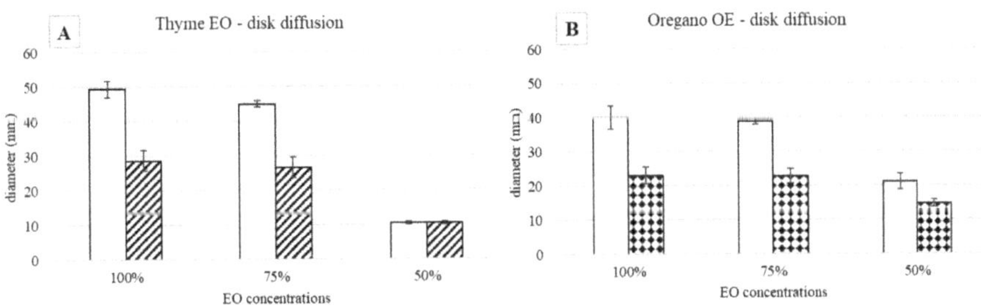

Figure 1. Agar disk diffusion test against *S. epidermidis* incubated at 37 °C: halo diameters measured after 24 (white bars) and 48 (drawn bars) h of incubation in the presence of (**A**) thyme and (**B**) oregano EOs.

As regards the thyme EO, it was able to influence bacterial growth at all the tested concentrations (Figure 1A). Looking at the changes of the halo diameters between 24 and 48 h of incubation, it is possible to observe that for the highest EO concentrations, the diameters decreased in a similar way, namely 41.9% for 100% EO and 40.9% for 75% EO, reaching, at the end of the incubation period comparable values, 28.6 mm and 26.5 mm respectively, which was not proportional to the EO concentration. On the contrary, in the presence of 50% EO, the diameter remained unchanged, i.e., equal to 10.4 mm, a value significantly lower with respect to that measured with the highest concentrations. Concerning the oregano EO, all the three concentrations allowed to measure inhibition halos, which varied between 24 and 48 h of incubation (Figure 1B). As observed for thyme EO, the effect due to 100% and 75% EO was very similar, and the respective diameters diminished by about the same percentage, namely 42.5% and 41.3%, reaching at 48 h 23 mm and 22.7 mm, respectively. In the case of oregano EO, for the 50% concentration, a decrease in halo diameter (30%) was also observed: at 48 h of incubation, the value was 14.7 mm. As an example, in Figure 2, it is possible to observe the decrease of the halo diameter in the presence of 100% thyme and oregano EOs.

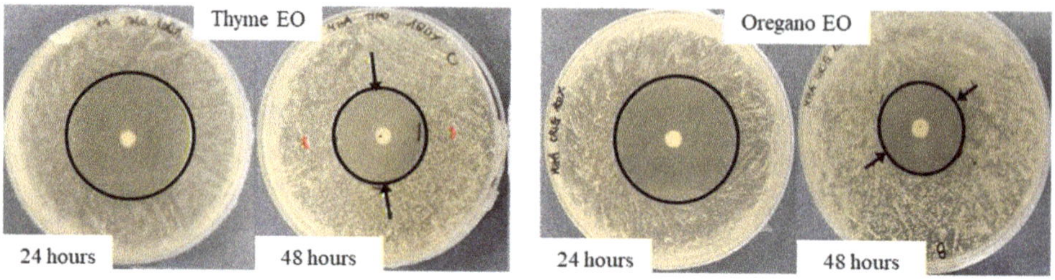

Figure 2. Variation of the inhibition halo diameter from 24 to 48 h, for the disk diffusion test, in the presence of 100% thyme or oregano EO, against *S. epidermidis*. Arrows indicate the variation direction.

2.2.2. Test with a Gram-Negative Bacterium: *E. coli*

The agar diffusion test was also carried out against *E. coli* grown at the optimal temperature of 28 °C. Differently from the results obtained in the presence of *S. epidermidis*, the haloes did not vary between 24 and 48 h of incubation; for this reason, only the results at 48 h are shown. Moreover, in all the tests performed in the presence of *E. coli*, a double halo was clearly visible, consisting in an inner portion, where the bacteria are absent, surrounded by a circular crown of "faint" microbial growth (Figure 3). According to the indications of [22] for the Enterobacteriaceae grown on Mueller–Hinton agar, the sum of the two inhibition haloes has to be considered as inhibition zone. In view of a possible dependence of the faint growth from the EO diffusion in the agar, the circular crown measures (mm) for each inhibition halo diameter are also reported.

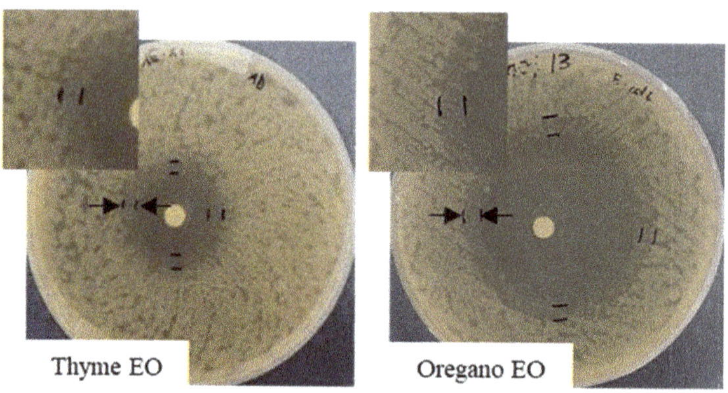

Figure 3. "Faint" microbial growth, shown between arrows and enlarged in the photo details, for *E. coli* growth in the presence of EOs in the disk diffusion assay.

Thyme EO, tested at 28 °C at 100 and 75%, allowed to obtain comparable results against *E. coli* (28.3 mm and 27.8 mm, respectively, Figure 4A). At the 50% concentration, the efficacy of thyme EO was lower, namely 24.3 mm, but comparable with respect to the higher concentrations. As regards the oregano EO, the efficacy at 100 and 75% was similar: 28 mm and 27 mm. At the same time, at 50%, the inhibition was less than half (12 mm).

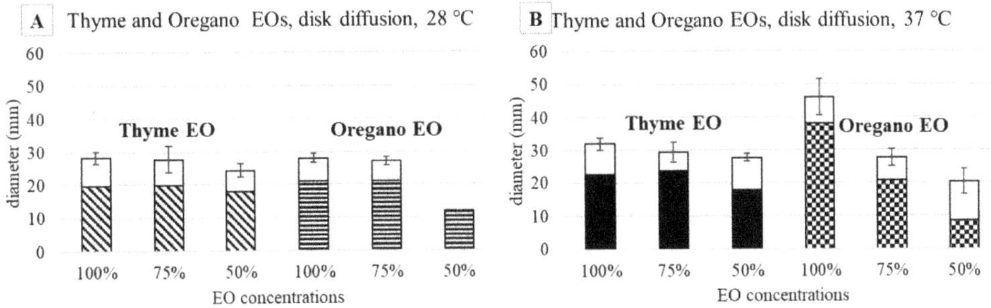

Figure 4. Agar diffusion test against *E. coli* incubated at 28 °C (**A**) and 37 °C (**B**): halo diameters measured after 48 h of incubation in the presence of thyme EO (oblique striped and black bars) and oregano EO (horizontal striped and checked bars). The white top portions of the bars represent the zones of faint bacterial growth.

The two EOs were also tested against *E. coli* grown at 37 °C (Figure 4B), the same incubation temperature of *S. epidermidis*, and the obtained results were compared with those at 28 °C. It is evident that at 37 °C, the inhibition was higher, independently from the EO used, in particular at 100% (32 mm and 46 mm for thyme and oregano, respectively).

2.3. Disk Volatilization Tests

The antibacterial properties of thyme and oregano volatile components were detected by means of disk volatilization test carried out in Petri dishes. In this case, the test was conducted with two different EO volumes, namely 3 and 10 μL, and paper disk diameters, namely 5 and 10 mm, respectively. The inhibition zone diameters were always measured at 24 and 48 h; in the tests with the higher EO volume, in the presence of *S. epidermidis*, the incubation was prolonged till 168 h, and the inhibition halo was evaluated each 24 h.

2.3.1. Test with a Gram-Positive Bacterium: *S. epidermidis*

As previously reported for disk diffusion tests, also in this case, between 24 and 48 h of incubation, a progressive reduction of the inhibition zone was observed.

As it is shown in Figure 5A,B, both EOs were able to influence *S. epidermidis* growth in a concentration-dependent way. In the first 24 h, in all the concentrations tested, the behavior of the inhibition halo was similar, with the measured diameters being equal to 26 mm, 20 mm, and 16 mm for thyme and 21.3 mm, 18 mm, and 15.3 mm for oregano EO, respectively. At 48 h, for both EOs, a bacterial growth recovery was observed, and the inhibition halo present at 24 h disappeared. In Figure 6, it is possible to identify two different zones: an outer portion with a normal bacterial growth and an inner one with a lower CFU number. For thyme EO, at 100% and 75%, the inner zones were 8.3 and 7.6 mm, corresponding, respectively, to 32 and 38%. For thyme at 50%, the bacterial growth completely covered the inhibition halo observed at 24 h. In the presence of oregano EO, the inner portions were equal to 50% in all the cases (10.7, 8.9, and 7.8 mm for 100, 75, and 50% EO, respectively).

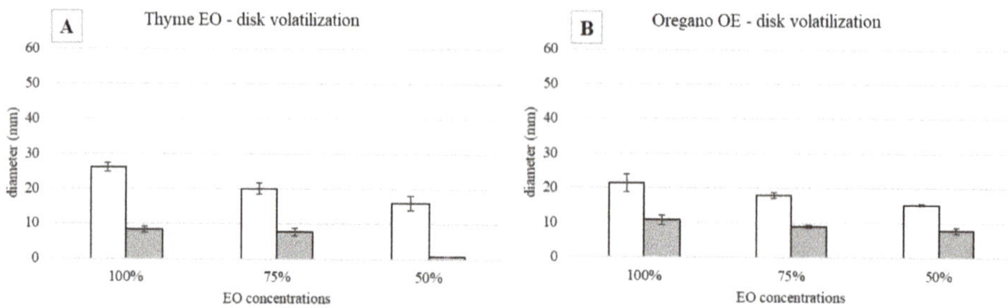

Figure 5. Disk volatilization test against *S. epidermidis* incubated at 37 °C: halo diameters measured after 24 (white bars) and 48 (grey bars) h of incubation in the presence of (**A**) thyme and (**B**) oregano EO (3 µL).

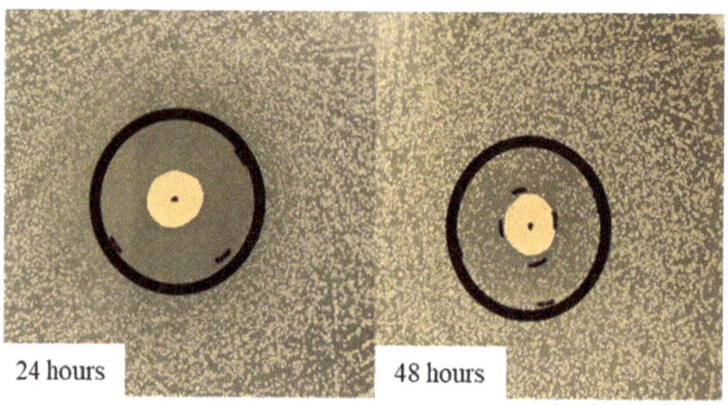

Figure 6. Variation of the inhibition halo diameter, from 24 to 48 h of incubation, for the disk volatilization test in the presence of 100% thyme EO against *S. epidermidis*.

The disk volatilization test conducted against *S. epidermidis* with 3 µL of EOs on 5 mm Ø paper disks (0.13 $\mu L_{EO}/mm^2$) gave a defined inhibition halo only in the first 24 h. To improve the inhibitory effect and to check how long it would be effective, the test was realized with 10 µL of 100, 75, and 50% EO on a 10 mm disk, maintaining a comparable ratio $volume_{EO}$/paper disk area (0.15 $\mu L_{EO}/mm^2$), and the bacterial growth was prolonged for 168 h.

As regards the thyme EO, at the two highest concentrations, a progressive halo reduction was measured until the 144th h, and then, stabilization of the inhibition was registered until the 168th hour (Figure 7A). At the end of the incubation, haloes were still high; in particular, that of 100% EO, i.e., 30.4 mm, was comparable to that obtained with 75% after 48 h (32.8 mm). Conversely, the 50% EO resulted as efficacious only in the first 24 h of treatment.

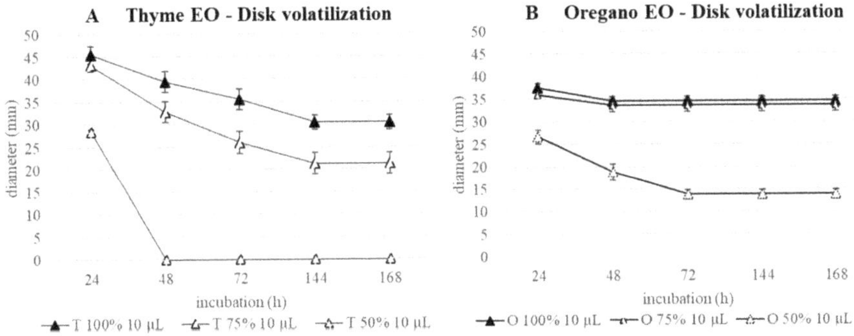

Figure 7. Disk volatilization test against *S. epidermidis*: results obtained with 10 µL of thyme (**A**) and oregano (**B**) EOs during 168 h of incubation.

Considering 100 and 75% oregano EO, the curves were overlapped, with an equal slope between 24th and 48th h (Figure 7B). After that, the stabilization of the haloes was maintained until the end of the incubation, when 34.6 and 33.2 mm were measured. A different trend was obtained for EO 50%, characterized by a reduction of the inhibition halo till the 72nd h, followed by its stabilization. The final halo was 13.7 mm, which is 2.5 times lower than those measured with the highest EO concentrations.

The antimicrobial efficacy of oregano appears consistently superior to that of thyme at all the tested concentrations.

2.3.2. Tests with a Gram-Negative Bacterium: *E. coli*

The antibacterial effect of the volatile phase of thyme and oregano EOs was also evaluated against *E. coli* grown at both 28 °C and 37 °C, utilizing 3 µL of EO on a paper disk of 5 mm Ø. Only 100% oregano EO was effective in the vapor phase; at 28 °C and 37 °C, comparable inhibition haloes (8.4 and 8.5 mm, respectively) were measured. The results obtained at 37 °C are reported in Table 1B and compared with those of *S. epidermidis*.

Table 1. Comparison of the inhibition zones (mm) measured after 48 h of incubation at 37 °C in the presence of thyme or oregano EOs against *S. epidermidis* and *E. coli*. (**A**) Agar disk diffusion; (**B**) disk volatilization.

(A)	Thyme EO %			(B)	Thyme EO %		
	100	75	50		100	75	50
S. epidermidis 3 µL	28.6	26.5	10.4	*S. epidermidis* 3 µL	8.3	7.6	0
				10 µL	39.5	32.8	0
E. coli 3 µL	32.0	29.5	27.7	*E. coli* 3 µL	0	0	0
				10 µL	38.5	35	19
	Oregano EO %				Oregano EO %		
	100	75	50		100	75	50
S. epidermidis 3 µL	23.0	22.7	14.7	*S. epidermidis* 3 µL	10.7	8.9	7.8
				10 µL	34.6	33.5	18.0
E. coli 3 µL	46.0	27.7	20.3	*E. coli* 3 µL	8.5	0	0
				10 µL	43	37.5	33

Considering the inhibition improvement obtained with a higher EO quantity (10 µL) against *S. epidermidis*, the same test was repeated against *E. coli* at 37 °C. After 48 h of incubation, an inhibition halo was measured for all the tested concentrations. The inhibition zones resulting from 100 and 75% thyme EO were similar, i.e., 38.5 and 35 mm, while that related to 50% was about halved, being equal to 19 mm. 100% Oregano EO allowed to obtain the highest inhibition halo, 43 mm, which is fivefold higher that that associated with 3 μL, while that related to 75% was slightly lower at 37.5 mm. Finally, 50% oregano EO showed an inhibition zone of 33 mm, comparable with those obtained with the highest concentrations of this EO. In Figure 8, an example of the obtained inhibition with 100% oregano EO, 3 and 10 μL, is shown.

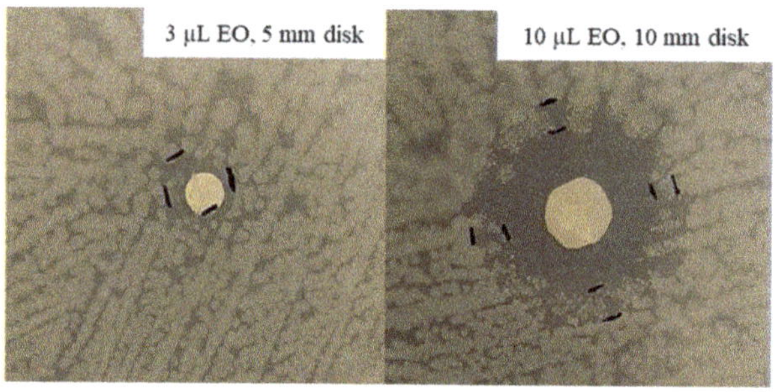

Figure 8. Disk volatilization test set-up with 100% oregano EO against *E. coli* after 48 h of incubation.

As far as the agar disk diffusion assay is concerned, considering the results obtained at the 48th h of incubation at 37 °C, both the EOs show a better antibacterial effect against *E. coli*; indeed, the inhibition haloes are always higher than those measured for *S. epidermidis* (Table 1A). The greatest differences were evidenced in the application of 100% oregano EO and 50% thyme EO. In the first case, the inhibition zone related to *E. coli* was double than that of *S. epidermidis*, and in the second one, a halo about three-fold higher for *E. coli* was observed. For all the other EO concentrations, differences in the efficacy against the two bacteria were less remarkable and in the range 10–25%.

As regard the application of the disk volatilization assay (Table 1B), both thyme and oregano EOs at 3 and 10 μL showed the capability to inhibit the growth of *S. epidermidis* when applied in the vapor phase, with the only exception represented by 50% thyme EO, for which the inhibition zone was absent also for the higher EO volume. The antibacterial effect of 3 μL EOs against *E. coli* was null except for 100% oregano. The inhibition effect was greatly improved for all the concentrations of both EOs, increasing the volume. The inhibition due to 10 μL thyme EO against both the bacteria was comparable; on the contrary, that related to oregano was always higher against *E. coli*.

3. Discussion

Thyme and oregano EOs are well-known for their antimicrobial efficacy due to their carvacrol and thymol constituents [9,11]. In the present work, as it has been reported, the same MIC value was obtained with thyme EO against both the bacteria. On the contrary, at the tested concentrations, an MIC was not identified for oregano EO. In any case, both EOs were applied in the following specific antimicrobial tests, i.e., disk diffusion and disk volatilization, because the EO activity can vary depending on the application modality, namely in the liquid or in the vapor phase.

As regards the agar disk diffusion test, when it was applied against the Gram-positive bacterium, it showed a decrease of the inhibition halo diameter between 24 and 48 h of incubation; this behavior could be explained by the "threshold EO effect"; i.e., if the EO concentration is below this value, bacteria are allowed to grow [23]. On the contrary, this decrease was not evidenced for the Gram-negative strain, for which the inhibition was already stable after 24 h of incubation [24].

The disk volatilization test allowed to verify the antibacterial activity of the phenolic EO compounds due to the evaporation at 37 °C [25]. Both thyme and oregano EO were able to inhibit *S. epidermidis* growth in the first 24 h. After that, the inhibition halo was covered by a new bacterial growth, which was poor with respect to that on the rest of the agar surface, probably due to an EO concentration below the threshold value. The obtained results confirmed that the definition of the threshold concentration is of great importance because, when exposed to EO sub-lethal concentrations, bacteria can adapt to the presence of EOs in a similar manner to that of the antibiotic resistance, as previously reported by [26]. The antimicrobial properties of EO vapors depend, at the same time, on the relative volatility and the antimicrobial properties of their constituents [27,28]; the higher EO volume applied probably allowed to overcome the threshold value of carvacrol and thymol, the main active components of the two EOs [25]. Concerning *E. coli*, it showed a high resistance against the lowest volume (3 μL) of both EOs: in fact, only the maximum oregano EO concentration was inhibiting. When the higher EOs volume (10 μL) was applied, at all the concentrations, an inhibition was observed, probably in relation to an EO quantity above the threshold value.

Generally, in the literature, Gram-positive bacteria are reported to be more sensitive than Gram-negative ones regardless of the applied EO [29]; the results obtained in our work with thyme and oregano suggest that the antimicrobial properties of the EOs are mostly related to the individual susceptibility of the strain and change in relation to both the applied test (disk diffusion or disk volatilization) and EO concentration [24].

From the obtained results, it is clear that, with the EO volume being equal and with the paper disk diameter and the bacterial inoculum concentration, the inhibition obtained by both disk diffusion and disk volatilization methods were different. The detected efficacy after 48 h of incubation was always higher in the presence of a direct contact between the microorganism and the EO (the disk diffusion assays) independently of the tested oil and concentration.

In the case of the disk diffusion assay, the EO inhibitory effect is due to both the EO liquid phase in direct contact with the bacterial cells and the EO vapors inside the free head space; consequently, the haloes are higher than those obtained with the disk volatilization tests. Diameters measured at 48 h of incubation in the disk volatilization test are always lower than those obtained in the disk diffusion one. This observation could be explained by the fact that, in the last case, the measured inhibition halo was the result of the effect due to volatile compounds and those present in the liquid phase. Considering all the above observations, the application of both agar disk diffusion and disk volatilizations tests is mandatory.

The tests applied in the present work are the most frequently found in the literature due to their easy set-up and rapidity of results [29]. They are based on the principle of the Kirby–Bauer assay, which is usually utilized for antibiotic resistance studies [16]. The number of scientific reports about EO efficacy against clinical isolates, such as the Gram-positive *B. subtilis*, *S. aureus*, and *L. monocytogenes* and the Gram-negative *E. coli*, *S. typhimurium*, *P. aeruginosa*, and *Campylobacter* spp., is high in comparison with applications against non-pathogenic bacteria [29]. Taking in mind that the bacterial sensitivity to EOs depends on both the oil characteristics and the type of microorganism tested, it is clear that pathogenic clinical strains and non-pathogenic ones could differ in sensitivity against the same EO [30].

The comparison between results obtained for pathogenic and non-pathogenic strains, although interesting, is not easy to be conducted; in fact, since the tested EO and the bacterial strain were equal, differences in the test set-up are represented by the EO volume, the paper disk diameter, and the CFU/mL of the inoculum. In analyzing the set-up, realized in recent times, from 2019 to 2021, it can be evidenced that microbial inoculum can vary from 10^5 to 10^8 CFU/mL [6,31–36]. The EO quantity can broadly differ from a minimum of 5 μL to a maximum increased up to four times [23,32,37,38]. Moreover, the CFU/mL and EO volume can be variously combined, bringing to different ratios "EO concentration in test area/CFU number". This parameter is essential in the comparison of the EO efficacy. The number of EO-impregnated disks positioned in the Petri dish is another experimental condition that can vary: we demonstrated (see Figure 9) that is fundamental to put a single paper disk in each dish in order to avoid the additive effect dependent on the disk number; in most of the work, there may be three to five in each dish [23,37,38].

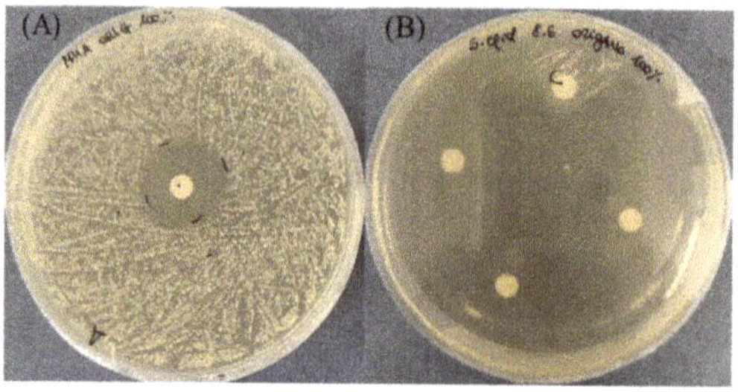

Figure 9. Inhibition effect due to a single (**A**) or three paper disks (**B**) impregnated with 100% oregano EO against *S. epidermidis*. In (**B**), a control disk with TEGO 1.5% (labeled "C") was present.

4. Materials and Methods

4.1. Microorganisms and Media

The tested standard strains, *Staphylococcus epidermidis* ATCC 12228 and *Escherichia coli* ATCC 8739, came from the Belgian Coordinated Collections of Micro-organisms (BCCM). They were maintained at +4 °C or cultivated at +37 °C on Mueller–Hinton agar (CM0337, Oxoid, Hampshire, UK) in aerobic conditions.

As indicated in the following chapters, in some antibacterial tests, *E. coli* was cultivated at 28 °C, using the same cultural medium. Mueller–Hinton broth (CM0405, Oxoid, Hampshire, UK) was utilized for the microdilution assays in well plates.

4.2. Essential Oils (EOs)

Commercial essential oils (EOs) from thyme (*Thymus vulgaris* EO, OE0970) and oregano (*Origanum vulgaris* leaf EO, OE0375) were purchased from Witt Italia Spa Company, Poirino, Italy. They were applied pure (100%) or diluted (75% v/v and 50% v/v) using a 1.5% solution of Polysorbate 20 (TEGO® SML 20, Waltham, MA, USA). This solution was also used for the positive controls to check the potential interaction with bacterial growth.

4.3. Preliminary Test—Microdilution in Broth

The microdilution test was carried out in sterile, 96-well microplates according to CLSI standard method [35]. Thyme or oregano EOs were dissolved in sterile 1.5% TEGO to obtain a 15 µg/mL stock solution. Then, 100 µL of 2X Mueller–Hinton broth was poured in each well, while in the first column, 100 µL of the stock solution was added. Serial two-fold dilutions were directly prepared in the wells, obtaining the following concentrations: 7.5, 3.75, 1.875, 0.938, 0.469, 0.234, 0.117, 0.059, and 0.0285 µg/mL. A standardized inoculum was prepared in Mueller–Hinton broth to obtain, in each well, a final bacterial concentration equal to 5×10^5 CFUmL^{-1}. The total tested volume in each well was 200 µL. Biotic controls were set up with inoculated Mueller–Hinton broth together with un-inoculated abiotic controls for each tested concentration of EO; biotic and abiotic controls were also prepared with the cultural medium added with the 1.5% TEGO alone. Microplates were incubated at 37 °C in agitation at 150 rpm. After 24 h, MIC values were identified as the lowest EO concentrations that showed no bacterial growth as checked by the naked eye.

4.4. Antimicrobial Tests

In all the antibacterial tests, the inoculum was prepared using the direct colony suspension method. Three colonies, coming from a 24 h old culture grown on solid medium, were withdrawn and suspended into 5 mL of 0.85% NaCl to obtain a cell density equal to 1×10^8 CFU/mL; this last density was further diluted, using the same saline solution, to reach the final concentration of 1×10^5 CFU/mL. All the tests were performed in 90 mm Ø Petri dishes (Polystyrene, PS) filled with 20 mL of Mueller–Hinton agar, giving a 10 mm high head space corresponding to a free volume of 63.62 cm^3 (Figure 10).

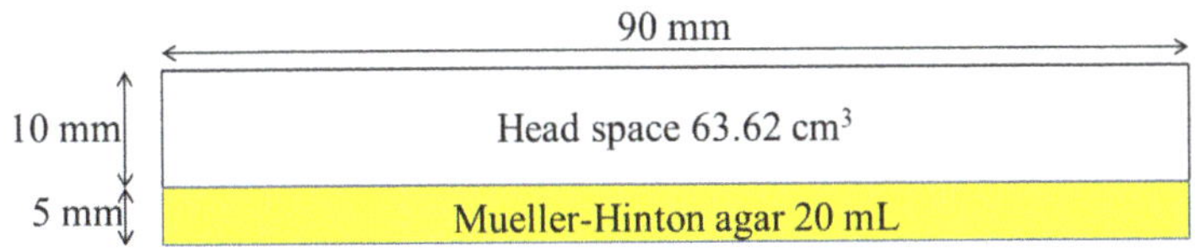

Figure 10. Dimensions of the Petri dishes filled with a fixed quantity of Mueller–Hinton agar, used for all the antibacterial tests.

4.4.1. Agar Disk Diffusion Test

The antimicrobial susceptibility testing for thyme and oregano EOs was carried out by applying the "Agar disk diffusion method" [39] using a single filter paper disc (Whatman N°1, 5 mm diameter) in each Petri dish. First, 100 µL suspensions of *S. epidermidis* or *E. coli*, 1.0×10^5 CFU/mL, were spread over the surface of the Mueller–Hinton agar plates. One paper disc was gently placed in the center of each plate and then soaked with 3 µL of 100, 75, or 50% EO, or with 1.5% Polysorbate 20 (TEGO) for the control. Plates were sealed off with Parafilm® (Neenah, WI, USA) and enveloped with PVC film to prevent EO vapor losses.

After 24 and 48 h of incubation, the inhibition zones at the two perpendicular diameters, as shown in Figure 11A, were measured by means of a ruler; the edges of the zones were read at the point of complete inhibition as judged by the naked eye. Each antibacterial test was performed in triplicate.

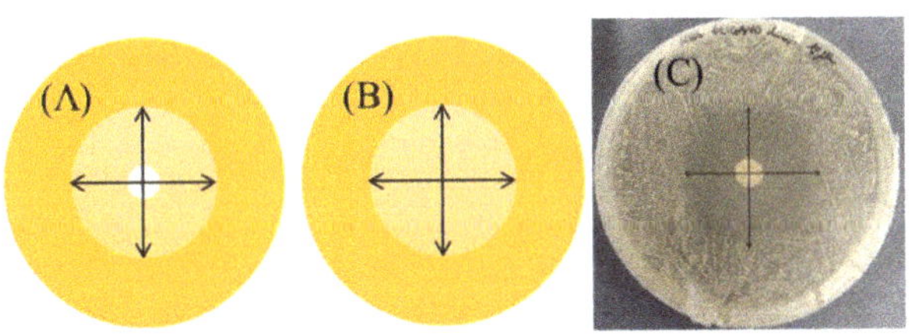

Figure 11. Inhibition zones measured (mm) at the two perpendicular diameters for the agar disk diffusion method (**A**) and the disk volatilization assay (**B**). (**C**) shows a real case measurement.

4.4.2. Disk Volatilization Test

The disk volatilization assay was set up to test the antibacterial efficacy of the two EOs in vapor phase. To this purpose, a single filter paper disk was attached to the lid of the Petri dish by means of a bi-adhesive tape. Used disks had a diameter of 5 or 10 mm and were soaked, respectively, with 3 µL or 10 µL of 100, 75, or 50% EO or 1.5% TEGO. The obtained ratio "EO volume/disk area" were similar and, respectively, equal to 0.13 and 0.15 $\mu L_{EO}/mm^2$. An amount of 100 µL of 1.0×10^5 CFU/mL bacterial suspension was spread over the surface of Mueller–Hinton agar. Once set up, Petri dishes sealed with Parafilm® (Neenah, WI, USA) M and enveloped with PVC film were incubated inverted on top of the lid.

After 24 and 48 h of incubation, the inhibition zones on the agar surface below the imbibed paper disk were measured at the two perpendicular diameters at the point of complete inhibition as judged by the naked eye, Figure 11B. In some experiments, as indicated in the Results section, diameter measurements were carried out until the 168th h of incubation. Each trial was conducted in triplicate.

5. Conclusions

In the present work, *S. epidermidis* and *E. coli*, belonging to Biosafety Level 1, were chosen as indicators of the EO efficacy against a Gram-positive and a Gram-negative bacterium. The effect of commercial thyme and oregano EOs was tested by means of microdilution in broth, agar diffusion, and disk volatilization tests. As regards the first test, an equal MIC value was found against *S. epidermidis* and *E. coli* in the presence of thyme EO. Concerning the agar disk diffusion test, both bacteria were inhibited by all the tested EO concentrations. The inhibition obtained in the disk diffusion assays was higher than that in disk volatilization test; in the first case, the antimicrobial effect is due to both the EO components in the liquid and in the vapor phase.

The comparison of the obtained results with those present in the literature was not so easy; consequently, it can be concluded that when an assessment is needed, it is necessary to interpret the data with a high attention in relation to the applied analytical method used. In fact, even though standard methods are usually applied, numerous modifications are brought to adapt the set-up to the specific case study. Moreover, it is mandatory to evaluate the threshold value of the EOs concentration in the real conditions of application.

Author Contributions: Conceptualization, D.F. and F.B.; methodology, D.F. and F.B.; formal analysis, C.M. and D.F.; investigation, C.M., F.B. and D.F.; data curation, F.B. and D.F.; writing—original draft preparation, F.B., D.F. and C.M.; writing—review and editing, C.M., F.B. and D.F.; supervision, F.B. and D.F. All authors have read and agreed to the published version of the manuscript.

Funding: This research received no external funding.

Institutional Review Board Statement: Not applicable.

Informed Consent Statement: Not applicable.

Data Availability Statement: Not applicable.

Acknowledgments: Authors wish to thank Chiara Gallo and Diego Burdizzo for their contribution in the experiment realization during their master thesis work.

Conflicts of Interest: The authors declare no conflict of interest.

References

1. Mondello, F.; Girolamo, A.; Vito, M. Sostanze naturali e antibiotico resistenza. *Natural 1* **2020**, 71–79.
2. Aziz, Z.; Ahmad, A.; Setapar, S.; Karakucuk, A.; Azim, M.M.; Lokhat, D.; Rafatullah, M.; Ganash, M.; Kamal, M.A.; Ashraf, G.M. Essential Oils: Extraction Techniques, Pharmaceutical and Therapeutic Potential—A Review. *Curr. Drug Metab.* **2018**, *19*, 1100–1110. [CrossRef] [PubMed]
3. Valdivieso-Ugarte, M.; Gomez-Llorente, C.; Plaza-Díaz, J.; Gil, Á. Antimicrobial, Antioxidant, and Immunomodulatory Properties of Essential Oils: A Systematic Review. *Nutrients* **2019**, *11*, 2786. [CrossRef] [PubMed]
4. Dhifi, W.; Bellili, S.; Jazi, S.; Bahloul, N.; Mnif, W. Essential Oils' Chemical Characterization and Investigation of Some Biological Activities: A Critical Review. *Medicines* **2016**, *3*, 25. [CrossRef]
5. Fokou, J.B.H.; Dongmo, P.M.J.; Boyom, F.F. Essential Oil's Chemical Composition and Pharmacological Properties. In *Essential Oils—Oils of Nature*; El-Shemy, H.A., Ed.; IntechOpen: London, UK, 2020. [CrossRef]
6. Alibi, S.; Selma, W.B.; Ramos-Vivas, J.; Smach, M.A.; Touati, R.; Boukadida, J.; Navas, J.; Mansour, H.B. Anti-oxidant, antibacterial, anti-biofilm, and anti-quorum sensing activities of four essential oils against multidrug-resistant bacterial clinical isolates. *Curr. Res. Trans. Med.* **2020**, *68*, 59–66. [CrossRef] [PubMed]
7. Esmael, A.; Hassan, M.G.; Amer, M.M.; Abdelrahman, S.; Hamed, A.M.; Abd-Raboh, H.A.; Foda, M.F. Antimicrobial activity of certain natural-based plant oils against the antibiotic-resistant acne bacteria Saudi. *J. Biol. Sci.* **2020**, *27*, 448–455.
8. Nieto, G. A Review on Applications and Uses of Thymus in the Food Industry. *Plants* **2020**, *9*, 961. [CrossRef]
9. Burt, S. Essential oils: Their antibacterial properties and potential applications in foods-a review. *Int. J. Food Microbiol.* **2004**, *94*, 223–253. [CrossRef]
10. Silva, A.S.; Tewari, D.; Sureda, A.; Suntar, I.; Belwal, T.; Battino, M.; Nabavi, S.M.; Nabavi, S.F. The Evidence of Health Benefits and Food Applications of *Thymus vulgaris* L. *Trends Food Sci. Technol.* **2021**, *117*, 218–227. [CrossRef]
11. Rostro-Alanis, M.J.; Báez-González, J.; Torres-Alvarez, C.; Parra-Saldívar, R.; Rodriguez-Rodriguez, J.; Castillo, S. Chemical Composition and Biological Activities of Oregano Essential Oil and Its Fractions Obtained by Vacuum Distillation. *Molecules* **2019**, *24*, 1904. [CrossRef]

12. Pontes-Quero, G.M.; Esteban-Rubio, S.; Pérez Cano, J.; Aguilar, M.R.; Vázquez-Lasa, B. Oregano Essential Oil Micro- and Nanoencapsulation with Bioactive Properties for Biotechnological and Biomedical Applications. *Front. Bioeng. Biotechnol.* **2021**, *9*, 703684. [CrossRef] [PubMed]
13. Van de Vel, E.; Sampers, I.; Raes, K. A review on influencing factors on the minimum inhibitory concentration of essential oils. *Critic. Rev. Food Sci. Nutr.* **2019**, *59*, 357–378. [CrossRef] [PubMed]
14. Balouiri, M.; Sadiki, M.; Ibnsouda, S.K. Methods for in vitro evaluating antimicrobial activity: A review. *J. Pharm. Anal.* **2016**, *6*, 71–79. [CrossRef] [PubMed]
15. Hulankova, R. The Influence of Liquid Medium Choice in Determination of Minimum Inhibitory Concentration of Essential Oils against Pathogenic Bacteria. *Antibiotics* **2022**, *11*, 150. [CrossRef]
16. Hudzicki, J. Kirby-Bauer Disk Diffusion Susceptibility Test Protocol. *Am. Soc. Microbiol.* **2009**, *15*, 55–63.
17. Reyes-Jurado, F.; Navarro-Cruz, A.R.; Ochoa-Velasco, C.E.; Palou, E.; López-Malo, A.; Ávila-Sosa, R. Essential oils in vapor phase as alternative antimicrobials: A review. *Crit. Rev. Food Sci. Nutr.* **2020**, *60*, 1641–1650. [CrossRef]
18. Thielmann, J.; Muranyi, P.; Kazman, P. Screening essential oils for their antimicrobial activities against the foodborne pathogenic bacteria *Escherichia coli* and *Staphylococcus aureus*. *Heliyon* **2019**, *5*, e01860. [CrossRef]
19. Friedman, M.; Henika, P.; Mandrell, R. Bactericidal Activities of Plant Essential Oils and Some of Their Isolated Constituents against Campylobacter jejuni, *Escherichia coli*, *Listeria monocytogenes*, and *Salmonella enterica*. *J. Food Protect.* **2002**, *65*, 1545–1560. [CrossRef]
20. Matuschek, E.; Brown, D.F.J.; Kahlmeter, G. Development of the EUCAST disk diffusion antimicrobial susceptibility testing method and its implementation in routine microbiology laboratories. *Bacteriology* **2013**, *20*, O255–O266. [CrossRef]
21. *CLSI Document MO2-A11*; Performance Standards for Antimicrobial Disk Susceptibility Tests, Approved Standard. 11th ed, Clinical and Laboratory Standards Institute (CLSI): Wayne, PA, USA, 2012.
22. EUCAST. *Reading Guide*; Version 2.0; The European Committee on Antimicrobial Susceptibility Testing: Växjö, Sweden, 2012.
23. Saranraj, P.; Durga Devi, V. Essential oils and its antibacterial properties—A review. *Life Sci. Arch.* **2017**, *3*, 994–1011. [CrossRef]
24. Ambrosio, C.M.S.; Ikeda, N.Y.; Miano, A.C.; Saldaña, E.; Moreno, A.M.; Stashenko, E.; Contreras-Castillo, C.J.; da Gloria, E.M. Unreveling the selective antibacterial activity and chemical composition of citrus essential oils. *Sci. Rep.* **2019**, *9*, 17719. [CrossRef] [PubMed]
25. Wang, T.H.; Hsia, S.M.; Wu, C.H.; Ko, S.Y.; Chen, M.Y.; Shih, Y.H.; Shieh, T.M.; Chuang, L.C.; Wu, C.Y. Evaluation of the Antibacterial Potential of Liquid and Vapor Phase Phenolic Essential Oil Compounds against Oral Microorganisms. *PLoS ONE* **2016**, *11*, e0163147. [CrossRef] [PubMed]
26. Melo, A.D.; Amaral, A.F.; Schaefer, G.; Luciano, F.B.; de Andrade, C.; Costa, L.B.; Rostagno, M.H. Antimicrobial effect against different bacterial strains and bacterial adaptation to essential oils used as feed additives. *Can. J. Vet. Res.* **2015**, *79*, 285–289. [PubMed]
27. Antih, J.; Houdkova, M.; Urbanova, K.; Kokoska, L. Antibacterial Activity of *Thymus vulgaris* L. Essential Oil Vapours and Their GC/MS Analysis Using Solid-Phase Microextraction and Syringe Headspace Sampling Techniques. *Molecules* **2021**, *26*, 6553. [CrossRef] [PubMed]
28. Chouhan, S.; Sharma, K.; Guleria, S. Antimicrobial Activity of Some Essential Oils-Present Status and Future Perspectives. *Medicines* **2017**, *4*, 58. [CrossRef] [PubMed]
29. Ouedrhiri, W.; Balouiri, M.; Bouhdid, S.; Moja, S.; Chahdi, F.O.; Taleb, M.; Greche, H. Mixture design of *Origanum compactum*, *Origanum majorana* and *Thymus serpyllum* essential oils: Optimization of their antibacterial effect. *Ind. Crops Prod.* **2016**, *89*, 1–9. [CrossRef]
30. Mutlu-Ingok, A.; Devecioglu, D.; Dikmetas, D.N.; Karbancioglu-Guler, F.; Capanoglu, E. Antibacterial, Antifungal, Antimycotoxigenic, and Antioxidant Activities of Essential Oils: An Updated Review. *Molecules* **2020**, *25*, 4711. [CrossRef]
31. Mutlu-Ingok, A.; Firtin, B.; Karbancioglu-Guler, F. Chemical composition and comparative antibacterial properties of basil essential oil against clinical and standard strains of *Campylobacter* spp. *ACTA Pharm. Sci.* **2019**, *57*, 183. [CrossRef]
32. Jaber, H.; Oubihi, A.; Ouryemchi, I.; Boulamtat, R.; Oubayoucef, A.; Bourkhiss, B.; Ouhssine, M. Chemical Composition and Antibacterial Activities of Eight Plant Essential Oils from Morocco against *Escherichia coli* Strains Isolated from Different Turkey Organs. *Biochem. Res. Int.* **2021**, 6685800. [CrossRef]
33. Brożyna, M.; Paleczny, J.; Kozłowska, W.; Chodaczek, G.; Dudek-Wicher, R.; Felińczak, A.; Gołębiewska, J.; Górniak, A.; Junka, A. The Antimicrobial and Antibiofilm In Vitro Activity of Liquid and Vapour Phases of Selected Essential Oils against *Staphylococcus aureus*. *Pathogens* **2021**, *10*, 1207. [CrossRef]
34. Fazeli-Nasab, B.; Shahraki-Mojahed, L.; Sohail-beygi, G.; Ghafari, M. Evaluation of Antimicrobial Activity of Several Medicinal Plants Against Clinically Isolated *Staphylococcus aureus* from Humans and Sheep. *Gene Cell Tissue* **2022**, *9*, e118752. [CrossRef]
35. Gonzalez, K.; Johnson, A.; Gonsalves, V.; Santos, A. The Effect of Thyme Essential Oil on *Escherichia coli*. *FASEB J.* **2021**, *35*. [CrossRef]
36. Kryvtsova, M.; Salamon, I.; Koscova, J.; Bucko, D.; Spivak, M. Antimicrobial, antibiofilm and biochemichal properties of Thymus vulgaris essential oil against clinical isolates of opportunistic infections. *Biosyst. Divers.* **2019**, *27*, 270–275. [CrossRef]
37. Queiroga, M.C.; Pinto Coelho, M.; Macedo Arantes, S.; Potes, M.E.; Martins, M.R. Antimicrobial Activity of Essential Oils of Lamiaceae Aromatic Spices Towards Sheep mastitis-Causing *Staphylococcus aureus* and *Staphylococcus epidermidis*. *J. Essent. Oil-Bear. Plants* **2018**, *21*, 1155–1165. [CrossRef]

38. Helal, I.M.; El-Bessoumy, A.; Al-Bataineh, E.; Joseph, M.; Rajagopalan, P.; Chandramoorthy, H.C.; Ben Hadj Ahmed, S. Antimicrobial Efficiency of Essential Oils from Traditional Medicinal Plants of Asir Region, Saudi Arabia, over Drug Resistant Isolates. *BioMed Res. Int.* **2019**, *2019*, 8928306. [CrossRef]
39. *CLSI Document M07-A9*; Methods for Dilution Antimicrobial Susceptibility Tests for Bacteria That Grow Aerobically. Approved Standard—Ninth Edition. Clinical and Laboratory Standards Institute: Wayne, PA, USA, 2012.

antibiotics

MDPI

Article

The Application of Ultrasonic Waves and Microwaves to Improve Antihyperglycaemic and Antimicrobial Activities of *Marrubium vulgare* Extracts

Aleksandra Gavarić [1], Jelena Vladić [1], Jelena Vujetić [2], Dragan Radnović [3], Ana Volarić [3], Jelena Živković [4], Katarina Šavikin [4] and Senka Vidović [1,*]

1 Faculty of Technology, University of Novi Sad, 21000 Novi Sad, Serbia
2 Institute of Food Technology, University of Novi Sad, 21000 Novi Sad, Serbia
3 Faculty of Sciences, University of Novi Sad, 21000 Novi Sad, Serbia
4 Institute for Medicinal Plants Research Dr. Josif Pančić, 11000 Belgrade, Serbia
* Correspondence: senka.vidovic@uns.ac.rs; Tel.: +381-21-485-3731

Abstract: Having scarce information about ultrasound assisted extraction (UAE) and microwave assisted extraction (MAE) of white horehound (*Marrubium vulgare* L.), the idea has emerged to determine the optimal process parameters for the maximization of polyphenols and to compare the efficiency of these green extraction technologies. The optimal UAE parameters are temperature of 73.6 °C, extraction time of 40 min and ultrasound power of 30.3 W/L, while the optimal MAE parameters are 63.8% ethanol, extraction time of 15 min and microwave power of 422 W. Extract obtained at optimal UAE parameters shows the highest antihyperglycemic activity (α-amylase inhibition: 50.63% and α-glucosidase inhibition: 48.67%), which can potentially be explained by the presence of chlorogenic acid and quercetin, which were not identified in the macerates. The most sensitive bacterial strain to optimal ultrasonic extract is *Bacillus cereus*, whereas the most sensitive fungal strain is *Saccharomyces cerevisiae*.

Keywords: *Marrubium vulgare*; ultrasound extraction; microwave extraction; antihyperglycaemic activity; antimicrobial activity

1. Introduction

White horehound (*Marrubium vulgare* L.) is a grey-leaved perennial herb belonging to the Lamiaceae family, distributed throughout the Eurasia and northern Africa zones [1]. There are contradictory literature data on the hypoglycemic activity of horehound. According to one source, aqueous horehound extract did not significantly reduce blood glucose levels [2], while according to another source, its administration induced a significant reduction in glucose levels in rats [3]. The variation in the results is most likely a consequence of the collection of plant material from different localities, which greatly affects the quality and quantity of the secondary metabolites, together with the use of different parts of the plant and different extraction methods. Several studies have shown that polyphenol-rich extracts can be a major cause of antihyperglycemic activity in animals and humans, most likely through the inhibition of α-amylase and/or α-glucosidase [4,5]. Oral hypoglycemic drugs used to treat diabetes have serious side effects, such as weight gain and gastrointestinal disorders [6]. Therefore, studies of potential insulin sensitizers, such as chlorogenic acid, which stimulate insulin action similar to the therapeutic action of metformin, are necessary [7].

The wide spectrum of solid/liquid extractions is available for the extraction and isolation of new functional ingredients. However, some common techniques are inconvenient due to inefficient time and elevated temperature, leading to the thermal degradation of phenolic compounds [8]. Therefore, employment of green extraction technologies is suitable to overcome these obstacles and improve the extraction yield and the quality of the obtained extracts. In line with that statement, some researchers investigated the application of a pulsed electric field as a pretreatment step for the intensification of the horehound essential oil isolation. They concluded that a pulsed electric field improves the extraction rate of the essential oil by 2–3 fold [9]. Another environment-friendly, efficient extraction technique is ultrasound-assisted extraction (UAE), the application of which has increased in recent decades due to the several disadvantages associated with conventional extraction techniques, such as high capital investment, large consumption of toxic organic solvents and their residues in the extract and energy expenditure. In addition, ultrasound is relatively easy to use, versatile, flexible and requires low investment as a result of a simple principle of UAE, which is based on cavitation effects causing the rupture of plant cell walls, thus increasing the contact area between the solid and solvent [10]. As opposed to traditional methods, in microwave assisted extraction (MAE), the heat and mass gradients act in the same direction (from inside outwards), with faster heating occurring inside the solids, where the dissolution takes place [11]. Microwaves generated by a magnetron interact with water and other polar molecules, causing their heating as the molecular dipoles try to orient themselves in the direction of the electromagnetic field. Part of electromagnetic radiation is thus converted into molecular motion and dissipated as heat. MAE affords much shorter extraction time, higher extraction yield and 5–10 fold less solvent consumption in comparison to conventional extraction [12].

In this study, the main goal was to identify the optimal UAE and MAE parameters responsible for enhanced extraction of polyphenols from horehound herba in order to deliver high-quality extracts with significant antihyperglycaemic and antimicrobial activities. The Box–Behnken experimental design, with three factors at three levels, was applied in order to provide exhaustive extraction of polyphenols and reduce the number of experimental runs.

2. Results and Discussion

2.1. Extraction Yield

Among the recent research papers interested in the valorization of horehound extracts obtained by UAE and MAE, those focusing on marrubiin are predominant [13–15]. In this study, the extraction yield obtained by MAE varied in the range 13.74–22.61%, and was slightly higher than the yield in the UAE, which varied from 12.91 to 20.08%. Compared with the extraction yield in the maceration with 50% ethanol, i.e., MAC (11.55%), both UAEopt (17.92%) and MAEopt (16.30%) extraction yields, were higher. Other researchers also applied Soxhlet extraction (18 h) of the aerial parts of horehound with ethanol as solvent and obtained a yield of 11.27% [13]. As opposed to 18 h of extraction, 6.22 min of MAE provided a yield of 20.48%. In addition, the S/L ratio in MAE was optimized at 1:32 (m/V), suggesting lower solvent consumption compared to Soxhlet extraction (1:50, m/V). Another study concluded that the most favorable MAE conditions in terms of extraction yield were temperature of 40 °C, 20% ethanol as a solvent and extraction time of 15 min [14]. The extraction yield (14.2%) and concentration of marrubiin (0.91%) were significantly improved at the optimized UAE conditions (ultrasound power 467 W, extraction time of 47 min and S/L ratio 1:33, m/V) as compared to the conventional method [15].

2.2. Total Phenolic Content

Experimentally obtained TP in horehound extracts generated by UAE varied from 73.66 to 99.30 mg GAE/g, depending on the applied extraction conditions. In our study, the lowest TP yield was observed after 60 min of extraction at a temperature of 40 °C and at an ultrasonic power of 60 W/L. Generally, low TP yields (73.66–83.89 mg GAE/g) were obtained using temperature of 40 °C, while higher TP yields (90–99.30 mg GAE/g) were obtained using 80 °C. The highest TP yield (99.30 mg GAE/g) in horehound extract was obtained at 80 °C after 40 min of extraction and at an ultrasound power of 42 W/L. These results are in accordance with a previous study, in which it was reported that the highest TP in sage ultrasonic extract was also obtained at 80 °C, while all UAE extracts obtained at

40 °C had significantly lower TP [16]. The highest TP yield from wild garlic was obtained at 80 °C using the same 50% ethanol concentration [17]. This suggests that temperature could be appointed as the most influential parameter in UAE.

In the case of MAE, TP varied in the range 81.94–117.58 mg GAE/g. It could be confirmed that both UAE and MAE ensured a remarkable increase in TP yield compared to S/L extraction with 30, 50 and 70% ethanol (63.77 mg GAE/g, 73.68 mg GAE/g and 70.90 mg GAE/g, respectively). The highest TP yield was obtained using 50% ethanol for 25 min of extraction at a microwave power of 600 W. Comparing the maximal TP yields obtained by UAE and MAE, it could be seen that MAE provides 15% higher TP. This difference could be attributed to the intense cell destruction provided by MAE. In another study, 80% methanol was used for MAE of horehound leaves, setting the process parameters as follows: temperature of 60 °C, extraction time of 10 min and microwave power of 800 W. The TP of 6.02 mg GAE/g was determined to be significantly lower than the TP (86.05 mg GAE/g) obtained in the present study for 15 min of extraction at 800 W [1].

2.3. Total Flavonoid Content

Experimentally obtained values of TF observed in horehound extracts created by UAE and MAE exploitation are presented in Tables 1 and 2, respectively. The TF in horehound extracts obtained by UAE ranged between 44.59 and 53.19 mg CE/g, which is slightly higher than the TF yield (42.51 mg CE/g) obtained by S/L extraction lasting for 24 h. The highest TF was obtained at 80 °C after 40 min extraction at an ultrasound power of 42 W, as was the case with TP, suggesting a solid correlation between the influence of UAE parameters and the monitored responses, TP and TF.

The TF observed in MAE extracts ranged between 49.76 and 65.80 mg CE/g. Again, the TF yield in MAE was slightly higher than in UAE, replicating the pattern noticed in TP. The maximal TF in MAE was obtained using 70% ethanol for 35 min of extraction at microwave power of 600 W. A TF yield of 45.21 mg CE/g was obtained at a temperature of 60 °C, extraction time of 10 min and microwave power of 800 W [1]. This is slightly lower than the TF yield (54.70 mg CE/g) obtained in present work for 15 min of extraction at 800 W.

Table 1. BBD matrix with natural UAE parameters and experimentally observed values of TP, TF, IC_{50} and EC_{50} values.

	Independent Variables			Investigated Responses				
Run Order	Temperature (°C)	Extraction Time (min)	Ultrasonic Power (W/L)	Y (mg/mL)	TP (mg GAE/g)	TF (mg CE/g)	IC_{50} (mg/mL)	EC_{50} (mg/mL)
1	60	60	42	15.92	85.10	50.42	0.0172	0.0593
2	60	40	60	16.02	87.66	52.40	0.0180	0.0566
3	80	40	42	18.48	99.30	53.19	0.0218	0.0575
4	60	60	42	15.76	76.36	49.84	0.0178	0.0591
5	60	80	60	17.42	80.10	48.58	0.0177	0.0576
6	40	80	42	15.16	78.94	44.97	0.0215	0.0561
7	80	60	60	20.08	92.39	50.93	0.0256	0.0636
8	40	40	42	12.91	76.00	49.03	0.0199	0.0480
9	60	60	42	16.90	82.45	44.67	0.0178	0.0557
10	40	60	60	15.35	73.66	49.08	0.0207	0.0505
11	60	60	42	15.95	82.15	51.10	0.0164	0.0562
12	60	40	24	15.19	79.85	50.51	0.0170	0.0524
13	80	60	24	17.95	94.57	44.59	0.0193	0.0566
14	60	80	24	17.15	77.58	49.15	0.0222	0.0569
15	40	60	24	13.61	83.89	50.35	0.0197	0.0427
16	80	80	42	19.11	90.00	48.25	0.0217	0.0568
17	60	60	42	16.22	86.99	52.97	0.0218	0.0606

Table 2. BBD matrix with natural MAE parameters and experimentally observed values of TP, TF, IC_{50} and EC_{50} values.

	Independent Variables			Investigated Responses				
Run Order	Extraction Time (min)	Ethanol Conc. (%)	Microwave Power (W)	Y (mg/mL)	TP (mg GAE/g)	TF (mg CE/g)	IC_{50} (mg/mL)	EC_{50} (mg/mL)
1	35	50	400	18.29	107.08	56.05	0.0216	0.0671
2	15	50	400	18.20	106.85	57.97	0.0197	0.0635
3	15	70	600	13.74	102.58	65.54	0.0192	0.0475
4	25	30	400	18.26	93.33	59.58	0.0188	0.0630
5	15	50	800	18.70	86.05	54.70	0.0171	0.0636
6	25	50	600	17.26	92.89	57.92	0.0198	0.0659
7	35	50	800	20.36	81.94	52.10	0.0275	0.0651
8	25	50	600	19.07	109.13	52.42	0.0159	0.0726
9	25	50	600	19.65	82.28	49.98	0.0212	0.0677
10	25	70	800	16.36	94.00	57.30	0.0240	0.0590
11	25	30	800	22.30	94.36	49.76	0.0164	0.0776
12	35	30	600	22.61	86.69	53.46	0.0129	0.0790
13	25	50	600	18.95	89.36	52.96	0.0186	0.0657
14	25	70	400	14.64	96.04	62.78	0.0195	0.0528
15	15	30	600	20.69	82.29	50.93	0.0178	0.0735
16	35	70	600	14.33	117.58	65.80	0.0259	0.0445
17	25	50	600	18.16	116.94	54.58	0.0175	0.0633

2.4. Antioxidant Activity

The antioxidant properties of horehound methanol extracts were investigated using DPPH assay and the results revealed a strong activity with IC_{50} value in the range 8.24–12.42 μg/mL [18]. The IC_{50} value for horehound was reported to be 0.0386 mg/mL [1], which is twice lower than the IC_{50} value (0.017 mg/mL) obtained in present study for 15 min of extraction at 800 W. Others used a central composite design to optimize the MAE of horehound in order to maximize its antioxidant activity. The optimized conditions were microwave power of 539 W, irradiation time of 373 s and S/L ratio of 1:32 (m/V). They reported an IC_{50} value of 0.066 mg/mL [13], which is out of the IC_{50} value interval (0.027–0.013 mg/mL) obtained in seventeen MAE runs conducted in our study.

2.5. Model Fitting

Experimental results of the investigated responses (Y, TP, TF, IC_{50} and EC_{50}) obtained under different UAE (temperature, extraction time, ultrasonic power) and MAE (extraction time, ethanol concentration, ultrasonic power) conditions using BBD are presented in Tables 1 and 2, respectively.

Results were fitted to a second-order polynomial model (Equation (13)) and multiple regression coefficients were generated for all five responses using the method of least squares. Analysis of variance (ANOVA) was employed in order to check the fitness of the applied models and the *p*-values of regression coefficients for each investigated response are summarized in Table 3.

Table 3. ANOVA of the fitted second-order polynomial models.

Ultrasound Assisted Extraction		**Microwave Assisted Extraction**	
	Extraction Yield		
	***p*-value**		***p*-value**
Model	0.0002 *	**Model**	0.0054 *
X_1-Temperature	<0.0001 *	X_1-Extraction time	0.2208
X_2-Extraction time	0.0034 *	X_2-Ethanol concentration	0.0001 *
X_3-Ultrasonic power	0.0105 **	X_3-Microwave power	0.0339 **
$X_1 \times X_2$	0.1566	$X_1 \times X_2$	0.5696
$X_1 \times X_3$	0.7143	$X_1 \times X_3$	0.5051
$X_2 \times X_3$	0.5972	$X_2 \times X_3$	0.3367
X_1^2	0.2930	X_1^2	0.8479
X_2^2	0.9427	X_2^2	0.1481
X_3^2	0.2470	X_3^2	0.7798
Lack of fit	0.3136	**Lack of fit**	0.2446
	Total phenols content		
	***p*-value**		***p*-value**
Model	0.0423 **	**Model**	0.0024 *
X_1-Temperature	0.0013 *	X_1-Extraction time	0.6941
X_2-Extraction time	0.2320	X_2-Ethanol concentration	0.0008 *
X_3-Ultrasonic power	0.8710	X_3-Microwave power	0.0006 *
$X_1 \times X_2$	0.2040	$X_1 \times X_2$	0.9955
$X_1 \times X_3$	0.3880	$X_1 \times X_3$	0.6239
$X_2 \times X_3$	0.5638	$X_2 \times X_3$	0.4306
X_1^2	0.0931 ***	X_1^2	0.0238 **
X_2^2	0.7544	X_2^2	0.0246 **
X_3^2	0.7782	X_3^2	0.0137 **
Lack of fit	0.3594	**Lack of fit**	0.0692 ***
	Total flavonoids content		
	***p*-value**		***p*-value**
Model	0.0195 ***	**Model**	0.0396 **
X_1-Temperature	0.6171	X_1-Extraction time	0.8377
X_2-Extraction time	0.0123 **	X_2-Ethanol concentration	0.0024 *
X_3-Ultrasonic power	0.1637	X_3-Microwave power	0.0281 **
$X_1 \times X_2$	0.2324	$X_1 \times X_2$	0.7070
$X_1 \times X_3$	0.0047 *	$X_1 \times X_3$	0.9099
$X_2 \times X_3$	0.2107	$X_2 \times X_3$	0.4765
X_1^2	0.0145 **	X_1^2	0.4200
X_2^2	0.6597	X_2^2	0.0485 **
X_3^2	0.1588	X_3^2	0.7988
Lack of fit	0.4961	**Lack of fit**	0.0590 ***
	IC_{50} value		
	***p*-value**		***p*-value**
Model	0.0006 *	**Model**	0.0432 **
X_1-Temperature	0.1235	X_1-Extraction time	0.0605 ***
X_2-Extraction time	0.2852	X_2-Ethanol concentration	0.0091 *
X_3-Ultrasonic power	0.0512 ***	X_3-Microwave power	0.4196
$X_1 \times X_2$	0.2903	$X_1 \times X_2$	0.0367 **
$X_1 \times X_3$	0.0029 *	$X_1 \times X_3$	0.1003
$X_2 \times X_3$	0.0054 *	$X_2 \times X_3$	0.1696
X_1^2	<0.0001 *	X_1^2	0.3658
X_2^2	0.1935	X_2^2	0.5369
X_3^2	0.0421 **	X_3^2	0.1437
Lack of fit	0.2875	**Lack of fit**	0.3580

Table 3. *Cont.*

Ultrasound Assisted Extraction		Microwave Assisted Extraction	
	EC$_{50}$ value		
	***p*-value**		***p*-value**
Model	0.0458 **	**Model**	0.0460 **
X_1-Temperature	0.0037 *	X_1-Extraction time	0.6595
X_2-Extraction time	0.1828	X_2-Ethanol concentration	0.0010 *
X_3-Ultrasonic power	0.0559 ***	X_3-Microwave power	0.2885
$X_1 \times X_2$	0.1967	$X_1 \times X_2$	0.4941
$X_1 \times X_3$	0.8936	$X_1 \times X_3$	0.8581
$X_2 \times X_3$	0.5826	$X_2 \times X_3$	0.4932
X_1^2	0.0792 ***	X_1^2	0.4893
X_2^2	0.7284	X_2^2	0.2220
X_3^2	0.2764	X_3^2	0.9648
Lack of fit	0.1248	**Lack of fit**	0.0708 ***

* highly significant ($p < 0.01$); ** significant ($0.01 < p < 0.05$); *** moderately significant ($0.05 < p < 0.10$); ***p*-value**, or probability value, is a number describing how likely it is that your data would have occurred by random chance; regression model exhibits **lack-of-fit** ($p < 0.01$) when it fails to adequately describe the functional relationship between the experimental factors and the response variable.

The coefficient of multiple regression (R^2) was used as the first indicator of the model adequacy. Descriptive statistics was in accordance with ANOVA, since R^2 was particularly high for Y, TP, TF, IC$_{50}$ and EC$_{50}$ (0.9668, 0.8349, 0.8717, 0.9567, 0.8304, respectively) obtained by UAE. The similar situation was observed with Y, TP, TF, IC$_{50}$ and EC$_{50}$ obtained by MAE, where the observed R^2 were 0.9141, 0.9334, 0.8386, 0.8337 and 0.8302, respectively. The relatively low (<12%) coefficient of variance for all responses suggested good reproducibility of the investigated systems. Good adequacy of the polynomial models for UAE indicated by descriptive statistics was confirmed by highly significant *p*-values (<0.001) for extraction yield and IC$_{50}$, while it was approved by significant *p*-values (<0.05) for TP, TF and EC$_{50}$ (Table 3). Good adequacy of the polynomial models for MAE indicated by descriptive statistics was also confirmed by highly significant *p*-values (<0.01) for extraction yield and TP, while it was approved by significant *p*-values (<0.05) for TF, IC$_{50}$ and EC$_{50}$ (Table 3). Moreover, proper model fitness has also been confirmed by insignificant lack of fit ($p > 0.05$) for all of the applied models. Method of least squares was used for calculation of regression coefficients in Equation (13), which provided descriptive model equations (Equations (1)–(10)), obtained by UAE and MAE:

$$Y = 16.15 + 2.32X_1 + 0.78X_2 + 0.62X_3 \quad (1)$$

$$TP = 0.083 + 7.97 \cdot 10^{-3}\, X_1 + 4.14 \cdot 10^{-3}\, X_1^2 \quad (2)$$

$$TF = 0.051 - 1.40 \cdot 10^{-3}\, X_2 + 2.40 \cdot 10^{-3}\, X_1X_3 - 1.86 \cdot 10^{-3}\, X_1^2 \quad (3)$$

$$IC_{50} = 0.017 + 5.84 \cdot 10^{-4}\, X_3 + 1.58 \cdot 10^{-3}\, X_1X_3 - 1.40 \cdot 10^{-3}\, X_1X_3 + 3.33 \cdot 10^{-3}\, X_1^2 + 8.51 \cdot 10^{-4}\, X_3^2 \quad (4)$$

$$EC50 = 0.058 + 4.64 \cdot 10^{-3}\, X_1 + 2.49 \cdot 10^{-3}\, X_3 - 3.07 \cdot 10^{-3}\, X_1^2 \quad (5)$$

$$Y = 18.62 - 3.1X_2 + 1.04X_3 \quad (6)$$

$$TP = 0.083 + 8.36 \cdot 10^{-3}\, X_2 - 8.87 \cdot 10^{-3}\, X_3 + 5.91 \cdot 10^{-3}\, X_1^2 + 5.87 \cdot 10^{-3}\, X_2^2 + 6.72 \cdot 10^{-3}\, X_3^2 \quad (7)$$

$$TF = 0.054 + 4.71 \cdot 10^{-3}\, X_2 - 2.82 \cdot 10^{-3}\, X_3 + 3.36 \cdot 10^{-3}\, X_2^2 \quad (8)$$

$$IC_{50} = 0.019 + 1.77 \cdot 10^{-3}\, X_1 + 2.83 \cdot 10^{-3}\, X_2 + 2.89 \cdot 10^{-3}\, X_1X_2 \quad (9)$$

$$EC50 = 0.067 - 0.011X_2 \quad (10)$$

where, X_1, X_2 and X_3 are temperature, extraction time and ultrasonic power in the case of UAE (Equations (1)–(5)), while they represent extraction time, ethanol concentration and microwave power in the case of MAE (Equations (6)–(10)). Predictive model equations (Equations (1)–(10)) interpreted reduced Equation (13), since the coefficients of variables with inferior influence could be neglected.

2.6. *Process Parameters Influencing UAE and MAE*

In UAE, the linear temperature term ($p < 0.0001$) is dominant over other parameters in the context of the influence on the extraction yield. According to the degree of influence, the second most dominant is a linear term of the extraction time, which showed a very significant ($p < 0.01$) influence on the extraction yield (Figure 1). In MAE, only the linear term of the ethanol concentration ($p < 0.001$) showed a markedly significant effect on the extraction yield (Figure 1). According to the ANOVA results from Table 3, it can be observed that in the UAE, the linear temperature term ($p < 0.01$) shows a significant effect, while the square temperature term ($p < 0.1$) shows a moderately significant effect on TP.

In the case of MAE, the most influential parameters were the linear terms of ethanol concentration and microwave power ($p < 0.001$), while their quadratic terms had a significant effect ($0.01 < p < 0.05$) on TP. In the case of UAE, the linear term of the extraction time ($p < 0.1$) showed a moderately significant effect on TF, while the linear member of the interaction between temperature and ultrasound power showed a markedly significant effect ($p < 0.005$). In MAE, both the linear and square terms of ethanol concentration ($p < 0.1$) showed a moderately significant effect on the TF.

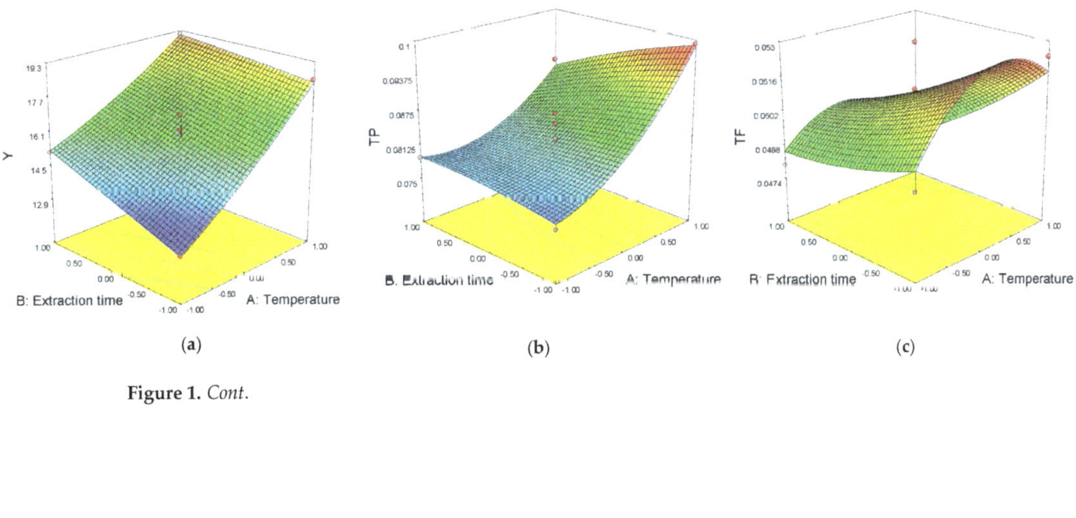

(a) (b) (c)

Figure 1. *Cont.*

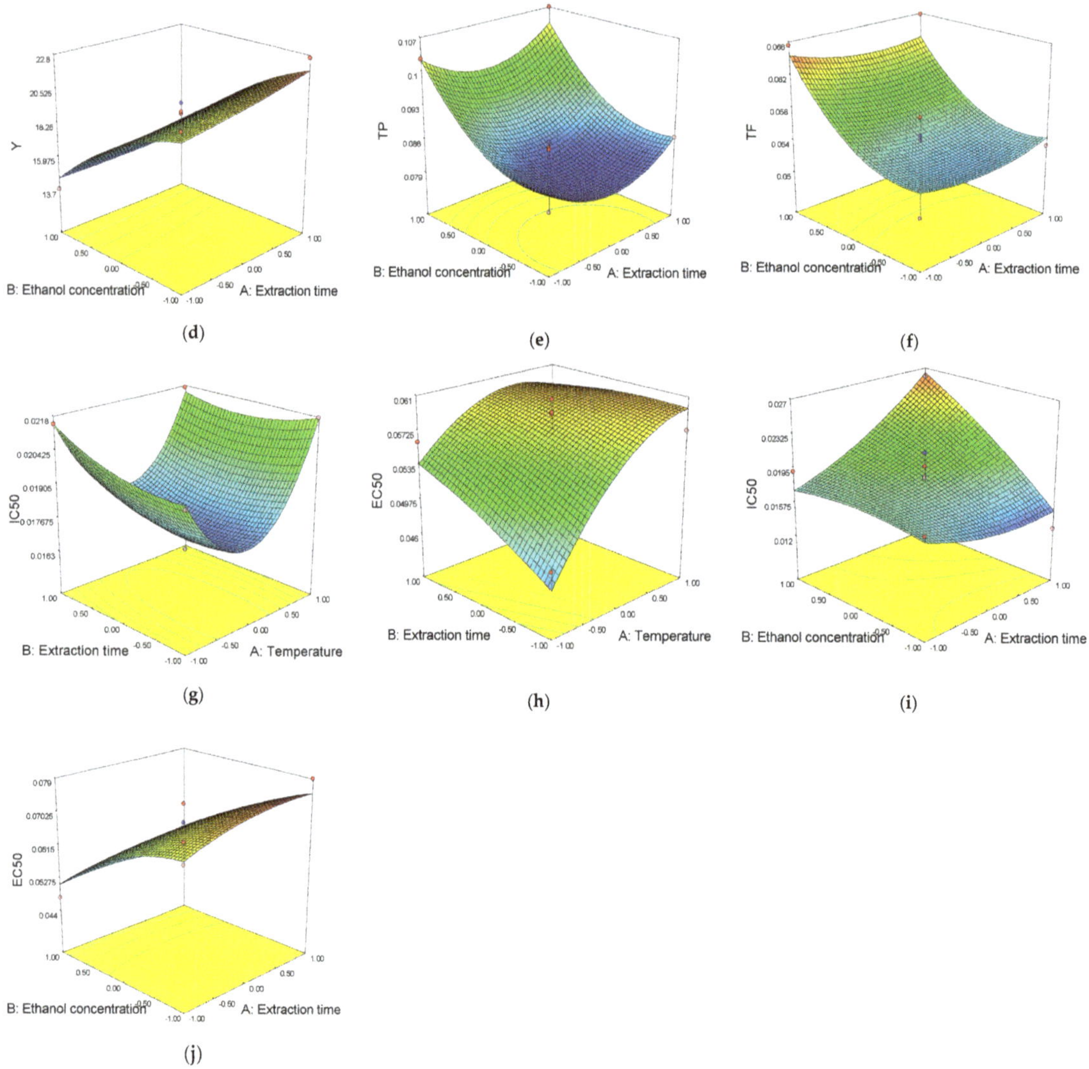

Figure 1. Response surface plots showing combined effects of temperature and extraction time on Y, TP, TF, IC_{50} and EC_{50} in UAE extracts (**a–c**,**g**,**h**) and combined effects of extraction time and ethanol concentration on Y, TP, TF, IC_{50} and EC_{50} in MAE extracts (**d–f**,**i**,**j**).

2.7. Phenolic Acids

In the extracts obtained by maceration, the prevalent flavonoid compounds are the glycosides quercetin, rutin and hyperoside. The content of rutin alters in range 20.41–236.93 μg/mL, while hyperoside varies in range 2.71–25.58 μg/mL. The most dominant compound in all macerates is rutin. The relatively low content of ferulic acid (8.39 μg/mL), rutin (30.63 μg/mL) and hyperoside (5.78 μg/mL) in MAC-W extract can be explained by the use of water as a solvent, which has low selectivity. The MAC showed the highest content of ferulic and *p*-coumaric acid, as well as rutin and hyperoside, compared to other macerates (Table 4).

Table 4. HPLC-DAD analyses of ethanol, water, UAEopt and MAEopt horehound extracts.

Sample	Content (µg/mL)						
	Ferulic Acid	*p*-Coumaric Acid	Caffeic Acid	Rutin	Hyperoside	Chlorogenic Acid	Quercetin
96% EtOH	5.05	6.67	6.43	20.41	2.71	n.d.	n.d.
70% EtOH	21.38	23.89	13.86	190.43	13.05	n.d.	n.d.
50% EtOH (MAC)	35.86	30.60	18.10	236.93	25.58	n.d.	n.d.
30% EtOH	25.02	29.49	35.26	87.51	11.39	n.d.	n.d.
MAC-W	8.39	tr	tr	30.63	5.78	n.d.	n.d.
UAEopt	1.34	4.75	0.26	49.59	19.06	33.11	34.88
MAEopt	1.07	4.26	tr	34.01	14.71	23.23	30.05

Abbrevation: tr, traces; n.d., not detected.

Chlorogenic acid and quercetin were not detected in any of the tested macerates. The eight phenolic acids and five flavonoids were identified in the ethyl acetate fraction of horehound [19]. Among the flavonoid aglycones present in the ethyl acetate fraction, apigenin, luteolin, kaempferol, quercetin and hyperoside were the most dominant. The detected phenolic acids were caffeic, ferulic and *p*-coumaric acid. The contents of caffeic (0.12 mg/g), ferulic (0.52 mg/g) and *p*-coumaric (0.06 mg/g) acids are significantly lower than their contents in MAC (caffeic acid (1.10 mg/g), ferulic acid (2.17 mg/g) and *p*-coumaric acid (1.85 mg/g)). According to the HPLC results (Table 4), UAEopt proved to be richer in phenolic acids compared to MAEopt, with a higher content of chlorogenic acid as well as the flavonoid rutin.

If the chemical profiles of UAEopt, MAEopt and MAC are compared, it can be concluded that UAEopt and MAEopt contain significantly fewer cinnamic acid derivatives and are richer in chlorogenic acid (UAEopt: 33.11 µg/mL and MAEopt: 23.23 µg/mL) and quercetin (UAEopt: 34.88 µg/mL and MAEopt: 30.05 µg/mL), which were not identified in the macerates. The content of rutin in UAEopt (49.59 µg/mL) and MAEopt (34.01 µg/mL) is significantly lower compared to that in MAC (236.93 µg/mL), most likely due to the hydrolysis of rutin to its aglycone quercetin, using these extraction techniques. In that context, some researchers examined the stability of 40 phenolic compounds in the ultrasonic extract obtained at temperature of 70 °C and concluded that rutin degradation (22.3%) and *p*-coumaric acid degradation (10.2%) occurred [20]. The least degradation is present in hyperoside whose contents in UAEopt (19.06 µg/mL) and MAEopt (14.71 µg/mL) extracts are similar to each other and slightly lower than MAC.

Others examined the degradation of seven phenolic acids under the influence of ultrasound in various commonly used extractants. Ferulic and *p*-coumaric acids have been shown to be stable in all extractants, while caffeic has undergone degradation, and the degree of degradation varies depending on the extractant used. The concentration of caffeic acid in ethanol extract after the UAE was reduced by 8.9%, while in the aqueous extract, the concentration was reduced by only 1%. From these results, it become apparent that the stability of phenolic acids in the UAE is also affected by the type of extractant used [21]. In this study, the chlorogenic acid content in UAEopt (1.84 µg/mg) and MAEopt (1.43 µg/mg) extracts is lower than its content in the aqueous extract [3]. Although the UAE is often used to extract phenolic acids due to higher extraction yields and shorter extraction time, the cavitation effect may be responsible for the degradation of flavonoids and carotenoids. A slight degradation of rutin has been observed in the UAE, although this compound possesses a sugar moiety that can potentially protect the molecule from degradation. Rutin degradation using UAE has also been previously described, and this phenomenon has been explained by the reaction of rutin with highly reactive hydroxyl radicals formed during UAE in a water-containing solvent, while glycosides were stable under the given conditions [22].

In MAE, the influences of a different microwave power (160–500 W) and an extraction time (1–10 min) on flavonoid degradation were examined. The increase in microwave power and time caused greater degradation of these compounds. The least degradation was observed for rutin and naringin, while significant degradation was observed for myricetin, kaempferol, ramnetin and quercetin. In this study, the extraction time of 15 min and the microwave power of 422 W caused an intensification of the extraction process due to higher pressure and temperature. Elevated temperature simultaneously results in improved extraction efficiency and a degradation of thermolabile compounds, which is indicated by a weaker profile of phenolic compounds compared to UAEopt. The stability of 22 phenolic compounds was investigated during the MAE with methanol as a solvent in the temperature range 50–175 °C and it was concluded that caffeic, *p*-coumaric and ferulic acids are stable at temperatures up to 100 °C, while at 125 °C they are subject to significant degradation. Of the cinnamic acid derivatives the most stable compound of the tested is ferulic acid, which is subject to degradation of 10.9% at 150 °C, while caffeic acid suffered a degradation of 16.3% at the same temperature. The most stable compound with the least number of substituents was found to be *p*-coumaric acid, which did not undergo degradation at 175 °C [23]. Also, in this work, *p*-coumaric acid underwent a lower degree of degradation compared to ferulic and caffeic acids.

2.8. Process Optimization

In this research, in the case of UAE, the optimal process parameters for investigated responses (Y, TP, TF, IC_{50} and EC_{50}) were temperature of 73.6 °C, extraction time of 40 min and ultrasound power of 30.3 W/L. Whilst in the case of MAE, the optimal process parameters for all five responses were ethanol concentration of 63.8%, extraction time of 15 min and microwave power of 422 W. It could be observed from Table 5 that MAE ensures slightly higher yields of polyphenols, while antioxidant activities, expressed by two in vitro assays, of both UAEopt and MAEopt, are rather similar.

In order to confirm the predictive mathematical models, validation was performed by separate extractions at optimal parameters for UAE and MAE. According to the results, it could be concluded that the experimentally obtained values were in line with the predicted results.

Table 5. Estimated optimal UAE and MAE parameters.

Extraction Method	Optimized Conditions	Predicted Responses	Observed Responses
UAE	Temperature: 73.6 °C Extraction time: 40 min Ultrasonic power: 30.3 W/L	Y = 16.93% TP = 91.48 mg GAE/g TF = 50.07 mg CE/g IC_{50} = 0.0181 mg/mL EC_{50} = 0.0564 mg/mL	Y = 16.90% TP = 109.62 mg GAE/g TF = 53.36 mg CE/g IC_{50} = 0.0189 mg/mL EC_{50} = 0.0623 mg/mL
MAE	Ethanol concentration: 63.8% Extraction time: 15 min Microwave power: 422 W	Y = 15.76% TP = 110.04 mg GAE/g TF = 62.45 mg CE/g IC_{50} = 0.0191 mg/mL EC_{50} = 0.0545 mg/mL	Y = 16.66% TP = 110.26 mg GAE/g TF = 54.86 mg CE/g IC_{50} = 0.0180 mg/mL EC_{50} = 0.0555 mg/mL

2.9. Antihyperglycaemic Activity

In this study, in vitro inhibitory potential of horehound ethanolic extracts (UAEopt, MAEopt and MAC) for the enzymes α-amylase and α-glucosidase was investigated. The inhibitory potential of horehound extracts for α-amylase has the following order: UAEopt > MAEopt > MAC (Figure 2). According to the results, UAEopt and MAEopt extracts show similar inhibitory activity against α-amylase (50.63 ± 0.05% and 48.58 ± 0.04%), which is significantly higher compared to MAC (21.38 ± 0.05%). Total α-amylase inhibition expressed via acarbose equivalent for UAEopt, MAEopt, and MAC is 81.37; 75.69 and 0.33 μg/mL, respectively. It can be concluded that UAEopt inhibits α-amylase the same order of magnitude as acarbose (80 μg/mL).

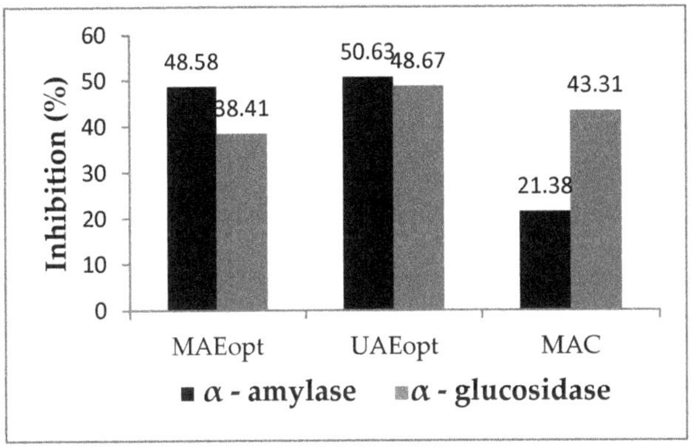

Figure 2. Inhibitory potential of horehound extracts for α-amylase and α-glucosidase.

The investigated UAEopt, MAEopt and MAC differ significantly in their chemical compositions, with UAEopt and MAEopt being richer in chlorogenic acid and quercetin. It was also shown that chlorogenic acid possesses antihyperglycemic potential in rats with induced diabetes [24]. Chlorogenic acid is known to lower blood glucose and inhibit glucose-6-phosphatase, a key enzyme that catalyzes the final step of glycogenolysis and gluconeogenesis, the two major metabolic pathways responsible for the release of glucose from the liver [25]. Previous experimental data show that chlorogenic acid stimulates glucose uptake into liver cells and regulates excessive glucose production by inhibiting this enzyme, thus controlling glycemic status in type 2 diabetes. Quercetin is also recognized as a flavonol that improves glycemic control and reduces diabetic nephropathy [26]. This aglycone of rutin reduces blood glucose concentrations and increases insulin release in rats with induced diabetes [27].

The inhibitory potential for α-glucosidase is weaker compared to α-amylase and has the following order: UAEopt > MAC > MAEopt (Figure 2). As in the case of α-amylase, UAEopt shows the highest antihyperglycemic activity (48.67 ± 0.04%), which can potentially be explained by the presence of chlorogenic acid (33.11 μg/mL) and quercetin (34.88 μg/mL). The total inhibition of α-glucosidase expressed via acarbose equivalent for UAEopt, MAEopt and MAC is 26.10; 18.60 and 22.18 μg/mL, respectively. It can be concluded that UAEopt inhibits α-glucosidase by the same order of magnitude as acarbose (27 μg/mL).

2.10. Antimicrobial Activity

The problem of microbial resistance continues to rise, despite the fact that there is a wide palette of antibiotics on the market, due to the uncontrolled use of these drugs against many infectious diseases [28]. Horehound essential oil is already recognized as a potential antimicrobial agent, but other extracts are still not identified. In order to gain an insight into the antimicrobial activity of horehound ethanolic extracts, minimum inhibitory concentration (MIC) values were determined for eleven pathogens. The differences in MIC values obtained for Gram-positive (Gr^+) and Gram-negative (Gr^-) bacterial strains are shown in Table 6.

Table 6. Antimicrobial activity (MIC and MBC values) of horehound extracts.

Strain	MIC Value (mg/mL)			MBC Value (mg/mL)		
	MAEopt	MAC	UAEopt	MAEopt	MAC	UAEopt
Escherichia coli ATCC 11775	25.00	25.00	25.00	25.00	50.00	25.00
Klebsiella pneumoniae ATCC 31488	25.00	25.00	12.50	25.00	25.00	25.00
Proteus mirabilis ATCC 12453	12.50	25.00	25.00	25.00	50.00	25.00
Pseudomonas aeruginosa ATCC 9027	25.00	25.00	25.00	25.00	50.00	50.00
Staphylococcus aureus ATCC 25923	12.50	12.50	12.50	25.00	25.00	25.00
Staphylococcus epidermidis JR-07	6.25	12.50	12.50	25.00	50.00	25.00
Micrococcus luteus JR-10	12.50	12.50	12.50	50.00	50.00	50.00
Bacillus cereus ATCC 11778	3.13	6.25	3.13	6.25	6.25	6.25
Bacillus subtilis PY79	12.50	12.50	12.50	>50.00	>50.00	>50.00
Candida albicans ATCC 10231	12.50	6.25	12.50	25.00	25.00	25.00
Saccharomyces cerevisiae ATCC 9763	≤0.05	0.20	≤0.05	≤0.05	1.56	≤0.05

It was shown that Gr^+ bacteria are more sensitive to the action of all three extracts compared to Gr^- bacteria because MIC values for Gr^+ vary in the range 3.13–12.50 mg/mL, and for Gr^- in the range 12.50–25.00 mg/mL. The different susceptibilities of Gr^+ and Gr^- bacteria are a consequence of the different structure of the cell wall. Gr^- bacteria are surrounded by a thin layer of peptidoglycan encircled by an outer membrane made up of lipopolysaccharides, while Gr^+ bacteria lack an outer membrane. Thus, the outer membrane represents a barrier that limits the diffusion of active ingredients [29]. The most sensitive bacterial strain to UAEopt and MAEopt extracts is *Bacillus cereus*, which is confirmed by the MIC value (3.13 mg/mL) which is twice lower than the one for MAC.

In the case of antifungal activity, the essential oil of horehound was tested on four strains of fungi, while horehound methanol extract was tested on *Candida albicans* [30]. Horehound methanol extract showed moderate to significant antibacterial activity in five out of the six bacterial organisms tested compared to standard ciprofloxacin. The study showed that the horehound methanol extract is very effective against *B. subtilis*, *S. epidermidis*, *S. aureus* (Gr^+) and *C. albicans*, and moderately effective against *P. vulgaris* and *E. coli*, while in the case of *P. aeruginosa* (Gr^-), it is inefficient. The lowest MIC value of 100 mg/mL was achieved in most of the tested bacteria (*B. subtilis*, *S. aureus* and *S. epidermidis*) and in the fungus *Candida albicans*, while the highest MIC of 400 mg/mL was achieved in *E. coli* and *P. vulgaris*, which showed moderate sensitivity [31]. In this study, the MIC values (12.50 mg/mL) of UAEopt and MAEopt for strains of *B. subtilis*, *S. aureus* and *S. epidermidis* are about 8-fold lower than the MIC values of methanol extract of horehound, indicating that UAEopt and MAEopt are significantly more potent for these strains.

One of the selected strains for testing the antimicrobial activity of UAEopt and MAEopt is *S. aureus*. The results showed that this strain was equally sensitive to UAEopt, MAEopt and MAC (MIC = 12.5 mg/mL). In the case of yeasts, *Saccharomyces* is multiple times more sensitive (MIC $\leq$ 0.05 mg/mL) to the action of UAEopt and MAEopt compared to *Candida albicans*, while inhibition of *S. cerevisiae* growth requires about 4-fold higher MAC concentration (MIC = 0.20 mg/mL). The *Saccharomyces* is considered an important industrial microorganism widely used in the production of food and alcoholic beverages, as well as being a source of yeast-derived β-glucans. Despite its numerous beneficial applications, *S. cerevisiae* can also act as a human opportunistic pathogen causing a variety of infections, especially in immunocompromised individuals [32]. The minimum bactericidal concentration (MBC) values were also determined for eleven pathogens (Table 6). In the case of MAC, the MBC value is at least twice as high as the MIC for a given bacterial or fungal strain. In the case of UAEopt, MIC and MBC have the same values for the following Gr^- strains: *E. coli* (25 mg/mL), *Proteus mirabilis* (25 mg/mL) and for the yeast *Saccharomyces* (≤0.05 mg/mL). In the case of MAEopt, MIC and MBC have the same values for the following Gr− strains: *E. coli* (25 mg/mL), *Klebsiella pneumoniae* (25 mg/mL), *Pseudomonas aeruginosa* (25 mg/mL) and for the yeast *Saccharomyces* (≤0.05 mg/mL).

3. Materials and Methods

3.1. Plant Material

M. vulgare was bought from the local supplier of cultivated plants "Chamomilla" (Banatski Karlovac, Serbia). The aerial parts of *M. vulgare* were air-dried in thin layers, collected in the paper bags, and stored at a room temperature. Afterwards, the dried *M. vulgare* herba was grounded in a domestic blender and the mean particle size (0.28 mm) of herbal material was determined using vibration sieve sets (CISA, Cedaceria, Spain).

3.2. Chemicals

Reagents used in the methods, 1,1-Diphenyl-2-picryl-hydrazyl-hydrate (DPPH), Folin-Ciocalteu and (±)-Catechin were purchased from Sigma (Sigma-Aldrich Chemie GmbH, Sternheim, Germany). The following reagents were also purchased from Sigma-Aldrich Chemie: iron (III)-chloride, potassium hexacyanoferrate (III), sodium hydrogen phosphate anhydrous, sodium dihydrogen phosphate and trichloroacetic acid. Gallic acid was purchased from Sigma (St. Luis, MO, USA). α-Amylase from porcine pancreas, α-glucosidase from *Saccharomyces cerevisiae*, 4-Nitrophenyl α-D-glucopyranoside and acarbose were obtained from Sigma (St Louis, MO, USA). All other chemicals and reagents were of analytical grade.

3.3. Conventional Solid/Liquid Extraction

Conventional solid/liquid (S/L) extraction was performed in order to determine experimental domain for the ethanol concentration used in the optimization scheme and to compare the yields of polyphenols obtained by conventional and green extraction techniques. The S/L ratio was 1:10. Distilled water and different concentrations of ethanol (30, 50 and 70%) were used. Extractions were performed in a shaker with temperature control (KS 4000i, IKA, Staufen, Germany) at 25 °C for 24 h with 150 rpm shaking speed. After extraction, the obtained extracts were filtrated through filter paper. The extracts were collected into glass vials and stored at 4 °C prior to analysis.

3.4. Ultrasound-Assisted Extraction (UAE)

In all UAE experimental runs, 10 g of sample was mixed with 100 mL of 50% ethanol in 250 mL glass flasks. Selection of optimal ethanol concentration (50%) was based on the highest polyphenol yield obtained by conventional extraction performed with a wider range of ethanol concentrations (30, 50, 70 and 96%). UAE was performed in a sonication water bath (EUP540A, Euin-struments, France). Temperature (40, 60 and 80 °C), extraction time (40, 60 and 80 min) and ultrasonic power (24, 42 and 60 W/L) were independent variables which were set by the control panel of the instrument. In order to prevent evaporation of the extraction solvent, condenser was added on the flask during extraction. Flasks were always positioned at the same distance from the transducer in the ultrasonic bath in order to provide constant ultrasonic power. After extraction, extracts were filtered through filter paper, collected into glass vials, sealed and stored at 4 °C prior to analysis.

3.5. Microwave-Assisted Extraction (MAE)

Mono-mode MAE was performed in a homemade setup consisting of a microwave oven (NN-E201W, Panasonic, Osaka, Japan) and appropriate glass apparatus with round flask attached to a condenser. In all MAE experimental runs, 10 g of horehound was mixed with 100 mL of extraction solvent in 250 mL round glass flasks. The flask was then placed in the microwave oven and extraction was performed. Flasks were always positioned at the same distance from the magnetron. Ethanol concentration (30, 50 and 70%), extraction time (15, 25 and 35 min) and irradiation power (400, 600 and 800 W) were independent variables. After the extraction, crude extracts were filtered through filter paper under vacuum, collected into glass vials, sealed and stored at 4 °C prior to analysis.

3.6. Analysis of Bioactive Compounds

3.6.1. Total Phenols Content

The content of total phenolic compounds (TP) in horehound extracts was determined by the Folin–Ciocalteu procedure [33]. The absorbance was measured at 750 nm. TP was expressed as mg of gallic acid equivalent per g of dry weight of extract (mg GAE/g). All experiments were performed in triplicate.

3.6.2. Total Flavonoids Content

The total flavonoids content (TF) was determined using aluminum chloride colorimetric assay [34], using catechin as a standard compound. The absorbance was measured at 510 nm. The content of total flavonoids was expressed as mg of catechin equivalent per g of dry weight of extract (mg CE/g). All experiments were performed in triplicate.

3.6.3. DPPH Assay

The free radical scavenging activity of horehound extracts was determined using a simple and fast spectrophotometric method previously described elsewhere [35]. The absorbance was measured at 517 nm. Radical scavenging capacity (RSC (%)) was calculated according to Equation (11). Antioxidant activity was expressed as IC_{50} value, which represents the concentration of extract solution required for obtaining 50% of radical scavenging capacity.

$$\%RSC = 100 - ((A\_sample \times 100))/A\_control \quad (11)$$

where, A_sample is the absorbance of sample solution and A_control is the absorbance of control. All experiments were performed in three replicates.

3.6.4. FRAP Assay

The reducing power of horehound extracts was determined by a method previously described in the literature [36]. Various concentrations of extracts obtained were mixed with phosphate buffer (2.5 mL, 0.2 M, pH 6.6) and 2.5 mL of 1% potassium ferricyanide ($K_3Fe(CN)_6$). The mixture was incubated for 20 min at 50 °C. After incubation, 2.5 mL of a 10% trichloroacetic acid solution was added to the mixture and the mixture was centrifuged (Tehtnica Železniki, Slovenia) for 10 min at 3000 rpm (0.402× *g*). The obtained supernatant (2.5 mL) was mixed with bidestillated water (2.5 mL) and 0.1% $FeCl_3$ solution (0.5 mL). Absorbance was measured at 700 nm. Antioxidant activity was expressed as EC_{50} value (mg/mL), which represents the concentration of extract solution required for 50% reduction of Fe^{3+} ions in reaction mixture. All experiments were performed in triplicate, and results are expressed as mean values.

3.6.5. HPLC Analyses of Phenolic Acids

The content of phenolic acids in horehound extracts obtained at optimal UAE parameters (UAEopt) and at optimal MAE parameters (MAEopt) was analysed by Agilent 1200 Series HPLC with DAD detector (Agilent Technologies, Palo Alto, CA, USA) equipped with LiChrospher® 100 RP-18 column (250 × 4 mm, 5 μm). The binary mobile phase consisted of 0.17% water solution of formic acid (A) and acetonitrile (B). The injection volume of the sample was 10 μL and flow rate was 0.8 mL/min, while elution was performed with a gradient according to the following scheme: 0–53 min, 0–100% B. The detection wavelength was set at the range of 200–400 nm for phenolic acids. The examined samples were analyzed in three independent replicates. Identification of compounds was performed based on comparison of retention times and absorption spectra of unknown peaks with reference standards.

3.7. Antihyperglycaemic Activity

3.7.1. α-Amylase Inhibitory Potential (α-AIP)

The α-amylase inhibition assay was performed according to the relevant procedure [37] with minor modifications. Acarbose (a generic antidiabetic drug) was used as a positive control that inhibited α-amylase in a dose-dependent manner, providing a value of 80 μg/mL. Briefly, 100 μL of sample, positive control (2 mM acarbose) or negative control (distilled water) was added to 200 μL of α-amylase solution in 0.02 M sodium phosphate buffer (pH 6.9). The tubes were incubated at room temperature for 5 min. Thereafter, 200 μL of 1% starch solution (prepared in the same buffer) was added to each tube and incubated for 6 min. Finally, 100 μL of dinitrosalicylic acid (dye reagent) was added, and the tubes were placed in a water bath at 100 °C and incubated for 5 min. The distilled water (1600 μL) was added to the mixture, and an absorbance was measured at 540 nm (T80 UV-Vis Spectrophotometer, PG Instruments LTD, Leicester, UK) in triplicate. The percentage of inhibition was calculated according to the following equation:

$$\%\text{Inhibition} = (\Delta A\_control - \Delta A\_sample)/\Delta A\_control \times 100 \quad (12)$$

where, ΔA_control and ΔA_sample are differences in absorbance of the control and sample.

3.7.2. α-Glucosidase Inhibitory Potential (α-GIP)

The test for this method was previously described elsewhere [38]. Acarbose (positive control) inhibited α-glucosidase in a dose-dependent manner, providing a value of 27 μg/mL. In the cells of the microtiter plate (12 × 8), 100 μL 2 mmol/L 4-nitrophenyl-α-D-glucopyranoside in 10 mmol/L potassium phosphate buffer (pH 7.0) and 20 μL sample were measured. The reaction was initiated after the addition of 100 μL of enzyme solution. In parallel with the samples, control and blank samples were prepared and analyzed. Sample microtiter plates were incubated for 10 min at 37 °C, after which, the absorbance was measured at 405 nm (T80 UV-Vis Spectrophotometer, PG Instruments LTD, Leicester, UK) in three replicates, and the result was expressed as the mean value. The percentage of α-glucosidase inhibition was calculated according to the previously stated Equation (12).

3.8. Antimicrobial Activity

The nine bacterial strains were used for testing the antimicrobial activity of horehound extracts, of which *Bacillus cereus* ATCC 11778, *Staphylococcus aureus* ATCC 25923, *Bacillus subtilis* PY79, *Staphylococcus epidermidis* JR-07 and *Micrococcus luteus* JR-10 belong to Gr^+ bacteria, while *Escherichia coli* ATCC 11775, *Pseudomonas aeruginosa* ATCC 9027, *Proteus mirabilis* ATCC 12453 and *Klebsiella pneumoniae* ATCC 31488 belong to Gr^- bacteria. Additionally, two yeast strains, *Saccharomyces cerevisiae* ATCC 9763 and *Candida albicans* ATCC 10231, were used for determining antifungal activity. The microdilution method was applied according to the CLSI protocol [39]. Cultures were grown overnight at 37 °C (i.e., 30 °C for *Bacillus* and *Saccharomyces*) on nutrient agar for bacteria and Sabouraud maltose agar for yeasts. The antimicrobial activity of each extract was tested in duplicate for each strain.

3.9. Design of Experiments

To set up experimental conditions suitable to ensure an exhaustive extraction of horehound, a Box–Behnken experimental design (BBD) approach, with three factors at three levels, was adopted. In both UAE and MAE, the design consisted of seventeen randomized runs with five replicates at the central point. The investigated UAE variables were temperature (40, 60 and 80 °C), extraction time (40, 60 and 80 min) and ultrasonic power (24, 42 and 60 W/L), while the investigated MAE parameters were ethanol concentration (30, 50 and 70%), extraction time (15, 25 and 35 min) and microwave power (400, 600 and 800 W). Unfortunately, temperature in MAE was not selected as variable due to the technical limitations of the microwave oven. Each of the coded variables was forced to range from −1 to 1 in order to normalize the parameters so that they would all affect the response more evenly, and the units of the parameters are irrelevant [40]. The natural and coded values of independent UAE and MAE variables used in BBD are presented in Table 7.

Table 7. Experimental domain with natural and coded values of independent variables.

Extraction Method	Independent Variable	Factor Levels		
		−1	0	1
UAE	Temperature (°C)	40	60	80
	Extraction time (min)	40	60	80
	Ultrasonic power (W/L)	24	42	60
MAE	Extraction time (min)	15	25	35
	Ethanol concentration (%)	30	50	70
	Microwave power (W)	400	600	800

The response variables were fitted to the commonly used second-order polynomial model (Equation (13)) [41]:

$$Y = \beta_0 + \sum_{i-1}^{2} \beta iXi + \sum_{i-1}^{2} \beta iiXi^2 + \sum_{i<j=1}^{2} \beta ijXiXj \quad (13)$$

where, Y represents the response variable, X_i and X_j are the independent variables affecting the response, and β_0, β_i, β_{ii}, and β_{ij} are the regression coefficients for mean, linear, quadratic and cross-product terms. Optimal extraction conditions were determined considering total phenols and total flavonoid contents, and the antioxidant capacity was expressed by two in vitro assays (DPPH and FRAP), while selection of optimal conditions was based on desirability function, D (Derringer and Suich, 1980). Design-Expert v.7 Trial (Stat-Ease, Minneapolis, MN, USA) was used for multiple linear regression analysis. The fitness of the polynomial model equation is expressed by the coefficient of determination (R^2) and its statistical significance was confirmed by F-test at a probability (p) of 0.10 or 0.05. In order to verify the obtained empirical models, validation was performed by extracts preparation at optimized conditions. The confidence interval (95%) of the predicted values was compared with the experimentally observed Y, TP, TF, IC_{50} and EC_{50} in the optimized extracts.

4. Conclusions

The UAEopt proved to be slightly more abundant in phenolic acids compared to MAEopt, with a higher content of chlorogenic acid, as well as the flavonoid quercetin. The UAEopt shows the highest inhibitory potential, the order of magnitude of generic antidiabetic drug acarbose, for both α-amylase and α-glucosidase, which can potentially be explained by the presence of chlorogenic acid and quercetin, which were not identified in the macerates. The most sensitive bacterial strain to UAEopt is *B. cereus*. In addition, *Saccharomyces* is multiple times more sensitive to the action of UAEopt compared to *Candida albicans*, while inhibition of *S. cerevisiae* growth requires about four times higher MAC concentration. Thus, UAEopt, obtained at temperature of 73.6 °C, extraction time of 40 min and ultrasound power of 30.3 W/L, is the most superior extract in terms of antihyperglycaemic and antimicrobial activities. The future perspective of this study would be to tranform the liquid UAEopt extract into a more stable powder form and incorporate it as a component in an oral antihyperglycaemic drug. In respect to industrial applications, ultrasound-assisted extraction can be scaled-up in a more straightforward manner compared to microwave-assisted extraction.

Author Contributions: Conceptualization, A.G., S.V., J.V. (Jelena Vladić) and D.R.; methodology, S.V., J.V. (Jelena Vladić) and D.R.; formal analysis, A.G., J.V. (Jelena Vujetić), A.V. and J.Ž.; investigation, A.G., J.V. (Jelena Vujetić), A.V. and J.Ž.; writing—original draft preparation, A.G.; writing—review and editing, S.V., J.V. (Jelena Vladić) and K.Š. All authors have read and agreed to the published version of the manuscript.

Funding: This research was funded by the Program of Ministry of Education, Science and Technological Development of Republic of Serbia; Projects No. 451-03-68/2022-14/200134 and No. 451-03-68/2022-14/200125.

Data Availability Statement: Not applicable.

Conflicts of Interest: The authors declare no conflict of interest.

References

1. Amri, B.; Martino, E.; Vitulo, F.; Corana, F.; Kaâb, L.B.-B.; Rui, M.; Rossi, D.; Mori, M.; Rossi, S.; Collina, S. *Marrubium vulgare* L. Leave Extract: Phytochemical Composition, Antioxidant and Wound Healing Properties. *Molecules* **2017**, *22*, 1851. [CrossRef] [PubMed]
2. Herrera-Arellano, A.; Aguilar-Santamaría, L.; García-Hernández, B.; Nicasio-Torres, P.; Tortoriello, J. Clinical trial of *Cecropia obtusifolia* and *Marrubium vulgare* leaf extracts on blood glucose and serum lipids in type 2 diabetics. *Phytomedicine* **2004**, *11*, 561–566. [CrossRef] [PubMed]
3. Boudjelal, A.; Henchiri, C.; Siracusa, L.; Sari, M.; Ruberto, G. Compositional analysis and in vivo anti-diabetic activity of wild Algerian *Marrubium vulgare* L. infusion. *Fitoterapia* **2012**, *83*, 286–292. [CrossRef] [PubMed]
4. Apostolidis, E.; Kwon, Y.-I.; Shetty, K. Inhibitory potential of herb, fruit, and fungal-enriched cheese against key enzymes linked to type 2 diabetes and hypertension. *Innov. Food Sci. Emerg. Technol.* **2007**, *8*, 46–54. [CrossRef]
5. Hogan, S.; Zhang, L.; Li, J.; Sun, S.; Canning, C.; Zhou, K. Antioxidant rich grape pomace extract suppresses postprandial hyperglycemia in diabetic mice by specifically inhibiting alpha-glucosidase. *Nutr. Metab.* **2010**, *7*, 71. [CrossRef]
6. Marre, M. Before oral agents fail: The case for starting insulin early. *Int. J. Obes.* **2002**, *26*, S25–S30. [CrossRef] [PubMed]
7. McCarty, M.F. AMPK activation as a strategy for reversing the endothelial lipotoxicity underlying the increased vascular risk associated with insulin resistance syndrome. *Med. Hypotheses* **2005**, *64*, 1211–1215. [CrossRef] [PubMed]
8. Ince, A.E.; Şahin, S.; Şümnü, S.G. Extraction of phenolic compounds from melissa using microwave and ultrasound. *Turk. J. Agric. For.* **2013**, *37*, 69–75. [CrossRef]
9. Miloudi, K.; Hamimed, A.; Benmimoun, Y.; Bellebna, Y.; Taibi, A.; Tilmatine, A. Intensification of Essential Oil Extraction of the *Marrubium vulgare* Using Pulsed Electric Field. *J. Essent. Oil Bear. Plants* **2018**, *21*, 811–824. [CrossRef]
10. Tiwari, B.K. Ultrasound: A clean, green extraction technology. *TrAC Trends Anal. Chem.* **2015**, *71*, 100–109. [CrossRef]
11. Ciriminna, R.; Fidalgo, A.; Delisi, R.; Carnaroglio, D.; Grillo, G.; Cravotto, G.; Tamburino, A.; Ilharco, L.M.; Pagliaro, M. High-quality essential oils extracted by an eco-friendly process from different citrus fruits and fruit regions. *ACS Sustain. Chem. Eng.* **2017**, *5*, 5578–5587. [CrossRef]
12. Destandau, E.; Michel, T.; Elfakir, C. *Microwave-Assisted Extraction*; RSC Publishing: Cambridge, UK, 2013.
13. Mittal, V.; Nanda, A. Intensification of marrubiin concentration by optimization of microwave-assisted (low CO_2 yielding) extraction process for *Marrubium vulgare* using central composite design and antioxidant evaluation. *Pharm. Biol.* **2017**, *55*, 1337–1347. [CrossRef]
14. Martino, E.; Della Volpe, S.; Cavalloro, V.; Amri, B.; Kaab, L.B.B.; Marrubini, G.; Rossi, D.; Collina, S. The use of a microwave-assisted solvent extraction coupled with HPLC-UV/PAD to assess the quality of *Marrubium vulgare* L. (white horehound) herbal raw material. *Phytochem. Anal.* **2019**, *30*, 377–384. [CrossRef] [PubMed]
15. Nanda, A. Design Based Ultrasound-Assisted Extraction of *Marrubium vulgare* Linn and Comparative Evaluation of Extracts for Furan Labdane Diterpene (Marrubiin) Concentration and Antihypertensive Potential. *Curr. Bioact. Compd.* **2020**, *16*, 924–936. [CrossRef]
16. Zeković, Z.; Pintać, D.; Majkić, T.; Vidović, S.; Mimica-Dukić, N.; Teslić, N.; Versari, A.; Pavlić, B. Utilization of sage by-products as raw material for antioxidants recovery—Ultrasound versus microwave-assisted extraction. *Ind. Crops Prod.* **2017**, *99*, 49–59. [CrossRef]
17. Tomšik, A.; Pavlić, B.; Vladić, J.; Ramić, M.; Brindza, J.; Vidović, S. Optimization of ultrasound-assisted extraction of bioactive compounds from wild garlic (*Allium ursinum* L.). *Ultrason. Sonochem.* **2016**, *29*, 502–511. [CrossRef]
18. Yousefi, K.; Hamedeyazdan, S.; Torbati, M.; Fathiazad, F. Chromatographic Fingerprint Analysis of Marrubiin in *Marrubium vulgare* L. via HPTLC Technique. *Adv. Pharm. Bull.* **2016**, *6*, 131–136. [CrossRef]
19. Boulila, A.; Sanaa, A.; Ben Salem, I.; Rokbeni, N.; M'Rabet, Y.; Hosni, K.; Fernandez, X. Antioxidant properties and phenolic variation in wild populations of *Marrubium vulgare* L. (Lamiaceae). *Ind. Crops Prod.* **2015**, *76*, 616–622. [CrossRef]
20. Setyaningsih, W.; Saputro, I.E.; Palma, M.; Barroso, C.G. Stability of 40 phenolic compounds during ultrasound-assisted extractions (UAE). In *AIP Conference Proceedings*; AIP Publishing LLC: Melville, NY, USA, 2016.
21. Qiao, L.; Ye, X.; Sun, Y.; Ying, J.; Shen, Y.; Chen, J. Sonochemical effects on free phenolic acids under ultrasound treatment in a model system. *Ultrason. Sonochem.* **2013**, *20*, 1017–1025. [CrossRef]
22. Paniwnyk, L.; Beaufoy, E.; Lorimer, J.; Mason, T. The extraction of rutin from flower buds of *Sophora japonica*. *Ultrason. Sonochem.* **2001**, *8*, 299–301. [CrossRef]
23. Liazid, A.; Palma, M.; Brigui, J.; Barroso, C.G. Investigation on phenolic compounds stability during microwave-assisted extraction. *J. Chromatogr. A* **2007**, *1140*, 29–34. [CrossRef] [PubMed]

24. Karthikesan, K.; Pari, L.; Menon, V.P. Combined treatment of tetrahydrocurcumin and chlorogenic acid exerts potential anti-hyperglycemic effect on streptozotocin-nicotinamide-induced diabetic rats. *Gen. Physiol. Biophys.* **2010**, *29*, 23–30. [CrossRef] [PubMed]
25. Herling, A.W.; Burger, H.-J.; Schwab, D.; Hemmerle, H.; Below, P.; Schubert, G. Pharmacodynamic profile of a novel inhibitor of the hepatic glucose-6-phosphatase system. *Am. J. Physiol. Liver Physiol.* **1998**, *274*, G1087–G1093. [CrossRef]
26. Anjaneyulu, M.; Chopra, K. Quercetin, an anti-oxidant bioflavonoid, attenuates diabetic nephropathy in rats. *Clin. Exp. Pharmacol. Physiol.* **2004**, *31*, 244–248. [CrossRef]
27. Vessal, M.; Hemmati, M.; Vasei, M. Antidiabetic effects of quercetin in streptozocin-induced diabetic rats. *Comp. Biochem. Physiol. Part C Toxicol. Pharmacol.* **2003**, *135*, 357–364. [CrossRef]
28. Karuppiah, P.; Mustaffa, M. Antibacterial and antioxidant activities of Musa sp. leaf extracts against multidrug resistant clinical pathogens causing nosocomial infection. *Asian Pac. J. Trop. Biomed.* **2013**, *3*, 737–742. [CrossRef]
29. Pierozan, M.K.; Pauletti, G.F.; Rota, L.; Dos Santos, A.C.A.; Lerin, L.A.; Di Luccio, M.; Mossi, A.J.; Atti-Serafini, L.; Cansian, R.; Oliveira, J.V. Chemical characterization and antimicrobial activity of essential oils of salvia L. species. *Food Sci. Technol.* **2009**, *29*, 764–770. [CrossRef]
30. Zarai, Z.; Kadri, A.; Ben Chobba, I.; Ben Mansour, R.; Bekir, A.; Mejdoub, H.; Gharsallah, N. The in-vitro evaluation of antibacterial, antifungal and cytotoxic properties of *Marrubium vulgare* L. essential oil grown in Tunisia. *Lipids Health Dis.* **2011**, *10*, 161. [CrossRef]
31. Kanyonga, P.M.; Faouzi, M.A.; Meddah, B.; Mpona, M.; Essassi, E.M.; Cherrah, Y. Assessment of methanolic extract of *Marrubium vulgare* for anti-inflammatory, analgesic and anti-microbiologic activities. *J. Chem. Pharm. Res.* **2011**, *3*, 199–204.
32. Pérez-Cantero, A.; Thomson, P.; Paredes, K.; Guarro, J.; Capilla, J. Antifungal susceptibility of *Saccharomyces cerevisiae* and therapy in a murine model of disseminated infection. *Rev. Iberoam. Micol.* **2019**, *36*, 37–40. [CrossRef]
33. Kähkönen, M.P.; Hopia, A.I.; Vuorela, H.J.; Rauha, J.-P.; Pihlaja, K.; Kujala, T.S.; Heinonen, M. Antioxidant Activity of Plant Extracts Containing Phenolic Compounds. *J. Agric. Food Chem.* **1999**, *47*, 3954–3962. [CrossRef] [PubMed]
34. Markham, K.R. Flavones, flavonols and their glycosides. In *Methods in Plant Biochemistry*; Academic Press: Cambridge, MA, USA, 1989; Volume 1, pp. 197–235.
35. Espín, J.C.; Soler-Rivas, C.; Wichers, H.J. Characterization of the Total Free Radical Scavenger Capacity of Vegetable Oils and Oil Fractions Using 2,2-Diphenyl-1-picrylhydrazyl Radical. *J. Agric. Food Chem.* **2000**, *48*, 648–656. [CrossRef] [PubMed]
36. Oyaizu, M. Studies on products of browning reaction—Antioxidative activities of products of browning reaction prepared from glucosamine. *Jpn. J. Nutr. Diet.* **1986**, *44*, 307–315. [CrossRef]
37. Johnson, M.H.; Lucius, A.; Meyer, T.; de Mejia, E.G. Cultivar Evaluation and Effect of Fermentation on Antioxidant Capacity and in vitro Inhibition of α-Amylase and α-Glucosidase by Highbush Blueberry (*Vaccinium corombosum*). *J. Agric. Food Chem.* **2011**, *59*, 8923–8930. [CrossRef] [PubMed]
38. Chan, H.-H.; Sun, H.-D.; Reddy, M.V.B.; Wu, T.-S. Potent α-glucosidase inhibitors from the roots of *Panax japonicus* C. A. Meyer var. major. *Phytochemistry* **2010**, *71*, 1360–1364. [CrossRef]
39. CLSI. *Standards for Antimicrobial Susceptibility Testing. Seventh Informational Supplement CLSI Document M100-S17*; CLSI: Wayne, PA, USA, 2007.
40. Baş, D.; Boyacı, I.H. Modeling and optimization I: Usability of response surface methodology. *J. Food Eng.* **2007**, *78*, 836–845. [CrossRef]
41. Ferreira, S.L.C.; Bruns, R.E.; Ferreira, H.S.; Matos, G.D.; David, J.M.; Brandão, G.C.; da Silva, E.G.P.; Portugal, L.A.; dos Reis, P.S.; Souza, A.S.; et al. Box-Behnken design: An alternative for the optimization of analytical methods. *Anal. Chim. Acta* **2007**, *597*, 179–186. [CrossRef]

antibiotics

MDPI

Article

Phytogenic Blend Improves Intestinal Health and Reduces Obesity, Diabetes, Cholesterol and Cancers: A Path toward Customised Supplementation

Sung J. Yu [1], Yadav S. Bajagai [1], Friedrich Petranyi [1], Sara de las Heras-Saldana [2], Thi Thu Hao Van [1,3] and Dragana Stanley [1,*]

1 Institute for Future Farming Systems, Central Queensland University, Rockhampton, QLD 4702, Australia
2 Animal Genetics and Breeding Unit, University of New England, Armidale, NSW 2351, Australia
3 School of Science, RMIT University, Bundoora West Campus, Bundoora, VIC 3083, Australia
* Correspondence: d.stanley@cqu.edu.au; Tel.: +61-7-4923-2079

Abstract: Poultry production is among the most challenging industries for pathogen control. High animal density and abundance of faecal material demand strict biosecurity measures and continual vigilance in monitoring animal health parameters. Despite this vigilance, dealing with disease outbreaks is a part of farmers' routines. Phytogenic feed additives comprised of herbs, spices, essential oils, and oleoresins have potent antimicrobial and anti-inflammatory actions. Related studies are gaining substantial interest in human and animal health worldwide. In this study, a commercial blend phytogenic feed additive was supplemented to layers in an industrial free-range production system with 20,000 birds in both control and treatment groups. At the end of the trial, the ileum tissue was sampled for RNAseq transcriptomic analysis to study the host reaction to the supplement. Phytogenic supplement significantly inhibited four cholesterol-related pathways and reduced the Arteriosclerosis disease category towards improved cardiovascular health. The supplemented birds exhibited reduced disease susceptibility for 26 cancer categories with *p*-values in the range from 5.23×10^{-4} to 1.02×10^{-25}. Major metabolic shifts in Lipid metabolism in combination with Carbohydrate metabolism have resulted in a decrease in the Obesity category, altering the ratio of fat and carbohydrate metabolism toward lower fat storage.

Keywords: essential oils; antibiotics; cancer; lipid; cholesterol; phytogenic; RNAseq

1. Introduction

For decades, public awareness of the cross-resistance of pathogens to antibiotics had gradually increased and initiated a ban on in-feed antibiotic growth promoters (AGPs) in the livestock and poultry industry in many countries [1]. Restricting the use of antibiotics has brought an upsurge in the research focusing on alternative antimicrobial supplements and improved management and biosecurity methods to maintain productivity and welfare in the absence of antibiotics. Eliminating AGPs can potentially aggravate the danger of bacterial diseases and intestinal "dysbiosis" in birds [2]. Understanding the importance of the interplay between the host and gut microbiota is essential to achieve optimum gut microbiota balance and overall health [3].

Hosts' constant interaction with the beneficial microbiota in the gut plays a critical role in birds' growth and health [4,5]. There are numerous factors known to modify the intestinal microbiota profile, such as the nutrition [6,7], environmental factors [8,9], and age [10]. Among these, nutrition is a key factor influencing gut microbiota [5]. Plant-based antimicrobials often found in essential oils, also referred to as phytogenic feed additives (PFA), are being actively investigated as potential alternatives to antibiotics and used to improve birds' welfare and mitigate antimicrobial resistance.

Modern molecular techniques, such as RNA sequencing (RNA-seq), are becoming vital for investigating PFA's general mechanism in the hosts' organ health and disease predisposition. The ileum is in direct contact with altered microbiota and the supplemented PFA and is thus suitable tissue to investigate the transcriptomic impact of feed additives on the host gene transcription [11]. This region of the intestine is essential for pathogen infiltration and continually exposed to antigens and immunomodulatory agents from foods and bacteria [12].

Studies investigating transcriptomic effects of the PFA supplementation in birds reported elevated expression of antioxidant genes [13], increased endocytosis and autophagy [14], inhibition of steroid hormones [15], and an increase in fat and carbohydrate metabolism-related pathways [16]. The outcomes of these studies indicated a high level of PFA interference with disease and metabolism-related pathways and interference with the efficiency of numerous medical drugs and supplements [15].

In vitro studies have highlighted that PFAs have numerous benefits, including antifungal, antiviral, antibacterial, antimycotic, antiparasitic, anti-inflammatory, antioxidant, antitumor, and anti-toxigenic properties [17–19]. The antioxidant effects have several health benefits [20] by minimising the toxic effects of reactive oxygen species (ROS) in cells. Strong antioxidant activity was observed in the mixture of thymol and carvacrol [21,22]. This property possessed by some PFAs has greatly increased the levels of superoxide dismutase, glutathione peroxidase, and polyunsaturated fatty acids in the tissue [23], which delayed lipid oxidation, enhanced birds' performance and improved digestive enzymes and immune response [18]. These beneficial properties are related to the course of physiological reactions driven by the enzymes, hormones, and metabolic changes in cells, hence improving the health and performance of birds [24]. PFA-induced improvements included higher quality of the eggs produced, reduced mortality, reduced feed conversion ratio (FCR), and an increase in weight gain [25–28].

Here, we investigated the effects of a commercial PFA blend comprised of a mixture of essential oils from the *Myrtaceae* and *Asteraceae* plant families and saponins supplemented to commercial free-range layer birds. We have recently reported performance and microbiome, including functional metagenomic alterations, in the present study [28]. Birds supplemented with PFA had reduced mortality and lower number of dirty eggs, increased rate of lay, and increased average egg weight [28]. These performance benefits were particularly evident during a natural Spotty Liver Disease outbreak in these sheds. Functional analysis established a considerable functional alteration in the microbial community, with PFA reducing a range of microbial functions, including the production of essential vitamins, cofactors, energy, and amino acids [28]. PFA supplementation induced a phenotypic shift in the intestinal bacterial lipopolysaccharide (LPS) phenotype towards the less pathogenic form [28].

To our knowledge, this is the first ileum gene expression study based on this phytogenic blend in layer birds. A similar ileum transcriptomic study on the effects of different blends of phytogens has reported an increase in the range of beneficial roles such as vasculogenesis, homeostasis, engulfment of tumour cells, the function of muscle, autophagy, obesity, gut health immune system and much more [14]. Industry-based trials have less control over environmental and biosecurity conditions and usually come with a very high number of birds per shed, up to 100,000 birds, which causes issues with sample size. However, they provide insight into various stresses, natural disease outbreaks, and environmental extremes that could never be replicated in fully controlled research facilities.

In this manuscript, we will continue this investigation to examine the effect of prolonged use of this PFA blend on the ileum transcriptome and evaluate possible mechanisms contributing to reduced mortality, reduced diarrhoea and improved egg production we previously reported in these birds [28].

2. Materials and Methods

2.1. Animal Trial and Bird Management

The study was approved by the Animal Ethics Committee of Central Queensland University under approval number 0000022879.

The study was performed on a commercial layer farm in Queensland, Australia. Specialised Breeders Australia P/L (Bendigo, Victoria) provided the Lohman-Brown day-old chicks. The chicks were brooded and reared on grower sheds until they reached 16 weeks of age with ad libitum access to feed and water. After the rearing stage, birds were randomised and transferred separately into the production shed, with 20,000 birds each in the treatment and control group with ad libitum access to water and feed. The birds in the treatment and control group had no physical contact indoors or in the range.

The birds were fed with a standard layer diet as an unsupplemented control (Ctr) on one side of the shed or with PFA supplemented feed (Phy) in the other section. The ratio of the feed ingredients was changed over time to adjust for bird age and production stage, but all the same main ingredients were used throughout the production cycle. The feed was provided in the form of a mash only. The phytogenic product used was the feed additive Biostrong® Protect (Delacon Biotechnik GmbH, Engerwitzdorf, Austria). The PFA was supplemented at the recommended dose rate of 600 mg/kg. PFA blend comprised a mixture of essential oils from the *Myrtaceae* (myrtle family) and *Asteraceae* (daisy family) and saponins. The supplementation lasted from week 16 to week 40 of bird age. The birds were monitored for the next ten weeks until week 50. We aimed to evaluate the efficacy of PFA against Spotty Liver Disease common in this region of Australia during the hottest summer period. The supplementation period started just before the height of the summer in mid-September, and the sampling of the birds was at 30 weeks of age, aiming at the end of the peak of production stage and at the peak of summer heat, collected on 20th of December with the maximum daily temperature of 38 °C on the sampling day. Birds were randomly selected from different parts of the shed, rejecting the outlier birds.

Performance parameters measured regularly included the rate of lay (ROL, measured daily as eggs produced over the number of birds in the shed), cumulative mortality, body weight, feed conversion ratio (feed consumed per dozen of eggs), cumulative hen housed eggs (total number of eggs compared to the number of birds), GBD (grams of feed consumed per bird per day), egg weight, eggshell thickness, cumulative dirty eggs (rejected dirty eggs), yolk colour and Haugh units. Performance, microbiota and metagenomic functional analysis were separately presented in Yu et al., [28].

At 30 weeks of age, ten birds from each treatment were euthanised, and ileum tissue was collected for RNAseq analysis and histology. Ileum tissue for RNAseq was snap frozen in liquid nitrogen and stored at −80 °C, and for histology, it was stored in 10% neutral buffered formalin.

2.2. RNA Sequencing and Analysis

Around 100 mg of tissue samples were homogenised with 1 mL of TRIsure (Cat# BIO-38033, Bioline Meridian Bioscience, London, UK) by OMNI tissue homogeniser TH (OMNI International, Kennesaw, GA, USA) and centrifuged with phase separation by addition of 200 µL of chloroform. The Isolate II RNA Mini Kit (Bioline, CAT# BIO-52072) was used to clean up the RNA from the aqueous phase and isolate the RNA following the manufacturer's instructions. This method was used previously in other similar studies to isolate good quality RNA [29–32]. Extracted RNA was freeze-dried and shipped to the sequencing facility (Azenta Life Sciences, Beijing, China) in RNAstable tubes. TruSeq RNA Library Prep Kit v2 #RS-122-2001 (Illumina, San Diego, CA, USA) was used to prepare the library, which was sequenced with Illumina Novaseq 600 platform with 2 × 150 bp paired-end configuration. Sequence data is available on the NCBI Sequence Read Archive (SRA) database with accession number PRJNA887923.

The alignment of the sequences with the chicken genome and transcriptome analysis was done using CLC Genomic Workbench 21.0.3 (Qiagen, Hilden, Germany). The differential genes were selected using the DESeq2 R package, and further pathway investigation was done using Ingenuity Pathway Analysis (QIAGEN IPA, version 76765844). Genes included in IPA analysis were DESeq2 $p < 0.05$, with an absolute fold change of 1.2.

2.3. Histology

The ileum tissue samples were fixed in 10% neutral buffered formalin and embedded on paraffin wax. The histological sections were obtained by cutting thin tissue sections with a Microtome (Leica RM2135) and stained with Periodic Acid Schiff and Alcian Blue (PASAB) staining. Slides were scanned using Panoptiq™ software (ViewsIQ Inc., Vancouver, BC, Canada) and Nikon Eclipse Ci-L Plus biological microscope, and morphometric analysis was done using QuPath v0.3.0 software. Villus height (μm), crypt depth (μm), and the number of goblet cells were measured from 10 villi in each slide and from five slides per group. Statistical analysis of the measurements was done using GrpahPad Prism v9.

3. Results

3.1. Sequencing Quality and Differential Analysis

Ten samples, 5 for each group, were successfully sequenced with a total of 489.26 million raw sequences, with the largest sample of 58.7 million and the lowest sequenced sample of 41.4 million sequences. The raw sequence QC report is given in Figure S1 of Supplementary File S1. The sequences were all 150 nt long, with no ambiguous sequences and average quality scores ranging from 20 to 38 (Supplementary File S1).

Out of 16,666 mapped and expressed genes, differential analysis done in DESeq2 revealed 202 genes with $p < 0.01$ and 720 with $p < 0.05$. A total of 505 genes were imported into IPA analysis with $p < 0.05$ and absolute fold change > 1.2. Figure 1 shows the most significantly altered genes, while Figure S2 of Supplementary File S1 shows the box plots of the most significantly altered genes.

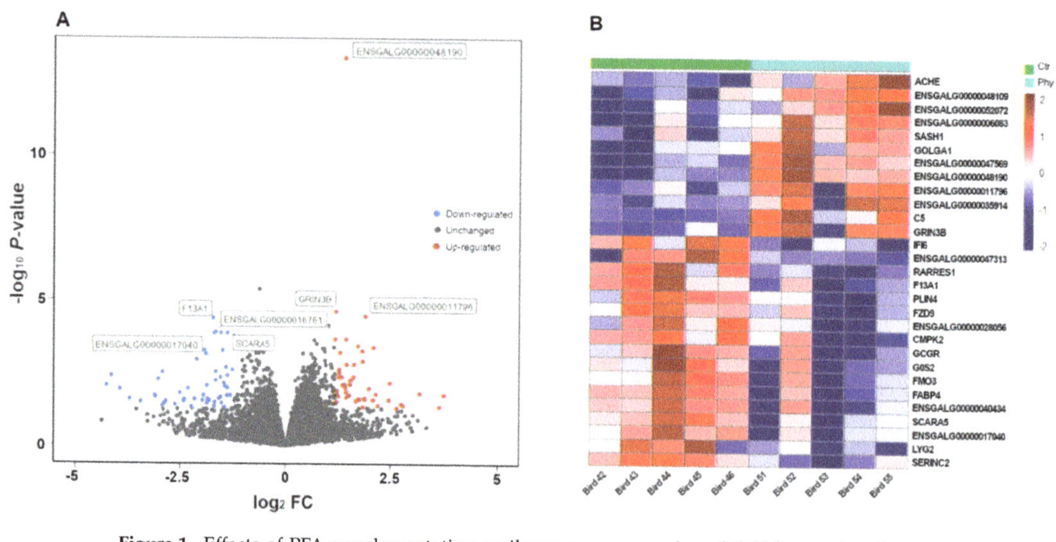

Figure 1. Effects of PFA supplementation on ileum gene expression. (**A**) Volcano plot of genes showing differentially expressed genes, red = upregulated, blue = downregulated, grey = unchanged. (**B**) Heatmap showing the most differentially expressed genes.

3.2. Pathway Analysis

Ingenuity Pathway Analysis (IPA, Qiagen, Germany) is based on more than 10 million manually curated gene expression-based annotations in the Ingenuity Knowledge Base (IKB). This software is widely used to discover networks, interactions, and novel regulators related to the uploaded gene lists. We used the Canonical Pathways function in IPA to identify pathways significantly altered by PFA ($p < 0.01$) and differentiate if the pathway was activated or inhibited due to PFA supplementation using z-score statistics.

PFA significantly inhibited four cholesterol pathways, including the Super-pathway of Cholesterol Biosynthesis, Cholesterol Biosynthesis I, Cholesterol Biosynthesis II (via 24, 25-dihydrolanosterol), and Cholesterol Biosynthesis III (via Desmosterol) (Figure 2). The significance values for the canonical pathways were calculated using the right-tailed Fisher's Exact Test to determine enrichment. The supporting data, including the altered gene list, is given in Table S1 of Supplementary File S1.

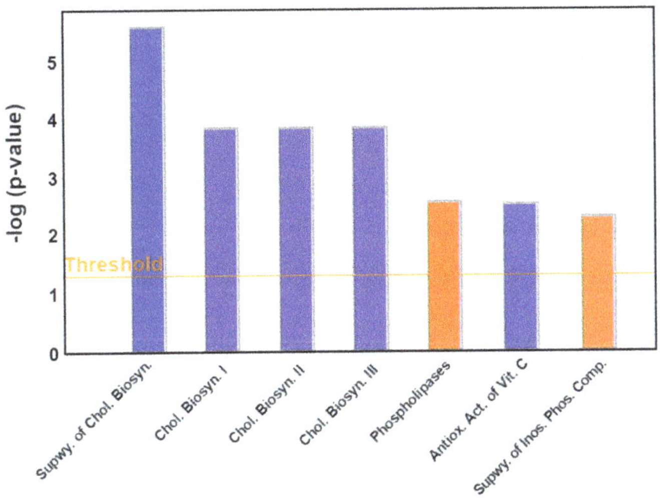

Figure 2. The most affected canonical pathways. The bars are coloured by z score, with blue indicating an inhibition and a negative z score ($z < -2$), and orange colour indicating activation ($z > 2$). The orange line shows $-\log$ (p-value) significance threshold of $p = 0.05$. An extended figure is provided in Supplementary File S1.

3.3. *Upstream Analysis*

The upstream analysis from IPA helps predict gene expression overlaps from the selected dataset with the IPK database. The upstream analysis identifies possible transcriptional regulators explaining investigated gene expression changes. The upstream regulators can be host transcription factors, but also any molecule that, based on the IPK expression database, has identical or reversed effects on a significant number of genes as the PFA treatment. The opposite, or reversed, effects on gene expression result in an inhibited regulator that can undo the effects of the treatment investigated, in this case, PFA. The identical transcriptional effects of the proposed regulator and PFA result in an activated regulator effect, suggesting that the regulator and PFA can enhance each other's action. In addition to host transcription factors, these molecules can be gene regulators from other host species, enzymes, micro-RNA, receptors, chemicals, and drugs, as long as they target a significant number of altered genes in the analysed dataset. This helpful feature allows us to identify possible drug interactions, or if an emerging disease is investigated, this feature could identify a range of existing developed drugs that can undo at least some effects of the disease.

Based on the IPA analysis, 17 regulators were most significantly overlapping with PFA transcriptomic effects ($p < 0.01$) in the same direction and thus highly significantly activated ($z > 2$). They included l-asparaginase, prostaglandin E2 and beta-carotene, drugs nelfinavir, calcitriol, arsenic trioxide, chemical toxicants pyridaben and maneb, cytokine OSM, enzymes POR, FBXW7 and PRKCD, transmembrane receptors IL6R and ITGB4 and other molecules shown in Table S2 of Supplementary File S1. The supplementary file shows all regulators and the genes regulated by both PFA and the regulator. Among the most activated regulators, l-asparaginase, nelfinavir, calcitriol, OSM, PRKCD, KDM5B, arsenic trioxide, beta-carotene, WT1, TEAD4, vorinostat, slirasib, tanespimycin, and sirolimus can treat cancers by their antineoplastic activity, prevention of metastasis, and suppression of tumour cells (IPK database) suggesting that PFA has considerably similar clinically significant anticancer properties.

The IPA analysis reported 24 predicted inhibited gene expression regulators that have the significant opposite effect ($p < 0.01$, $z < -2$) on the gene expression compared to PFA, with the remaining regulators shown in Table S2 of Supplementary File S1. These include exogenous chemicals linoleic acid, elaidic acid and inosine, registered drugs ezetimibe, norephedrine, rosuvastatin, genistein, clozapine, pitavastatin, isoquercitrin, rosiglitazone, transcription factors SIRT2, SIRT1, KLF15, SREBF1, CTNNB1, SREBF2, ESRRA and a transmembrane receptor LGR4. A complete list is given in Table S2 of Supplementary File S1. According to IPA database annotations, among these regulators, there were molecules or transcription factors highly related to lipid metabolism; SREBF2, SREBF1, SCAP, AKT1, INSR and RETN.

Based on the upstream regulator analysis data, prolonged supplementation of the PFA can interfere with a range of medical drugs, either enhancing their effects by amplifying gene expression changes caused by the drug, or in other cases, inhibiting the effects of some drugs by having the opposite effect on the high number of genes altered by this drug (Table 1).

Table 1. IPA upstream analysis identified possible PFA interference with known medical drugs. Drugs shown in the pink background are activated, and those in blue are inhibited by PFA. Descriptions were taken from the IPK database.

Drug	Description (IPK Database)
Vorinostat	Anticancer drug
1-2 Salirasib	Anticancer drug
1-2 Tanespimycin	Anticancer drug
1-2 Arsenic trioxide	Anticancer drug
1-2 Sirolimus	Anticancer drug; Immunosuppressant
1-2 Dimethyl sulfoxide	Anti-inflammatory agent
1-2 Nelfinavir	Antiviral drug
1-2 Calcitriol	Calcium regulator
1-2 Genistein	Angiogenesis inhibitor
1-2 Isoquercitrin	Anti-cachexia drug
1-2 Streptozocin	Anticancer drug
1-2 Methylprednisolone	Anti-inflammatory and immunosuppressive medication.
1-2 Norephedrine	Direct agonist of adrenergic receptors
1-2 17-alpha-ethinylestradiol	Estrogen used widely in birth control pills
1-2 Clozapine	Psychiatric medication, antipsychotic (schizophrenia)
1-2 Rosuvastatin	Statin medication used to prevent cardiovascular disease and treat abnormal lipids
1-2 Rosiglitazone	The antidiabetic drug, works as an insulin sensitiser
1-2 Pitavastatin	For high blood cholesterol
1-2 Clofibrate	For high blood cholesterol
1-2 Cerivastatin	For high blood cholesterol
1-2 Ezetimibe	For high blood cholesterol
1-2 Lovastatin	For high blood cholesterol

3.4. Regulatory Effects

The Regulator Effects analysis in IPA identified five predicted regulatory networks which combine multiple upstream regulators expressed in our dataset to identify the significant influence of their activation/inhibition in our dataset on the regulator-controlled disease and functions. The top-scoring network (Figure 3) shows how activation of POR and inhibition of ESRRA, SIRT1 and SREBF1 results in altered gene expression of 10 target genes, which affects the significant inhibition of synthesis of glucose, triglycerol and cleavage of fatty acids. This was tightly connected with the reduction of Type 2 diabetes signalling and the Adipogenesis pathway, contributing to reduced development and accumulation of adipose tissue (fat) across all body locations, both as subcutaneous fat and as depots.

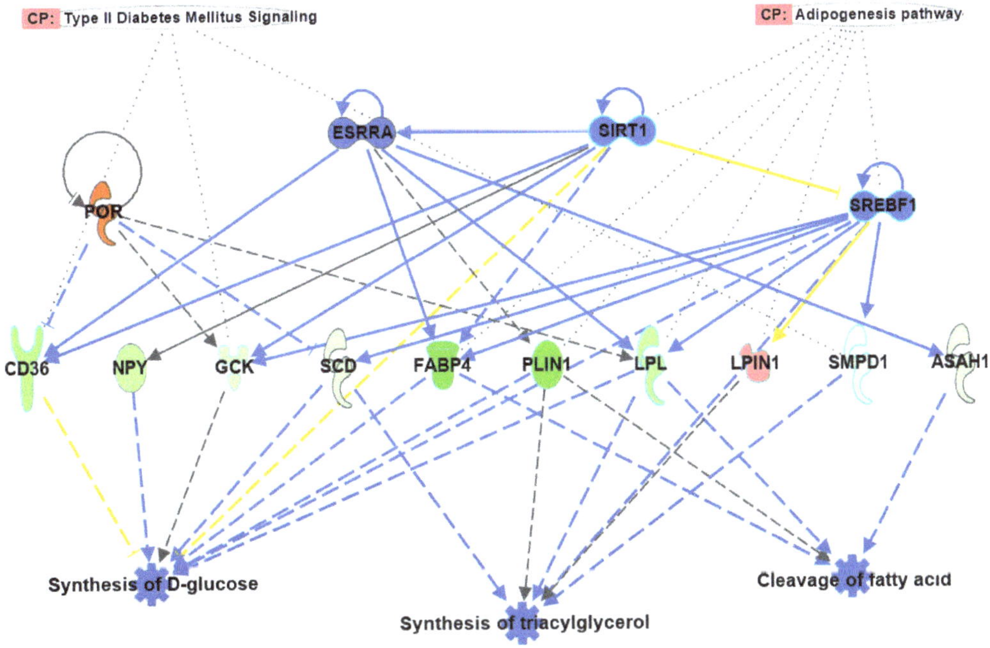

Figure 3. Chicken transcription factors predicted to control reduction in fat deposition and consequent reduction in type 2 diabetes signalling via alterations in glucose and fat metabolism.

3.5. Diseases and Functions

IPA's diseases and functions feature allows us to predict whether the PFA can increase or reduce susceptibility to diseases or alter significant metabolic functions by comparing PFA-altered genes to the IPK database. Complete data is provided in Table S3 of Supplementary File S1 and sorted by function for clarity of interpretation in Table S4 of Supplementary File S1.

The analysis identified clear trends in both PFA inhibited and activated diseases and functions. Inhibited diseases and functions are dominated by major categories Cancer, Carbohydrate metabolism, Cardiovascular disease, Organismal injury and abnormalities, Developmental disorder, Inflammatory response, Lipid metabolism and Nutritional disease. Activated categories were dominated by Amino acid metabolism, Cardiovascular disease, Cell movement and survival, Connective tissue inflammation, Quantity of glucagon, Quantity of blood cells and leucocytes, RNA virus infection and Lipid metabolism.

Categories with both activated and inhibited arms, such as 14 inhibited and five activated categories of Lipid metabolism, in combination would result in a faster turnover of steroids and triglycerols. In addition to this, seven inhibited categories of Carbohydrate metabolism would result in less glucose in the bloodstream; significantly altered and marginally activated Quantity of amino acids ($p = 3.33 \times 10^{-7}$), and a Quantity of glucagon ($p = 0.00065$), which is known to raise the concentration of glucose and fatty acids in the bloodstream all indicate major alterations of metabolism. In combination, all of these metabolic changes are predicted to result in reduced Weight gain and inhibited Obesity, which is among the most significantly inhibited categories, propelled by a faster turnover of glucose and fat and likely more muscle building. Cross-referencing this with the actual bird performance data (Table S3), the weight of the PFA-treated birds was consistently higher than the control from week 25 to the end of supplementation at 40 weeks (Figure 4) which persisted to the end of data monitoring at 50 weeks old Yu et al. [28].

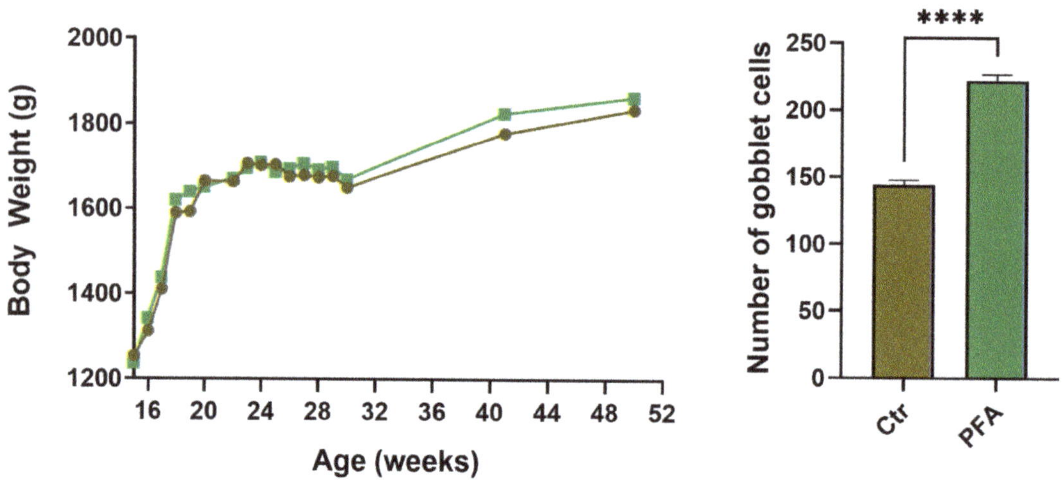

Figure 4. Bird body weight of the birds from the start of PFA supplementation and histological examination showing a significant increase in the number of ileum goblet cells (**** = $p < 0.0001$).

Twenty six cancer categories were significantly inhibited, including multiple types of gastrointestinal and digestive system-related cancers, a range of haematological cancers of different types of leucocytes, and a range of genitourinary cancers, like pelvic and breast cancer. While other categories, like lipid and carbohydrate metabolism, had some arms inhibited and others activated, all affected cancer categories were inhibited by PFA.

Another group of inhibited categories includes the reduction of developmental abnormalities, with the overall Perinatal death category amongst the most significant and most inhibited ($p = 1.96 \times 10^{-7}$, $z = -2.13$). Significantly reduced Inflammatory response ($p = 0.00033$) and Inflammation of the body cavity (ileum) is in agreement with the significantly increased Quantity of goblet cells category ($p = 5.73 \times 10^{-4}$, $z = 1.97$), Tables S4 and S5 of the Supplementary File S1. This is in agreement with our histology data that showed no change in villi and crypt morphology but showed a significant increase ($p < 0.0001$) in the number of goblet cells (Figure 4).

Hypothetically, based on the data from Supplementary Tables S4 and S5 and Figure 5, if we were to translate disease and function prediction findings to possible human use of this product, we would not recommend PFA to those suffering from seizures (increased by PFA, $p = 7.32 \times 10^{-5}$, $z = 2.23$), blood clots and formation of thrombus, those with issues with urination disorder or retroviral infections. We could recommend it to those with gastrointestinal inflammation, gastrointestinal and other cancers, obesity, pregnancy, and those who want to lose fat and gain muscle.

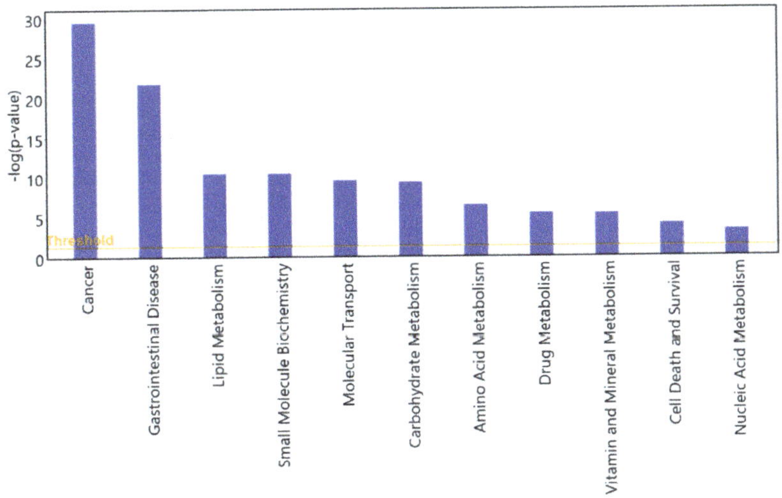

Figure 5. Major Disease and Function categories, most influenced by the supplementation of PFA. The PFA strongly inhibits a range of cancers and gastrointestinal diseases while altering the metabolism that mimics obesity reduction but practically results in heavier animals.

4. Discussion

Based on the upstream analysis, prolonged phytogenic supplementation demonstrated both activation and inhibition of the regulators specifically related to lipid metabolism and tumorigenesis. The synthesis of glucose and lipid biosynthesis are prominent metabolic processes associated with cancer metabolic reprogramming. This metabolic alteration is a prerequisite for the fast proliferation of cancer cells [33]. The Warburg effect, which is the increase in the use of aerobic glycolysis and glucose uptake, is the most significant metabolic alteration in the cancer [34], however, lipid metabolism also plays a vital role in the development of cancer cells. These cells harness lipid metabolism to acquire energy and cellular components for biological membranes, signalling molecules for survival, proliferation, metastasis, and invasion [35]. This may suggest that alterations in lipid and carbohydrate metabolism by PFA also play a role in predicted PFAs cancer-reducing capacity.

Two of the sterol regulatory element-binding transcription factors 1 and 2 (SREBF1 and SREBF2) were highly inhibited ($z = -2.21$ and -2.44) by the phytogenic supplementation. Together with SREBP-cleavage activating proteins (SCAP), they are crucial for maintaining cellular lipid homeostasis [36]; hence their aberrant activation is known to cause fatty liver disease, insulin resistance, obesity, and cancer development [37]. Obesity was also significantly decreased ($p = 4.02 \times 10^{-6}$, $z = -1.13$).

Similarly, nine categories of Lipid metabolisms were decreased in the Disease and Functional analysis. Notably, the metabolism and synthesis of sphingolipid (SL) were decreased. Sphingolipids with sphingosine-1-phosphate (S1P) and ceramide are important biomolecules with extensive effects on vital cellular processes, including programmed cell death, cell growth, and proliferation [38]. The perturbations of SL metabolism will change the responsible enzymatic pathways, which in turn can take part in the progression of various cancer cells such as colon [39] and breast cancer [40]. Nagahashi et al. (2016), through an in vitro experiment, demonstrated that cancer cells in breast cancer contain a higher amount of SL than in normal breast tissue [40]. Other lipid-related inhibited categories include Metabolism and Synthesis of triacylglycerol, Cleavage and Hydrolysis of fatty acids, Hydrolysis and Catabolism of lipid, and Lipolysis, which could have led to perturbation in the lipid metabolism preventing the tumour-adipose microenvironment. This is in agreement with phytogenic supplementation reducing the disease susceptibility for numerous cancer categories, including breast and colorectal cancers.

Various anticancer upstream regulators or drugs were activated (upstream analysis), suggesting that they have similar effects to PFA. The activated drug nelfinavir is the most potent anticancer drug inhibiting 60 cancer cell lines derived from nine different tumour types [41]. In in vivo experiment done by Gills, Lopiccolo and Dennis [41], nelfinavir inhibited tumour growth and upregulated markers of endoplasmic reticulum stress, apoptosis, and autophagy. This drug was clinically tested and used to treat patients with breast cancer [42], thyroid cancer [43], and renal cancer [44]. Similarly, vorinostat, an antineoplastic drug actively used in current medicine, was also activated. This is an inhibitor of class I and II of histone deacetylases [45], which have promising effects as anticancer agents inhibiting the proliferation of cancer cells in breast cancer [46], renal cancer [47], and pancreatic cancer [48]. Aside from drugs, calcitriol, the most active metabolite of vitamin D, was upregulated, which has significant antineoplastic activity in various cancers by regulating multiple signalling pathways, including inhibition of proliferation associated with cell cycle arrest, induction of apoptosis, and reduction in invasiveness and angiogenesis [49]. Beta-carotene, a natural nutrient widely found in vegetables and fruits and known to be beneficial to human health, was also activated. Like the phytogenic products, beta-carotene has a clear role in antioxidant, immune-related functions, and cell gap junction-related functions [50] and has been explored by many researchers to treat gastric cancers [51] and to decrease the proliferation of colon [52] and prostate cancer cells [53].

There were several other less explored molecules or regulators with anticancer properties upregulated by PFA in this study. Although plant-derived natural products have demonstrated outstanding anticancer properties to effectively suppress early and intermediate stages of carcinogenesis in their pure form [17,54,55], their pharmacological potential is impeded by their poor penetration into cells, poor bioavailability, narrow therapeutic index, rapid uptake by normal tissues, and low aqueous solubility [56]. To alleviate this problem, synergistic studies on facilitating nanoparticles have shown improvements in treating cancer by greater stability and solubility of phytogenic compounds with enhanced tissue targeting and cellular uptake [56].

An increase in Weight loss ($p = 7.26 \times 10^{-5}$, z = 2.499) and a decrease in Weight gain ($p = 6.70 \times 10^{-6}$, z = −2.007) were among the most affected annotations in the category of Nutritional disease. There were 15 of 20 genes with expression change direction consistent with an increase in Weight loss, including the *DGAT2* genes. Diacylglycerol O-Acyltransferase 2 (DGAT2) is a critical catalysing enzyme for triglyceride (TG) biosynthesis and storing fat [57], resulting in obesity in humans [58]. *DGAT2* is an essential marker gene to trace fat deposition for meat processing animals, and numerous studies have been done to elucidate the relationship between intramuscular fat content and meat quality [59–62]. Recently, a positive correlation of *DGAT2* genes with obesity has been reported [58].

Intriguingly, although several genes related to weight gain were downregulated in phytogen-treated birds, these birds were heavier than the birds on control diet (Figure 4). As presented and discussed above, lipid metabolism was affected by the inhibition of several functional categories, including Metabolism and Synthesis of triacylglycerol, which is the form in which fat is stored in the body. Therefore, a reduction in Obesity or Weight loss categories is most likely the result of less fat storage. Notably, the category Quantity of amino acid was significantly increased ($p = 3.33 \times 10^{-7}$, z = 1.187) in the PFA-supplemented group with upregulation of *SLC6A18* gene, which is the epithelial neutral amino acid transporter. This indicates that the higher body weight of PFA-supplemented birds compared to control birds was not due to an increase in fat but to an increase in lean muscle.

Results from the histology data (Figure 4) in conjunction with transcriptomic analysis have demonstrated a tremendous increase in the number of goblet cells in PFA-supplemented birds. Goblet cells secrete mucin responsible for generating the mucus layer to protect the gut against pathogen invasion [63]. Mucins are composed of highly hydrophilic gel-like glycoproteins that help prevent direct contact with pathogenic microorganisms [63]. A reduced amount of mucin layer could allow intestinal mucosal barrier dysfunction [64], causing an excessive immune response in the host and resulting in colitis [65] and diarrhoea [66]. This is in agreement with the lower amount of dirty eggs produced in the PFA-supplemented birds in the previous study [28] as dirty eggs are an indicator of diarrhoea and intestinal issues in birds. This could have been contributing factor in the improved performance of PFA-supplemented birds during the Spotty Liver Disease outbreak in this trial. Increasing goblet cells promotes a healthier intestinal mucosal layer and is ideal for maintaining gut immune homeostasis.

5. Conclusions

The effects of this PFA blend on ileum gene expression show substantial benefits on the gastrointestinal system. It is also beneficial for controlling high blood pressure, obesity, diabetes, atherosclerosis, and cholesterol levels. This PFA can cause weight loss by altering the ratio of fat and carbohydrate metabolism toward lower fat storage. This could be a useful feature in the pig finisher growth stage. An increase in the number of goblet cells reduced inflammation levels in the ileum, suggested by significantly decreased Inflammation of body cavity disease category, and by a reduced number of dirty eggs.

Based on predicted disease profiles, this PFA would be beneficial for overall intestinal health but should be avoided in flocks infected with poultry retroviral infections: the avian leukosis/sarcoma virus (ALSV), reticuloendotheliosis virus (REV), and lymphoproliferative disease virus (LPDV) of turkeys. Transcriptomic data allows us to understand overall effects, including other indications of when it would be beneficial to use or avoid the product. This type of comprehensive mechanistic research investigation is a step toward a shed personalised treatment selection based on the burning issues in each farm and production system. A better understanding of PFAs' actions can maximise their benefits and make the first steps toward the customised farm, shed or production system supplementation.

Supplementary Materials: The following supporting information can be downloaded at: https://www.mdpi.com/article/10.3390/antibiotics11101428/s1, Table S1: Differentially abundant pathways, Table S2: Upstream analysis results, Table S3: Bird performance data, Table S4: Significantly affected disease categories, Table S5: Significantly affected disease categories sorted by disease, Figure S1: Sequencing report for raw sequences per sample, Figure S2: Top differentially expressed genes

Author Contributions: CRediT author statement: S.J.Y.: Investigation, Methodology, Formal analysis, Writing—Original Draft. Y.S.B.: Investigation, Methodology, Formal analysis, Project administration, Writing—Review & Editing. F.P.: Investigation, Methodology, Writing–Review & Editing. S.d.l.H.-S.: Formal analysis, Writing—Review & Editing. T.T.H.V.: Methodology, Writing—Review & Editing. D.S.: Conceptualisation, Methodology, Formal analysis, Funding acquisition, Writing—Review & Editing. All authors have read and agreed to the published version of the manuscript.

Funding: This research was funded by the Central Queensland University Merit Grant scheme under the project funding number RSH/4200.

Institutional Review Board Statement: The animal study protocol was approved by the Institutional Review Board of the Animal Ethics Committee of Central Queensland University, under approval number 0000022879.

Informed Consent Statement: Not applicable.

Data Availability Statement: All sequencing data are publicly available in NCBI SRA database under project number PRJNA887923 (https://www.ncbi.nlm.nih.gov/bioproject/887923).

Acknowledgments: The data was analysed using the Marie Curie High-Performance Computing System at Central Queensland University. We acknowledge and appreciate Jason Bell's help in all aspects of High-Performance Computing.

Conflicts of Interest: The authors declare no conflict of interest.

References

1. Ricke, S.C.; Dittoe, D.K.; Richardson, K.E. Formic acid as an antimicrobial for poultry production: A review. *Front. Vet. Sci.* **2020**, 7. [CrossRef] [PubMed]
2. Paiva, D.M.A. Necrotic enteritis: Applications for the poultry industry. *J. Appl. Poult. Res.* **2014**, 23, 557–566. [CrossRef]

3. Lee, J.Y.; Tsolis, R.M.; Baumler, A.J. The microbiome and gut homeostasis. *Science* **2022**, *377*, eabp9960. [CrossRef] [PubMed]
4. Rinttilä, T.; Apajalahti, J. Intestinal microbiota and metabolites—Implications for broiler chicken health and performance. *J. Appl. Poult. Res.* **2013**, *22*, 647–658. [CrossRef]
5. Yadav, S.; Jha, R. Strategies to modulate the intestinal microbiota and their effects on nutrient utilization, performance, and health of poultry. *J. Anim. Sci. Biotechnol.* **2019**, *10*, 2. [CrossRef]
6. Oviedo-Rondón, E.O.; Hume, M.E.; Barbosa, N.A.; Sakomura, N.K.; Weber, G.; Wilson, J.W. Ileal and caecal microbial populations in broilers given specific essential oil blends and probiotics in two consecutive grow-outs. *Avian Biol. Res.* **2010**, *3*, 157–169. [CrossRef]
7. Thompson, K.; Burkholder, K.; Patterson, J.; Applegate, T.J. Microbial ecology shifts in the ileum of broilers during feed withdrawal and dietary manipulations. *Poult. Sci.* **2008**, *87*, 1624–1632. [CrossRef]
8. Shi, D.; Bai, L.; Qu, Q.; Zhou, S.; Yang, M.; Guo, S.; Li, Q.; Liu, C. Impact of gut microbiota structure in heat-stressed broilers. *Poult. Sci.* **2019**, *98*, 2405–2413. [CrossRef]
9. Kers, J.G.; Velkers, F.C.; Fischer, E.A.J.; Hermes, G.D.A.; Stegeman, J.A.; Smidt, H. Host and environmental factors affecting the intestinal microbiota in chickens. *Front. Microbiol.* **2018**, *9*, 235. [CrossRef]
10. Han, Z.; Pielsticker, C.; Gerzova, L.; Rychlik, I.; Rautenschlein, S. The influence of age on *Campylobacter jejuni* infection in chicken. *Dev. Comp. Immunol.* **2016**, *62*, 58–71. [CrossRef]
11. Camp, J.G.; Frank, C.L.; Lickwar, C.R.; Guturu, H.; Rube, T.; Wenger, A.M.; Chen, J.; Bejerano, G.; Crawford, G.E.; Rawls, J.F. Microbiota modulate transcription in the intestinal epithelium without remodeling the accessible chromatin landscape. *Genome Res.* **2014**, *24*, 1504–1516. [CrossRef] [PubMed]
12. Mowat, A.M.; Agace, W.W. Regional specialization within the intestinal immune system. *Nat. Rev. Immunol.* **2014**, *14*, 667–685. [CrossRef] [PubMed]
13. Bastos, M.S.; Del Vesco, A.P.; Santana, T.P.; Santos, T.S.; de Oliveira Junior, G.M.; Fernandes, R.P.M.; Barbosa, L.T.; Gasparino, E. The role of cinnamon as a modulator of the expression of genes related to antioxidant activity and lipid metabolism of laying quails. *PLoS ONE* **2017**, *12*, e0189619. [CrossRef] [PubMed]
14. Bajagai, Y.S.; Petranyi, F.; Horyanto, D.; Batacan, R., Jr.; Lobo, E.; Ren, X.; Whitton, M.M.; Yu, S.J.; Kayal, A.; Stanley, D. Ileum transcriptional response to prolonged supplementation with phytogenic product containing menthol, carvacrol and carvone. *Heliyon* **2022**, *8*, e09131. [CrossRef]
15. Bajagai, Y.S.; Steel, J.C.; Radovanovic, A.; Stanley, D. Prolonged continual consumption of oregano herb interferes with the action of steroid hormones and several drugs, and effects signaling across the brain-gut axis. *Food Funct.* **2021**, *12*, 726–738. [CrossRef]
16. Sabino, M.; Capomaccio, S.; Cappelli, K.; Verini-Supplizi, A.; Bomba, L.; Ajmone-Marsan, P.; Cobellis, G.; Olivieri, O.; Pieramati, C.; Trabalza-Marinucci, M. Oregano dietary supplementation modifies the liver transcriptome profile in broilers: RNASeq analysis. *Res. Vet. Sci.* **2018**, *117*, 85–91. [CrossRef]
17. Sampaio, L.A.; Pina, L.T.S.; Serafini, M.R.; Tavares, D.D.S.; Guimaraes, A.G. Antitumor effects of carvacrol and thymol: A systematic review. *Front. Pharmacol.* **2021**, *12*, 702487. [CrossRef]
18. Hashemipour, H.; Kermanshahi, H.; Golian, A.; Veldkamp, T. Effect of thymol and carvacrol feed supplementation on performance, antioxidant enzyme activities, fatty acid composition, digestive enzyme activities, and immune response in broiler chickens. *Poult. Sci.* **2013**, *92*, 2059–2069. [CrossRef]
19. Barboza, J.N.; da Silva Maia Bezerra Filho, C.; Silva, R.O.; Medeiros, J.V.R.; de Sousa, D.P. An overview on the anti-inflammatory potential and antioxidant profile of eugenol. *Oxid. Med. Cell. Longev.* **2018**, *2018*, 3957262. [CrossRef]
20. Muanda, F.; Kone, D.; Dicko, A.; Soulimani, R.; Younos, C. Phytochemical composition and antioxidant capacity of three malian medicinal plant parts. *Evid. Based Complement. Alternat. Med.* **2011**, *2011*, 674320. [CrossRef]
21. Yanishlieva, N.V.; Marinova, E.M.; Gordon, M.H.; Raneva, V.G. Antioxidant activity and mechanism of action of thymol and carvacrol in two lipid systems. *Food Chem.* **1999**, *64*, 59–66. [CrossRef]
22. Omonijo, F.A.; Liu, S.; Hui, Q.; Zhang, H.; Lahaye, L.; Bodin, J.C.; Gong, J.; Nyachoti, M.; Yang, C. Thymol improves barrier function and attenuates inflammatory responses in porcine intestinal epithelial cells during Lipopolysaccharide (LPS)-induced inflammation. *J. Agric. Food Chem.* **2019**, *67*, 615–624. [CrossRef] [PubMed]
23. Youdim, K.A.; Deans, S.G. Effect of thyme oil and thymol dietary supplementation on the antioxidant status and fatty acid composition of the ageing rat brain. *Br. J. Nutr.* **2000**, *83*, 87–93. [CrossRef] [PubMed]
24. Vinus, R.D.; Sheoran, S.N.; Maan, N.; Tewatia, B. Potential benefits of herbal supplements in poultry feed: A review. *Pharm. Innov. J.* **2018**, *7*, 651–656.
25. Flees, J.J.; Ganguly, B.; Dridi, S. Phytogenic feed additives improve broiler feed efficiency via modulation of intermediary lipid and protein metabolism-related signaling pathways. *Poult. Sci.* **2021**, *100*, 100963. [CrossRef]
26. Wati, T.; Ghosh, T.K.; Syed, B.; Haldar, S. Comparative efficacy of a phytogenic feed additive and an antibiotic growth promoter on production performance, caecal microbial population and humoral immune response of broiler chickens inoculated with enteric pathogens. *Anim. Nutr.* **2015**, *1*, 213–219. [CrossRef]
27. Murugesan, G.R.; Syed, B.; Haldar, S.; Pender, C. Phytogenic feed additives as an alternative to antibiotic growth promoters in broiler chickens. *Front. Vet. Sci.* **2015**, *2*, 21. [CrossRef]
28. Yu, S.J.; Bajagai, Y.S.; Petranyi, F.; Stanley, D. Phytogen improves performance during Spotty Liver Disease by impeding bacterial metabolism and pathogenicity. *Appl. Environ. Microbiol.* **2022**, *88*, e00758-22. [CrossRef]

29. Willson, N.L.; Van, T.T.H.; Bhattarai, S.P.; Courtice, J.M.; McIntyre, J.R.; Prasai, T.P.; Moore, R.J.; Walsh, K.; Stanley, D. Feed supplementation with biochar may reduce poultry pathogens, including *Campylobacter hepaticus*, the causative agent of Spotty Liver Disease. *PLoS ONE* **2019**, *14*, e0214471. [CrossRef]
30. Connerton, P.L.; Richards, P.J.; Lafontaine, G.M.; O'Kane, P.M.; Ghaffar, N.; Cummings, N.J.; Smith, D.L.; Fish, N.M.; Connerton, I.F. The effect of the timing of exposure to *Campylobacter jejuni* on the gut microbiome and inflammatory responses of broiler chickens. *Microbiome* **2018**, *6*, 88. [CrossRef]
31. Schokker, D.; Veninga, G.; Vastenhouw, S.A.; Bossers, A.; de Bree, F.M.; Kaal-Lansbergen, L.M.T.E.; Rebel, J.M.J.; Smits, M.A. Early life microbial colonization of the gut and intestinal development differ between genetically divergent broiler lines. *BMC Genomics* **2015**, *16*, 418. [CrossRef] [PubMed]
32. Bajagai, Y.S.; Radovanovic, A.; Steel, J.C.; Stanley, D. The effects of continual consumption of *Origanum vulgare* on liver transcriptomics. *Animals* **2021**, *11*, 398. [CrossRef] [PubMed]
33. Baenke, F.; Peck, B.; Miess, H.; Schulze, A. Hooked on fat: The role of lipid synthesis in cancer metabolism and tumour development. *Dis. Model. Mech.* **2013**, *6*, 1353–1363. [CrossRef]
34. Vander Heiden, M.G.; Cantley, L.C.; Thompson, C.B. Understanding the Warburg effect: The metabolic requirements of cell proliferation. *Science* **2009**, *324*, 1029–1033. [CrossRef]
35. Bian, X.; Liu, R.; Meng, Y.; Xing, D.; Xu, D.; Lu, Z. Lipid metabolism and cancer. *J. Exp. Med.* **2021**, *218*, e20201606. [CrossRef] [PubMed]
36. Bengoechea-Alonso, M.T.; Ericsson, J. SREBP in signal transduction: Cholesterol metabolism and beyond. *Curr. Opin. Cell. Biol.* **2007**, *19*, 215–222. [CrossRef]
37. Shao, W.; Espenshade, P.J. Expanding roles for SREBP in metabolism. *Cell. Metab.* **2012**, *16*, 414–419. [CrossRef]
38. Hannun, Y.A.; Obeid, L.M. Sphingolipids and their metabolism in physiology and disease. *Nat. Rev. Mol. Cell. Biol.* **2018**, *19*, 175–191. [CrossRef]
39. Garcia-Barros, M.; Coant, N.; Truman, J.P.; Snider, A.J.; Hannun, Y.A. Sphingolipids in colon cancer. *Biochim. Biophys. Acta* **2014**, *1841*, 773–782. [CrossRef]
40. Nagahashi, M.; Tsuchida, J.; Moro, K.; Hasegawa, M.; Tatsuda, K.; Woelfel, I.A.; Takabe, K.; Wakai, T. High levels of sphingolipids in human breast cancer. *J. Surg. Res.* **2016**, *204*, 435–444. [CrossRef]
41. Gills, J.J.; Lopiccolo, J.; Dennis, P.A. Nelfinavir, a new anti-cancer drug with pleiotropic effects and many paths to autophagy. *Autophagy* **2008**, *4*, 107–109. [CrossRef] [PubMed]
42. Bruning, A.; Friese, K.; Burges, A.; Mylonas, I. Tamoxifen enhances the cytotoxic effects of nelfinavir in breast cancer cells. *Breast Cancer Res.* **2010**, *12*, R45. [CrossRef]
43. Jensen, K.; Bikas, A.; Patel, A.; Kushchayeva, Y.; Costello, J.; McDaniel, D.; Burman, K.; Vasko, V. Nelfinavir inhibits proliferation and induces DNA damage in thyroid cancer cells. *Endocr. Relat. Cancer* **2017**, *24*, 147–156. [CrossRef] [PubMed]
44. Okubo, K.; Isono, M.; Asano, T.; Sato, A. Panobinostat and nelfinavir inhibit renal cancer growth by inducing endoplasmic reticulum stress. *Anticancer Res.* **2018**, *38*, 5615–5626. [CrossRef]
45. Shirzad, M.; Taghdisi, M.H.; Dehdari, T.; Abolghasemi, J. Oral health education program among pre-school children: An application of health-promoting schools approach. *Health Promot. Perspect.* **2016**, *6*, 164–170. [CrossRef]
46. Wawruszak, A.; Borkiewicz, L.; Okon, E.; Kukula-Koch, W.; Afshan, S.; Halasa, M. Vorinostat (SAHA) and breast cancer: An overview. *Cancers* **2021**, *13*, 4700. [CrossRef] [PubMed]
47. Okubo, K.; Isono, M.; Miyai, K.; Asano, T.; Sato, A. Fluvastatin potentiates anticancer activity of vorinostat in renal cancer cells. *Cancer Sci.* **2020**, *111*, 112–126. [CrossRef]
48. Sanaei, M.; Kavoosi, F. Effect of vorinostat on INK4 family and HDACs 1, 2, and 3 in pancreatic cancer and hepatocellular carcinoma. *Res. Pharm. Sci.* **2021**, *16*, 260–268. [CrossRef]
49. Beer, T.M.; Myrthue, A. Calcitriol in cancer treatment: From the lab to the clinic. *Mol. Cancer Ther.* **2004**, *3*, 373–381. [CrossRef]
50. Paolini, M.; Abdel-Rahman, S.Z.; Sapone, A.; Pedulli, G.F.; Perocco, P.; Cantelli-Forti, G.; Legator, M.S. Beta-carotene: A cancer chemopreventive agent or a co-carcinogen? *Mutat. Res.* **2003**, *543*, 195–200. [CrossRef]
51. Chen, Q.H.; Wu, B.K.; Pan, D.; Sang, L.X.; Chang, B. Beta-carotene and its protective effect on gastric cancer. *World J. Clin. Cases* **2021**, *9*, 6591–6607. [CrossRef] [PubMed]
52. Lee, K.E.; Kwon, M.; Kim, Y.S.; Kim, Y.; Chung, M.G.; Heo, S.C.; Kim, Y. Beta-carotene regulates cancer stemness in colon cancer in vivo and in vitro. *Nutr. Res. Pract.* **2022**, *16*, 161–172. [CrossRef] [PubMed]
53. Dulinska, J.; Gil, D.; Zagajewski, J.; Hartwich, J.; Bodzioch, M.; Dembinska-Kiec, A.; Langmann, T.; Schmitz, G.; Laidler, P. Different effect of beta-carotene on proliferation of prostate cancer cells. *Biochim. Biophys. Acta* **2005**, *1740*, 189–201. [CrossRef] [PubMed]
54. Li, L.; He, L.; Wu, Y.; Zhang, Y. Carvacrol affects breast cancer cells through TRPM7 mediated cell cycle regulation. *Life Sci.* **2021**, *266*, 118894. [CrossRef]
55. Ahmad, A.; Ansari, I.A. Carvacrol exhibits chemopreventive potential against cervical cancer cells via caspase-dependent apoptosis and abrogation of cell cycle progression. *Anticancer Agents Med. Chem.* **2021**, *21*, 2224–2235. [CrossRef]
56. Vimala, K.; Kannan, S. Phyto-drug conjugated nanomaterials enhance apoptotic activity in cancer. *Adv. Protein Chem. Struct. Biol.* **2021**, *125*, 275–305. [CrossRef]

57. Brandt, C.; McFie, P.J.; Stone, S.J. Biochemical characterization of human acyl coenzyme A: 2-monoacylglycerol acyltransferase-3 (MGAT3). *Biochem. Biophys. Res. Commun.* **2016**, *475*, 264–270. [CrossRef]
58. Ning, T.; Zou, Y.; Yang, M.; Lu, Q.; Chen, M.; Liu, W.; Zhao, S.; Sun, Y.; Shi, J.; Ma, Q.; et al. Genetic interaction of DGAT2 and FAAH in the development of human obesity. *Endocrine* **2017**, *56*, 366–378. [CrossRef]
59. Mao, H.; Yin, Z.; Wang, M.; Zhang, W.; Raza, S.H.A.; Althobaiti, F.; Qi, L.; Wang, J. Expression of DGAT2 gene and its associations with intramuscular fat content and breast muscle fiber characteristics in domestic pigeons (*Columba livia*). *Front. Vet. Sci.* **2022**, *9*, 847363. [CrossRef]
60. Mao, H.G.; Dong, X.Y.; Cao, H.Y.; Xu, N.Y.; Yin, Z.Z. Association of DGAT2 gene polymorphisms with carcass and meat quality traits in domestic pigeons (*Columba livia*). *Br. Poult. Sci.* **2018**, *59*, 149–153. [CrossRef]
61. Zang, L.; Wang, Y.; Sun, B.; Zhang, X.; Yang, C.; Kang, L.; Zhao, Z.; Jiang, Y. Identification of a 13 bp indel polymorphism in the 3′-UTR of DGAT2 gene associated with backfat thickness and lean percentage in pigs. *Gene* **2016**, *576*, 729–733. [CrossRef] [PubMed]
62. Zhang, J.F.; Choi, S.H.; Li, Q.; Wang, Y.; Sun, B.; Tang, L.; Wang, E.Z.; Hua, H.; Li, X.Z. Overexpression of DGAT2 stimulates lipid droplet formation and triacylglycerol accumulation in bovine satellite cells. *Animals* **2022**, *12*, 1847. [CrossRef] [PubMed]
63. Birchenough, G.M.; Johansson, M.E.; Gustafsson, J.K.; Bergstrom, J.H.; Hansson, G.C. New developments in goblet cell mucus secretion and function. *Mucosal. Immunol.* **2015**, *8*, 712–719. [CrossRef]
64. Johansson, M.E.; Hansson, G.C. Is the intestinal goblet cell a major immune cell? *Cell Host Microbe* **2014**, *15*, 251–252. [CrossRef]
65. Van der Sluis, M.; De Koning, B.A.; De Bruijn, A.C.; Velcich, A.; Meijerink, J.P.; Van Goudoever, J.B.; Buller, H.A.; Dekker, J.; Van Seuningen, I.; Renes, I.B.; et al. Muc2-deficient mice spontaneously develop colitis, indicating that MUC2 is critical for colonic protection. *Gastroenterology* **2006**, *131*, 117–129. [CrossRef] [PubMed]
66. Jung, K.; Saif, L.J. Goblet cell depletion in small intestinal villous and crypt epithelium of conventional nursing and weaned pigs infected with porcine epidemic diarrhea virus. *Res. Vet. Sci.* **2017**, *110*, 12–15. [CrossRef] [PubMed]

antibiotics

MDPI

Review

Insight on Incorporation of Essential Oils as Antimicrobial Substances in Biopolymer-Based Active Packaging

Ana Tomić, Olja Šovljanski * and Tamara Erceg

Faculty of Technology Novi Sad, University of Novi Sad, Bulevar Cara Lazara 1, 21 000 Novi Sad, Serbia; anav@uns.ac.rs (A.T.); tamara.erceg@uns.ac.rs (T.E.)

* Correspondence: oljasovljanski@uns.ac.rs

Abstract: The increasing interest in microbiological food safety requires the development of sensitive and reliable analyses and technologies for preserving food products' freshness and quality. Different types of packaging systems are one of the solutions for controlling microbiological activity in foods. During the last decades, the development of biopolymer-based active packaging with essential oil incorporation systems has resulted in technologies with exceptional application potential, primarily in the food industry. There is no doubt that this principle can facilitate food status monitoring, reduce food waste, extend the shelf life, improve the overall quality of food, or indicate a larger problem during the storage, production, and distribution of foodstuffs. On the other hand, most antimicrobial packaging systems are in the development phase, while the sensitivity, selectivity, complexity, and, above all, safety of these materials are just some of the essential questions that need to be answered before they can be widely used. The incorporation of essential oils as antimicrobial substances in biopolymer-based active packaging holds significant promise for enhancing food safety, extending shelf life, and offering more sustainable packaging solutions. While challenges exist, ongoing research and innovation in this field are likely to lead to the development of effective and environmentally friendly packaging systems with enhanced antimicrobial properties.

Keywords: antimicrobial packaging system; antimicrobial incorporation; biopolymer matrix; food application; microbiological food safety

1. Introduction

Microbiological contamination is a significant concern in the food industry as it can lead to foodborne illnesses and the spoilage of products. There are several acute problems associated with microbiological contamination in the food industry: foodborne illness outbreaks, product recalls, regulatory compliance, consumer trust, economic loss, supply chain issues, etc. To address these acute problems, the food industry employs various strategies, including stringent sanitation practices, HACCP (Hazard Analysis of Critical Control Points) systems, regular testing and monitoring, and compliance with food safety regulations. Additionally, advances in food processing technologies as well as new packaging technologies are continuously being developed to mitigate microbiological contamination risks and improve food safety. On the other hand, the global production of plastics has gradually increased since plastics' industrialization in the 1950s, reaching 368 million tons in 2019, with the expectation that it will reach 1.1 billion tons by 2050 [1]. The packaging industry is one of the main consumers of conventional plastic due to its good mechanical and barrier properties, lightweight, low-cost petrochemical building blocks, and established processing methods. Despite the numerous advantages, non-degradable plastic packaging has a negative impact on the environment and human health. Production of conventional plastic requires non-renewable fossil fuels as feedstock, resulting in the depletion of their reserves and increased emissions of greenhouse gases (GHG) [2]. Furthermore, the manufacturing, processing, and burning of plastic materials require high energy consumption, leading to the increased release of volatile organic compounds (VOCs) and harmful gases [3]. The enormous conventional plastic production, followed by the low level of recycling and high resistance to biodegradation, has resulted in the accumulation of a large quantity of plastic waste in nature. Over 45% of plastic waste comes from packaging, and even 90% of this amount comes from food and beverage packaging (wrappers, bags, containers, etc.). The slow degradation along with UV irradiation and abrasion results in the generation of microplastics, which end up in all ecosystems and living beings, causing different harmful effects. These facts have led to a growing interest in the development and manufacturing of biodegradable packaging materials obtained from renewable resources. Biopolymers, such as proteins and polysaccharides obtained by extraction from animal and plant materials, are degraded in the natural environment through chemical and biological processes, especially by the metabolism of microorganisms [4].

Beside plastic waste, food waste and spoilage are globally recognized as environmental and economic problems that need an emerging solution. Only a small percentage of food is composted, and the rest of the unused food is the largest compound of solid municipal waste, which degrades, releasing methane and contributing to greenhouse emissions. The food can be spoiled in physical, chemical, biochemical, and microbial ways during distribution, storage, and consumption. It is estimated that the amount of wasted food per year can feed one-eighth of the world's population and answer the global challenge of meeting the increased need for food [5]. Packaging has a significant role in preventing and decreasing spoilage factors, acting as a barrier for water, gases, chemical, and microbiological agents, improving the safety of food, maintaining its quality, and extending the product's shelf life. Perishableness of food and long-term distribution have imposed a need for the development of active packaging that is able to inhibit microbial growth due to the presence of antimicrobial compounds incorporated in a polymer matrix, which should be biodegradable according to environmental and ecological demands. Synthetic antimicrobial and antioxidant agents are used in the food industry, but some of them can be harmful to humans, causing resistance or disorder of the microbiological flora. Those facts, along with a demand for the utilization of renewable resources, have launched essential oils (EOs) into the focus of the scientific public as biobased compounds with pronounced antimicrobial and antioxidative effects, edibility, and harmlessness for human health that are suitable for application in food packaging [6,7].

Therefore, the development of active biodegradable packaging with incorporated bio-based antimicrobial agents such as essential oils can address urgent challenges on a global level, such as reducing plastic and food waste and their harmful effects on the environment. This review includes information about biopolymer-based structures used for packaging systems and different approaches for the incorporation of essential oils in targeted structures. Additionally, the emergence of microbiological contamination in the food industry, the influence of the packaging system on the inactivation of microbiological contamination, the migration of the antimicrobial substance into the packaging system, and the proposal for comprehensive determination of the antimicrobial potential of biopolymer-based active packaging with incorporated essential oils were summarized.

2. Emergence of Microbiological Contamination in the Food Industry

Diseases caused by the consumption of contaminated food, called foodborne diseases, represent a challenge to the entire system of food production and supply. The food supply line represents the processes of growing, harvesting, transporting, storing, and preparing food in an unhygienic environment, often without adequate environmental control measures. Therefore, this indispensable route represents an infection path for humans. Foodborne microorganisms often cause acute illness in humans but also significant economic losses during food production and processing. It should be noted that some groups of the human population are more at risk than others, such as children, pregnant women, elders with low immune status, persons with cancer, on chemotherapy, or/and infected with HIV [8]. There are thought to be more than 30 pathogens that are known to cause illness if present in food. Based on the World Health Organization (WHO) data, priority food contaminants are pathogen bacteria such as *Campylobacter* spp., *Escherichia coli* O157 (STEC and VTEC), *Listeria monocytogenes*, *Salmonella* spp. (non-typhoidal strains), *Salmonella enteritica* serotype Typhi, *Shigella* spp., and *Yersinia enterocolitica*. The mentioned bacteria are monitored in numerous countries and by a large number of health organizations for the prevention of foodborne diseases, determining the source and place of outbreaks, etc. [9].

In the last decade, the global food and beverage industry has seen significant growth. Following this trend, this industry is predicted to be worth more than 5700 billion dollars by the end of 2025 [10]. The turnover of the food and beverage industry in the reports of the European Union (EU) is estimated at 956.2 billion euros, whereby, within the framework of this community, over four million people are employed, with an over 20% increase in exports every year. Globalization and the increasing need for food introduce new risks into the system in terms of food safety, and contaminated food can be a source of risk that can spread over larger geographic areas [11]. Consumption of food containing an infectious dose of one of the mentioned pathogens affects every sixth resident in economically developed countries [12]. In addition to the mentioned bacterial contaminants, norovirus is at the top of the ladder. In addition to it, non-typhoidal species of *Salmonella* bacteria, *S. aureus*, *C. perfringens*, and *Campylobacter* spp. are found in five prominent foodborne pathogens [13]. Based on reports from 27 EU member states and four states that are not members of this community, a total of 5196 outbreaks of foodborne diseases were recorded in 2013. Most diseases are caused by the occurrence of salmonellosis, viral diseases, and the occurrence of bacterial toxins in food, while almost 30% of reported cases had an unknown source [14]. The most frequently contaminated foodstuffs are eggs, RTE (ready-to-eat) food, fish, and fish products. For example, the EU reported a total of 82,694 confirmed cases of salmonellosis in 2013, resulting in a reporting rate of 20.4 cases per 100,000 population, with 59 deaths. Furthermore, outbreaks of listeriosis were recorded in this community every year, while the number of confirmed VTEC infections in humans increased over the last ten years [15].

Microbiological contamination can enter the food chain in a production environment (farm, orchard, pond, etc.), process environment (slaughterhouse, factory, packaging plant, etc.), preparation environment (kitchen, food service, etc.), and/or water used in any production-process phase [16]. Although food spoilage can be attributed to many sources, such as enzymatic decomposition, physico-chemical reactions, damage during transport, and the influence of rodents and other pests, microbiological contamination has a decisive and very important contribution to food spoilage. Some of the most common non-pathogenic bacteria that cause food spoilage are *Pseudomonas* spp. and lactic acid bacteria (LAB), which are often involved in the spoilage of dairy and meat products. What distinguishes microbiological contamination in the food industry is that bacteria easily resist adverse environmental conditions, including high pH, low temperatures, and anaerobic environmental conditions [16].

2.1. *Presence of Bacteria in Food*

Bacteria occupy a very important place among the microorganisms found in food. This is not only because many species can be present in food but also because of their fast growth and ability to use nutrients, as well as their ability to grow in different conditions (wide range of temperature, presence of air, pH, water activity). Various indicators of fecal contaminants, such as *E. coli*, *Salmonella* spp., *L. monocytogenes*, *Vibrio cholerae*, and *Pseudomonas* spp., were isolated from water used in cases of agricultural production [10]. Also, farmed poultry and livestock are the primary sources of pathogenic bacteria that are often associated with human infections. Pathogenic bacteria can be "transferred" from infected or contaminated meat and become part of the food chain. Cross-contamination of foodborne pathogens in the retail sector is also a major public health issue, contributing to the increased risk of foodborne illness outbreaks. RTE food, such as meat delicacies, cheese, and other perishable ingredients, is often the cause of contamination with the bacteria *L. monocytogenes*. It is considered that bacteria are the main cause of spoilage in most food products, which causes a great economic loss in the process of food storage and preservation [12].

The presence of bacteria in food products is a matter of great importance. Bacterial motility, adaptability, sporogenicity, toxin production, and cell wall structure dictate the treatments involved in food preparation and processing. Although there are many ways to group bacteria, from the point of view of the food industry, the following division is the most important: non-pathogenic, conditionally pathogenic, and pathogenic bacteria, whereby the controversy that the mentioned groups may or may not be the cause of food spoilage must be added to the discussion [17]. Pathogenic microorganisms are the source of foodborne epidemics and cause everything from mild disease symptoms to fatal outcomes. Although a significant number of bacteria can be present in food, *E. coli*, *Salmonella* spp., and *Clostridium botulinum* stand out in particular and are extensively studied by both the medical and scientific public. An unavoidable detail is the unpredictable nature of bacterial contamination due to the type of food in which they are found, the environment and storage conditions, and the possibility of toxin production. Some bacteria are found in food products as secondary contamination, while others live only in certain food environments, such as *C. botulinum*, which has been a problem for the canned food industry for decades due to its anaerobicity and sporogenicity [18]. Another example of this is *L. monocytogenes*, which represents a major risk in RTE foods containing smoked meats and sausages [19]. Non-pathogenic bacteria, although less harmful to humans, indirectly affect the world economy by limiting access to food. For this reason, methods to preserve and slow down the rate of food spoilage have been a subject of interest since the beginning of the modern understanding of the concept of healthy and safe nutrition.

The most common foodborne bacteria, coupled with food sources and health risks, are summarized in Table 1.

Table 1. Common foodborne bacteria.

Bacteria	Food Sources	Health Risks
Salmonella	Raw poultry, eggs	Gastroenteritis, fever
Escherichia coli	Undercooked beef, raw vegetables	Diarrhea, kidney failure
Listeria monocytogenes	Deli meats, soft cheeses	Listeriosis (severe illness)
Campylobacter	Raw or undercooked poultry	Diarrhea, cramps
Clostridium botulinum	Canned and low-acid foods	Botulism (paralysis)

2.2. Presence of Yeasts and Fungi in Food

Due to their ability to contaminate and degrade food products by producing extracellular enzymes, mycelial fungi and molds are of great importance in the microbiological contamination of food [20]. According to an estimate by the USDA Economic Research Service, about 96 billion kilograms of human food is discarded annually due to fungal contamination, with the largest share in the form of fresh fruits and vegetables (19.6%), milk and milk products (18.1%), grain products (15.2%), and sweeteners (12.4%). For example, in the fruit industry, post-harvest losses of 5 to 10% have been estimated when fungicides are used, and when fungicides are not used, losses amount to more than 50%. In the bakery industry, losses due to fungal contamination are up to 5%, which is over 23,000 tons of bread per year or 200 million pounds [21].

Among the fungi that appear as food contaminants, *Aspergillus* and *Penicillium* species stand out. In addition to them, *Mucor*, *Absidia*, and *Rhizopus* genera stand out. Apart from representatives of *Ascomycotina* and *Zygomycotina*, *xerophilic* fungi whose growth is characteristic under conditions of reduced water activity (aw) also occur as food contaminants. Representatives of this group of fungi are *Xeromyces* and *Vallemia* [21]. Representatives of the genus *Deuteromycotina* can also be food contaminants, with *Alternaria, Botrytis, Cladosporium,* and *Fusarium* species being the most prominent [17]. The most dominantly present foodborne yeasts and fungi are systematically present in Table 2.

Table 2. Common foodborne yeasts and fungi.

Microorganism	Food Sources	Health Risks
	Yeasts	
Saccharomyces cerevisiae	Bread, beer, wine	Generally non-pathogenic
Candida spp.	Found in milk products	Opportunistic infections
Zygosaccharomyces spp.	Found in fermented foods	Generally non-pathogenic
Debaryomyces spp.	Dairy products, fermented foods	Generally non-pathogenic
	Fungi	
Aspergillus spp.	Nuts, grains, dried fruits	Aflatoxin production
Penicillium spp.	Cheese, spoilage of various foods	Some species used in cheese production, allergenic spores
Fusarium spp.	Grains, cereals	Mycotoxin production
Botrytis cinerea	Fruits, vegetables	Allergenic spores
Rhizopus spp.	Fruits, vegetables, baked goods	Allergenic spores

Fungal contamination of food generally occurs first as contamination with spores that can be part of the sexual and asexual reproduction of fungi [22]. In favorable environmental conditions, spores break the resting phase, start germination, and create visible mycelia [20]. After a certain period, depending on the type of mold, food type, and storage conditions, the mycelium produces a series of conidia, and continuous development of the mold begins. This development is conditioned by environmental factors, but it is essentially impossible to prevent the spread of mold and food spoilage when favorable conditions for the initiation of the mold life cycle occur [22].

2.3. The Main Problem Related to the Presence of Microorganisms in Food

The presence of microorganisms in food is one of the main problems for the food industry, scientific community, and global economy. This problem appears to be a global issue because it represents a constant threat to health. As a consequence of the solution to this problem, the food industry must constantly develop and prepare procedures that minimize the occurrence and persistence of microbiological contamination in food [23]. This problem is also reflected in the fact that a large number of microorganisms can survive the effects of chemical agents allowed for use in food, as well as the physical and chemical procedures currently applied in the food industry to extend the shelf life [24]. Food safety depends to a large extent on appropriate government regulations, but also on the requirements and proper implementation of legal regulations, such as appropriate and constant training of people involved in food manipulation. The basic rules of food hygiene are essential, but they are still missing in many steps of food processing, such as the processes related to the slaughtering and processing of animal carcasses [25].

Modern methods for early detection of microbiological contamination include expensive genotyping and identifying the presence of microorganisms where possible and feasible in real-time [26]. However, a large number of food industries have introduced preventive measures for the occurrence of microbiological contamination. These procedures usually involve the use of antibiotics or alternative biocide compounds to suppress the growth of the microbiota. The long-term use of antibiotics leads to the emergence of bacterial resistance, creating a much bigger and longer-term problem for the food cycle in humans and animals. On the other hand, bacteria have the ability, after acquiring resistance, to suppress the effect of the antibiotic so that a critical intracellular concentration of the growth-inhibiting agent never accumulates [27].

In the last few decades, the resistance of microorganisms to antimicrobial agents has become a major environmental problem, and consequently, the number of broad-spectrum antimicrobial agents is decreasing. The acquired antimicrobial resistance, most microorganisms can transfer to new generations by simple, horizontal gene transfer. In addition, the abuse of antimicrobial agents, which is expressed in the veterinary and meat industries, has caused even specific antimicrobial agents to be no longer effective in the fight against pathogens in food. On the other hand, the pharmaceutical industry does not have a solution for the production of new antimicrobial agents, both due to the lack of sources and the high cost of production [27].

3. Biopolymer-Based Structures for Formation of Packaging Systems

Different materials have been used in food packaging, such as metal, glass, paper, and plastic. Environmental concerns and strivings to reduce the amount of solid waste, as well as consumers' requirements for increasing food safety, have imposed a need for the development of biodegradable active packaging [28]. The differences between classical and biodegradable food packaging, along with the adventages and limitations, are summarized in Table 3.

Table 3. Packaging types based on used material(s), advantages, and limitations.

	Comparation of Packaging Type		
	Classical Food Packaging	**Biodegradable Food Packaging**	
Used materials	Metal Glass Paper Conventional plastic	Based on synthetic polymers	Based on biopolymers obtained from plants, animals, and microorganisms
Properties	Non-biodegradable persists in environment—degrades very slow good barrier and mechanical properties low levels of interaction with packaged food	Biodegradable in nature possesses worse mechanical and barrier properties low weight and ability to be easily handled	
Advantages	Strong and durable, excellent food protection longer shelf life of food product widely available and versatile; some of them can be low weight (plastic, paper) low levels of interaction with packaged food	Environmentally friendly, reduces plastic pollution can be produced from renewable resources nontoxic reduces carbon emissions and amount of plastic waste low weight and ability to be easily handled; can be edible can be designed to prolong food product shelf-life [29]	
Limitations	Non-environmentally friendly; production leads to great energy consumption, fossil fuel depletion, and emissions of volatile organic compounds (VOC) limited recyclability for some materials; long-time of decomposition; increase the amount of solid waste generation production of microplastic (conventional plastic)	Poor barrier and mechanical properties; may require specific disposal conditions to biodegrade properly (polylactide, polyhydroxyalkanoate)	

Biopolymer-based structures for the encapsulation of essential oils can be divided into particles, fibers, and gels (Figure 1).

They usually have nanodimensions, which classify them as nanostructures. Different biopolymers have been utilized for the preparation of nanoparticles—vesicles with sizes up to 100 nm, intended for the encapsulation of essential oils in active packaging applications. Proteins and polysaccharides, individually or together (in the form of complexes), are used for obtaining nanoparticles. For the production of protein, polysaccharides, and protein/polysaccharides-based nanoparticles, different methods have been utilized, such as nanospray drying and complex coacervation. Different proteins and polysaccharides such as zein, gelatin, soy protein, whey protein, milk proteins, alginate, pectin, chitosan, pullulan, starch, cellulose, gellan gum, and maltodextrin have been successfully used for the formation of nanoparticles or nanocapsules intended for the incorporation of essential oils as antimicrobial agents in active packaging with the aim to achieve their compatibilization with hydrophilic biopolymer matrix and protect them from evaporation, thermal degradation, and oxidation during film processing and product storage [29,30]. The spray-drying technique enables the micro or nanoencapsulation of essential oils by dispersing them in an aqueous solution of film-forming biopolymer to obtain emulsion, which is pulled into the dryer through a nozzle providing small droplets. Improved thermal stability and controlled release of essential oils in active packaging formulations can be achieved by microencapsulation of essential oils by complex coacervation when two oppositely charged biopolymers make an electrostatic complex, which results in phase separation. As a result of neutralization, the dispersion is separated into two phases—one rich in biopolymer (coacervate) and the other with a low amount of biopolymer. This process implies the emulsification of essential oils in an aqueous solution of cationic and anionic biopolymers, adjustment of pH value, biopolymer ratio, concentration, and as a last step, washing, filtration, and centrifugation, ionic strength, temperature, and stirring speed. Different protein/polysaccharides and lipopolysaccharide combinations have been employed for the encapsulation of essential oils using the method of complex coacervation, such as gelatin/gum arabic, gelatin/sodium alginate, gelatin/pectin, sodium alginate/chitosan, milk protein/carboxymethyl cellulose, whey protein isolate/gum arabic, whey protein isolate/sodium carboxymethyl cellulose, whey protein isolate/sodium alginate, chitosan/kappa carrageenan, chitosan/gum arabic, chitosan/sodium carboxymethyl cellulose [31–40].

Nanofibers are obtained by a process that implies the conversion of biopolymer solution into nanofibers using electrohydrodynamic techniques such as electrospraying (low-density polymer solution) and electrospinning (high-density polymer solution). The fibers are formed under an electrical field passing through the syringe. The first step in the preparation of nanofiber-loaded essential oils implies the formation of EO emulsion in a hydrophilic biopolymer solution using usually non-ionic surfactants from the group of Triton X or Tween. Active packaging based on nanofibers obtained from chitosan, gelatine, alginate, zein, chitosan/gellan, tragacanth, and sodium alginate/polyvinyl alcohol with different EOs has been proven effective in the protection of food products against foodborne pathogens [41–46].

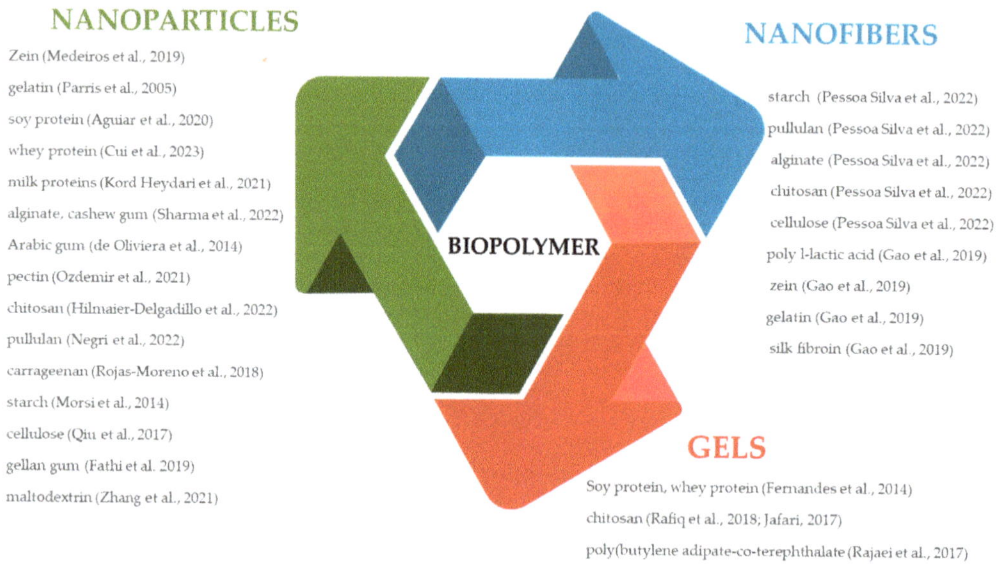

Figure 1. Biopolymer-based structures for encapsulation of essential oils [37,47–66].

3D networks are comprised of chemically or physically crosslinked hydrophilic or amphiphilic polymers, usually nano-sized (1–200 nm), called nanogels. According to affinity for certain solvents (water or hydrophobic ones), nanogels are divided into hydrogels and organogels. Hydrogels are obtained by the crosslinking of hydrophilic monomers or polymers, possess an affinity for water, and are suitable for the incorporation of hydrophilic compounds. On the other hand, organogels possess an affinity for a hydrophobic medium and are suitable for entrapping essential oils. Nanoorganogels have been proven to be promising systems for encapsulating and delivering EOs, improving their performance. They are obtained by a covalently crosslinked or self-assembly process. Nanogels based on chitosan/myristic acid and chitosan/benzoic acid have been shown to be efficient in the encapsulation of clove and rosemary essential oils, contributing to the better antimicrobial activity of active packaging toward food pathogens [47,48]. The high encapsulation efficiency of oregano essential oil was achieved using a procedure of ionic gelation to entrap EO into the alginate-based hydrogels. This kind of hydrogel is obtained using spray-drying and subsequent ionic gelation by dripping microcapsules in a calcium chloride solution. Poly(butylene adipate-co-terephthalate) (PBAT)/cassava starch films containing obtained microcapsules were produced by extrusion blow molding, which has demonstrated the high efficiency of obtained gels to protect encapsulated EO from thermal degradation [49]. Availability, biocompatibility, and the ability to encapsulate antimicrobial compounds and improve the applicative properties of biopolymer-based films make clay one of the most preferred nanomaterials. They consist of aluminosilicate layers with traces of organic matter, metals, and metal oxide, parallel-bonded due to secondary forces. Clay minerals are classified according to their chemical composition into three main categories: the first one with a silica/alumina ratio of 2:1 (montmorillonite, bentonite, etc.), the second with a silica/alumina/magnesium ratio of 2:1:1, and the third with silica/alumina ratio of 1:1 (kaolin, halloysite) [67]. The entrapping of EOs in montmorillonite and halloysite is carried out via the evaporation/adsorption procedure by directly mixing of EOs with clay minerals, avoiding high temperatures. The encapsulation of carvacrol, oregano, and cinnamon essential oils into halloysite-based nanocarriers incorporated into cardboard boxes has resulted in improved antimicrobial activity against foodborne pathogens. Active packaging has been successfully manufactured by the incorporation of montmorillonite-loaded

EOs into chitosan, poly(hydroxybutyrate-co-hydroxy valerate), hydroxypropyl methylcellulose, and alginate; bentonite–loaded EOs into chitosan, cassava starch, levan, and poly(ε-caprolactone); and kaolinite into poly(hydroxybutyrate-co-hydroxy valerate) [68].

Another example of a good carrier for antimicrobial substances are the cyclodextrins (CDs). CDs are cyclic oligosaccharides obtained as a result of the enzymatic conversion of starch by the action of the enzyme glycosyltransferase, produced by the bacteria *Bacillus* sp. and *Klebsiella*. The main types of cyclodextrins consist of 6, 7, and 8 glucopyranose units (α, β, γ) connected by a (1–4) glycosidic bond. The inner cavity of CDs is hydrophobic, while the outer side has an affinity toward the aqueous phase. With hydrophobic substances, such as essential oils, CDs form host-guest inclusion complexes via secondary forces, enabling their compatibilization with a hydrophilic biopolymer matrix. The procedure of preparation of inclusion complexes implies the dispersion of CDs and essential oil in an aqueous medium, stirring in mild conditions, and the filtration of obtained inclusion complexes [30]. Active packaging containing CDs can be prepared by solution casting (clove oil with chitosan/β-cyclodextrin citrate/oxidized nanocellulose biocomposite) [69], formation of edible coatings (chitosan-gelatine edible coating with β-cyclodextrin/lemongrass essential oil inclusion complex) [70], or CD-EO inclusion complexes can be directly subjected to the electrospinning technique to form a nanofibrous web with potential application in active packaging [71].

4. Antimicrobial Packaging as Control of Microbiological Activity in Food

The ideal antimicrobial biopolymer packaging should meet several important criteria. To begin with, all phases (components) in their production must, following legal regulations, meet the conditions of direct contact with food [72]. In addition, the procedure for incorporating the antimicrobial phase should be simple and economical, so that the final price of the active packaging would be attractive to the food industry [23]. Like any other packaging, this one must remain chemically stable for long-term use and storage and satisfy the function of a water and gas barrier. Also, packaging with antimicrobial action must not be subject to easy and rapid degradation (especially in the case of biopolymers) and should maintain its antimicrobial function during the entire packaging and storage process. No less important is the fact that this kind of packaging must not have a harmful effect on people's health when handling it or consuming the food that was packed in it. The antimicrobial component added to this type of active packaging must not exceed the maximum allowed amount of antimicrobial agent and be in accordance with the type of packaged food [73].

The basic division of packaging with antimicrobial action is biodegradable and non-degradable. Most synthetic polymers are not biodegradable, which is why they are often used as packaging materials. In addition, they are characterized by low cost, low density, internality, good protective properties, mechanical strength, a high degree of transparency, the ability to heat seal, and the possibility of labeling and printing [74]. The most commonly used synthetic packaging materials in the food industry are polyethylene, polypropylene, ethylene vinyl acetate, polystyrene, polyethylene terephthalate, and polyvinyl chloride. Synthetic biodegradable polymers such as polycaprolactone or polyvinyl alcohol are also used, which are still in the minority compared to non-degradable ones [73,75]. Additionally, this would mean that the use of packaging based on synthetic polymers has a negative impact on the environment via the creation of landfills, environmental pollution, and high levels of energy consumption during their production. For these reasons, the use of biopolymers and materials of natural origin is being sought, which are currently a more expensive but more environmentally friendly solution due to their biodegradability [76]. For example, the use of biopolymers from insufficiently used materials or agro-industrial and food by-products and waste is increasingly recommended, which would significantly reduce the costs of biopolymer packaging [77].

5. Incorporation of Essential Oil as the Antimicrobial Substance in the Biopolymer Matrix

Essential oils are hydrophobic liquids consisting of volatile aromatic compounds with diverse effects—antimicrobial, antioxidant, anti-inflammatory, analgetic, anti-depressive, relaxing, etc. They are highly recognized in the pharmaceutical industry and medicine, but also in the gastronomy and food packaging industries. EOs are obtained by extraction from different plant parts—seeds, stems, bark, buds, leaves, and flowers. The composition and yield are influenced by the conditions of plant growth and harvesting as well as extraction parameters (type, solvents, duration, etc.). Among different extraction methods for EO, steam distillation is the most widely used method, resulting in a high yield (above 93%) [78]. This method along, with Eos, gives a secondary product—hydrosol or hydrolat, which contains water-soluble compounds [79].

It can be summarized that essential oils play a crucial role in active packaging systems by virtue of their profound antimicrobial attributes, which synergistically enhance the protective capabilities of packaging materials against microbial threats. These oils, harnessed from botanical sources, contain a rich array of bioactive constituents, including phenols, terpenes, and aldehydes, that collectively exhibit potent inhibitory effects against a spectrum of microorganisms. The main compounds of essential oils belong to the class of monoterpenes, monoterpenoids, and phenylpropanoids (with alcohol or aldehyde functional groups) [80]. Those compounds have antimicrobial effects. EOs are recognized as safe by the U.S Food and Drug Administration (FDA) [81], which, along with their antimicrobial effects against foodborne pathogens and use as food flavors, make them suitable for food packaging applications. To be used in active food packaging, essential oils should show activity against foodborne pathogens, which cause food spoilage, but also foodborne illness in people, which can have serious consequences. This effect has been proven for a wide spectrum of essential oils, such as eugenol essential oil, ginger essential oil (*Zingiber officinale*), cinnamon oil, thyme oil (*Thymus vulgaris*), lemongrass oil (*Cymbopogon citratus*), oregano oil, tea tree oil (*Melaleuca alternifolia*), sage oil (*Salvia officinalis*), catnip essential oil (*Nepeta cataria*), *Satureja* Khuzestanica, *Helichrysum italicum*, mustard (*Brassica nigra*), etc. [63]. Mechanistically, essential oils disrupt cellular membranes, impede critical enzymatic processes, and intricately modulate microbial gene expression. This intricate interplay of multifaceted mechanisms underscores their ability to hinder microbial proliferation, ensuring extended shelf life and enhanced product safety in the context of biopolymer-based active packaging systems [82]. This integration not only capitalizes on the antimicrobial potential of essential oils but also leverages the innate biocompatibility of biopolymers, thus engendering a harmonious synergy. The compatibility of essential oils with biopolymers ensures a controlled and sustained release of their antimicrobial constituents, effectively extending the protective capabilities of the packaging throughout the product's shelf life. Moreover, the introduction of essential oils can mitigate the drawbacks associated with synthetic additives while addressing consumer preferences for natural and eco-friendly packaging solutions [83]. Different approaches have been developed for the incorporation of essential oils in a biopolymer matrix (direct incorporation, encapsulation), which depend on the compatibility of essential oils and biopolymers.

5.1. Direct Incorporation

When a biopolymer possesses a hydrophobic character, such as in the case of cellulose acetate [84], cellulose acetate/polycaprolactone diol [83,85], or polylactide [86], EOs can be directly and uniformly incorporated into the biopolymer matrix. Some researchers have carried out direct incorporation of essential oils into a hydrocolloid matrix (cassava starch/cellulose nanofiber, sago starch, starch/chitosan, chitosan/gelatine, neat chitosan, etc.) without the addition of amphiphilic molecules using a high-sheared homogenizer (over 10,000 rpm) [87–90]. However, this method can lead to the accumulation of essential oil on the surface of the film because of the differences in polarity between essential oil and hydrocolloids. That changes the kinetics of releasing active compounds to the food surface, decreases their activity, and can also lead to the EOs oxidation if they form a layer on the top surface of the film. However, some proteins (whey proteins) have an emulsifying effect, enabling the formation of a uniform dispersion of EOs in a hydrocolloid matrix [91].

In order to achieve complete incorporation (solubility) of essential oils into hydrocolloids—water-soluble proteins and/or polysaccharides matrix, controlled release of EOs, their protection against oxidation, thermal degradation, and evaporation—with the aim of ensuring uniform dispersion into a hydrocolloid matrix, it is necessary to encapsulate them using different approaches such as emulsification, liposome formation, entrapping in biopolymers and clay-based nanocarriers, as well as in cyclodextrins. The advantages and limitations of each method of incorporation of essential oils in a biopolymer matrix are given in Table 4.

Table 4. The advantages and limitations of each method of incorporation of essential oils in a biopolymer matrix.

Method	**Direct Incorporation**	**Emulsification**	**Liposomes Formation**
The main characteristics of method	Using low energy if biopolymers possess hydrophobic character [63–66]; using a high-sheared homogenizer for hydrocolloids [67–71]	Using high-speed stirring and emulsifying agent intended for the formation of oil in water emulsion [73–82]	Dissolution of phospholipids and EOs in an organic solvent to create a lipid solution; evaporation of solvent and formation of a lipid dispersion in distilled water; size adjustment by ultrasonication.
Advantages	Shorter time for the preparation of active packaging; no additional steps –simpler procedure; can be more cost-effective	Stabilization and protection of EOs; improve their solubility in aqueous environments, provide their uniform distribution and controlled release. Nanoemulsions ensure better bioavailability of antimicrobial compounds and improved optical properties of packaging. In comparison to emulsions, nanoemulsions provide better stability to environmental conditions such as pH, temperature, and shear forces.	Targeted delivery and improved bioavailability, along with protection of ingredients and reduced undesirable reactions.
Limitations	Possible accumulation of essential oil on the surface of the film; deterioration of EO properties (oxidation, thermal degradation);	Specialized equipment and careful formulation to obtain stable formulation; Use of synthetic surfactants that can be irritable.	Complex production, difficulties in achieving consistent and desired liposome sizes, as well as the potential impact on texture, appearance, and flavor of food.
Method	Biopolymer–Based Nanostructures	Cyclodextrins	Nanoclays
The main characteristics of method	- Spray-drying by dispersing of EO in an aqueous solution of biopolymer obtain emulsion, which is pulled into the dryer through a nozzle giving small droplets (nanoparticles); - Complex coacervation when two oppositely charged biopolymers make an electrostatic complex (nanoparticles); - Electrospinning–formation of EO emulsion in aqueous biopolymer solution and fibers are formation of the fibers under an electrical field, passing through the syringe; - Covalently or self-assembly cross-linking of hydrophilic monomers or polymers (nanogels).	Mixing of EO and cyclodextrins in distilled water, stirring, filtration, and drying.	Preparation of EO and nano clay solution in an appropriate solvent. Mixing the solutions and stirring
Advantages	- Controlled release of active compounds, enhanced stability of essential oils, improved mechanical properties and durability (nanoparticles); - Can provide excellent barrier properties against gases and liquids; can be engineered to meet special requirements to gradually release antimicrobial compounds; can be transparent, which is important for packaging with special optical demands (nanofibers); - Can help maintain moisture levels in packaged foods, preventing dehydration and preserving freshness, and can improve barrier properties of packaging against oxygen and contaminants ensuring the controlled release of antimicrobial compounds over time (nanogels).	Odor and flavor control; help to maintain the sensory quality of the packaged food; they ensure protection of Eos' degradation and their slow release over time.	Improvement of mechanical and barrier properties of packaging material.

Table 4. *Cont.*

Method	Direct Incorporation	Emulsification	Liposomes Formation
Limitations	- Difficulties in achieving of uniform distribution, high cost of manufacturing, and incorporation into the packaging (nanoparticles); - Challenging scalability, commercialization, poor mechanical properties, and the high cost of their production (nanofibers); - Low level of compatibility between gels and matrix which may require some adaptations (nanogels).	High price and limited solubility in water.	Can cause reduced transparency and migration into packaged food.

5.2. Emulsification

Encapsulation by emulsification is a simple method for the compatibilization of essential oils and hydrophilic biopolymers, which requires high mechanical energy incorporated in the system and the addition of amphiphilic molecules—emulsifiers or surfactants. After the formation of EO droplets in the aqueous medium under high-speed stirring, an emulsifying agent intended for the formation of oil-in-water emulsion is added. The droplet size is mostly between 20 and 200 nm; therefore, the obtained emulsion has the prefix nano [92]. Different researchers have used surfactants (oil in water)—synthetic, mostly non-ionic Tween 20 and Tween 80, and natural ones (soya lecithin). This procedure has been applied by researchers who developed active packaging by incorporating different essential oils into films based on gelatin [93], fish gelatin [94], gelatin-chitosan [95], chitosan [96], chitosan–carboxymethyl cellulose [97], carboxymethylcellulose [98], sodium alginate/carboxymethyl cellulose [99], methylcellulose [100], whey protein isolate [101], whey protein isolate incorporated with chitosan nanofibers [102], etc. This method consists of several steps, where the first implies the dissolution of surfactant into water and the addition of essential oils to form an emulsion, followed by the addition of the obtained emulsion/nanoemulsion to the water solution of biopolymers. The formed dispersion can then be subjected to the formation of nanofibers or films by the casting method, or, in the case of edible films, directly applied to the food surface. Also, the emulsification of essential oils into a biopolymer matrix can be performed by the subsequent addition of EO and emulsifier to the biopolymer solutions and the application of ultrasound after intensive homogenization [103]. Instead of surfactants, Feng and co-authors have used starch modified by octenyl succinate anhydride with amphiphilic character to make nanoemulsion, which was incorporated into a pullulan solution to obtain biodegradable films [104].

5.3. Liposomes Formation

Liposomes are vesicles that consist of a hydrophilic core and an amphiphilic—phospholipids-based bilayer. Liposomes are categorized according to their size and lamellarity, such as small unilamellar vesicles (SUV)—with sizes in the range between 20 and 100 nm; large unilamellar vesicles (LUV)—with sizes above 100 nm; and multilamellar vesicles (MLV)—sizes above 500 nm [105]. Hydrophobic compounds, such as essential oils have been incorporated into the lipid bilayer. A procedure for the encapsulation of thyme essential oil in a liposomal chitosan-based matrix has been carried out by Al-Moghazy et al. Multilamellar and unilamellar vesicles were prepared by dissolving lecithin and essential oil in the chloroform, forming dry film, and adding chitosan solution to form dispersion, which was then subjected to stirring and sonication [106].

6. Migration of the Antimicrobial Substance into the Packaging System

The basic property of most antimicrobial packaging is based on the migration of the antimicrobial substance from the packaging matrix to the packaged food and/or the space around the food. In contrast to microbiological contamination, the migration of the active compound from the matrix is a deliberate, targeted, and necessary process to achieve the antimicrobial effect and protection of the antimicrobial package. Only proper and controlled migration of the antimicrobial substance can inhibit or reduce the proliferation of microorganisms and delay food spoilage and expiration [107].

Unlike other types of active packaging materials where the migration of the target compound does not have to be efficient, this property of antimicrobial packaging is a critical point and is largely determined by the proper release of the antimicrobial compound from the active material. Only a gradual migration of the antimicrobial agent will maintain an effective antimicrobial concentration of the target substance in the packaging system during a longer period of storage [108]. Behind this concept is the fact that antimicrobial agents must reach each microbial cell and act on them, while other compounds, such as antioxidants, can be effective without direct contact with the product and without a gradual release from the packaging matrix. A properly designed antimicrobial packaging system can protect packaged food during the long-term process of transportation and storage, with a minimal concentration of the antimicrobial agent in the food product itself [107].

However, there is one important but expected drawback of antimicrobial packaging. In addition to the desired migration of the active compound, antimicrobial packaging can also release other low-molecular-weight substances into the food. Volatile substances, polymer additives, residual monomers, or oligomers that are not bound to the packaging matrix can migrate into the packaged food [109]. The migration of undesirable molecules can change the sensory acceptability of food or even pose a risk to the consumer. Therefore, European Regulation 10/2011/EU established a regulation that packaging material that poses any risk to the health of consumers must not be included in circulation. This regulation establishes global and specific limits for concentrations of substances that migrate from packaging to packaged food. In relation to active materials, antimicrobial packaging belongs to the packaging systems covered by this regulation [110].

The term "migration" refers to the transfer of low-molecular-weight compounds from the packaging matrix to the packaged food. In polymer packaging, the migration process is characterized by great complexity, which is strongly influenced by the interaction between the food components and the packaging material [109]. Bhunia et al. [111] explained the migration mechanisms, dividing them into four main steps:

1. Diffusion of the substance from the packaging matrix;
2. Desorption from the matrix surface;
3. Sorption of the substance in the contact space;
4. Desorption into food.

This migration mechanism can be twofold, depending on whether the packaged food is in direct contact with the packaging matrix or not (Figure 2). Namely, when a packaging system is established that contains an intermediate space between the polymer matrix and the food, we speak in indirect contact, and the migration mechanism is changed. In this case, there are additional steps in the migration mechanism that involve the diffusion of migrants into the interstitial space and mass transfer through the second contact surface to the food [112]. The phenomenon of migration includes two thermodynamic and kinetic parameters, namely the distribution coefficient and the diffusion coefficient [113]. The diffusion coefficient is determined by mass transfer due to the movement of molecules from an area of high concentration to an area of low concentration until equilibrium is established. The distribution coefficient refers to the concentration balance of the substance that migrates between the packaging and the packaged food. Both coefficients will depend on the properties of the material, the antimicrobial substance, and the packaged food. All substances present in the packaging system can migrate independently of the layer and the position they occupy. Therefore, the method of production of the packaging (polymer, properties, polarity, etc.), the characteristics of the antimicrobial substance (washability and polarity), the chemical and temporal interaction between the antimicrobial substance and the polymer matrix, the characteristics of the food (composition, pH value, and humidity), and environmental factors (temperature and relative humidity) must be examined before commercial use [113].

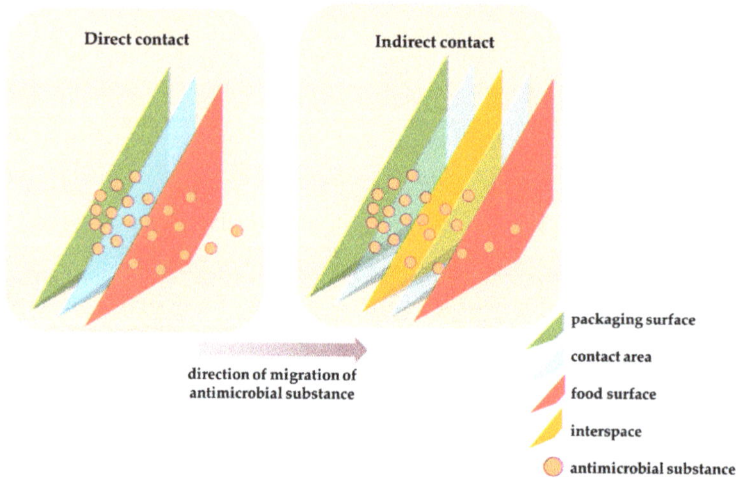

Figure 2. Direct and indirect contact between antimicrobial packaging and food sample.

For antimicrobial packaging to be effective, the active compound must be released at a minimum inhibitory concentration (MIC) level. However, this reference concentration will not only depend on the antimicrobial activity of the compound incorporated in the polymer matrix but also on the matrix itself, given that the interaction between them strongly affects the release of the active substance [114]. Therefore, the method of incorporating the active compound into the polymer matrix is extremely important. Also, when it comes to the mechanisms of migration and the interaction of the antimicrobial substance and the polymer matrix, the nature of the polymer used (natural or synthetic) plays an important role [114]. The effect of temperature and relative humidity on migration arrest is much greater in the case of biopolymer-based packaging systems compared to synthetic polymers due to the hydrophilic nature of some protein- and carbohydrate-based materials [115].

It is important to emphasize that multi-layer systems provide numerous advantages in terms of the migration of the active substance in the packaging. As for the migration process, the combination of different layers achieves a controlled release of the active compound from the packaging. From an industrial point of view, this combination can affect packaging costs, which can be another disadvantage of active packaging [114].

7. The Influence of the Packaging System on the Inactivation of Microbiological Contamination

In the last decades, materials for food packaging have been improved in several different aspects, such as the development and selection of the best packaging option, prolongation of the shelf life of food, meeting environmental requirements, etc. Modified atmosphere-, smart-, and active packaging have become essential in the improvement of food storage and protection conditions from processing and production processes, through handling and storage, to the final consumer and disposal [116]. Interestingly, about 25% of the total costs of the consumer food industry are packaging costs. It is the reason the incentive for the production of functional packaging with minimal costs and minimal impact on the environment is a priority for this century. Disciplines such as chemistry, microbiology, food science, and engineering must be involved in the production of any type of modern packaging to realize the prerequisite of an interdisciplinary base in the field of packaging materials technology [18].

Furthermore, packaging materials should not be seen as waste but as a resource. One of the best ways to achieve this result is by recycling. Many food companies have been much more interested in another way of using packaging materials: biodegradable packaging. However, a major problem is excessive costs in proportion to the amount of biodegradable material that has to be used [27]. Equally valuable are biopolymer materials that are increasingly used for the partial or complete production of packaging materials that are inert to the food matrix [26]. The time of use of food packaging is very short, so it is not economically convenient to spend a lot of money on the production of innovative materials only for the preservation and transportation of food with a short shelf life. The use of biodegradable or biopolymer materials could be a good alternative to reduce environmental impact. The choice of the most suitable packaging depends on several factors, primarily on the type of food that must be protected. Some of the most important properties of packaging are mechanical, physical-chemical, and optical properties, which play a key role in choosing the appropriate material [26,27,116,117].

Today's trends in developed countries related to fresh, minimally processed, easy-to-prepare, and RTE foods represent major challenges in terms of the microbiological safety and quality of these foods. A similar problem arises in the course of globalization, i.e., the distribution of food from centralized industrial systems to the whole world [15]. This flow of the food industry also means the production of food with an extended shelf life to ensure the global market. Consequently, the presence and potential of microbiological contamination are extremely high, reducing shelf life and increasing the risk of foodborne illness. Therefore, the entire food industry is directed towards innovative ways of inhibiting microbial growth in food while maintaining quality, freshness, safety, and expiration dates [118].

Although the primary idea of inactivating microbiological contamination was related to improvements in traditional food preservation methods (drying, heating, freezing, fermentation, salting, etc.), it was quickly realized that no single method is comprehensive and is not the right solution for inhibiting the growth of microorganisms and preventing food spoilage completely. One of the innovative strategies to extend the shelf life of food is the addition of antimicrobial substances to food, which has also had a limited effect given that most consumers want high-quality food without preservatives [119]. Also, the direct surface application of antimicrobial substances to food is restricted due to the rapid diffusion from the surface into the food mass, which causes only a momentary reduction of the microbial population [120]. However, this strategy was retained in the food industry but received a different performance. Namely, the research on antimicrobial agents of natural origin that prevent the growth of microorganisms is aimed at the use of special packaging systems with an antimicrobial effect to ensure increased food safety and quality [117].

As already mentioned, the primary function of packaging is related to the protection of food from external influences, mechanical force, and spoilage by environmental microorganisms, moisture, gases, dust, odors, etc. [117]. Also, the packaging is very important from the point of view of marketing and standardization because it can be used as an informative asset for consumers. Sung et al. [117] emphasize that in this way useful information is provided to consumers, and the product itself is made more usable and practical. On the other hand, the antimicrobial food packaging system is a modern concept of active packaging and represents one of the most perceptive concepts for food safety and quality [121].

Packaging with antimicrobial activity is reflected in a physical combination of two or more chemically different phases, where one of the phases is the matrix of the packaging, while the other phases are in the form of embedded substances with antimicrobial properties [122]. One important advantage of antimicrobial packaging is that it is a more effective system than directly adding an antimicrobial agent to food. The reason for this advantage is the time-limited and controlled release of the antimicrobial substance or the identical but direct contact with food, which is achieved by different methods of addition and retention of the phase in the basic matrix phase of the packaging [117].

In other words, the use of polymeric materials as a matrix phase (carrier) of antimicrobial agents has a consequent, threefold role, as presented in Figure 3 [120].

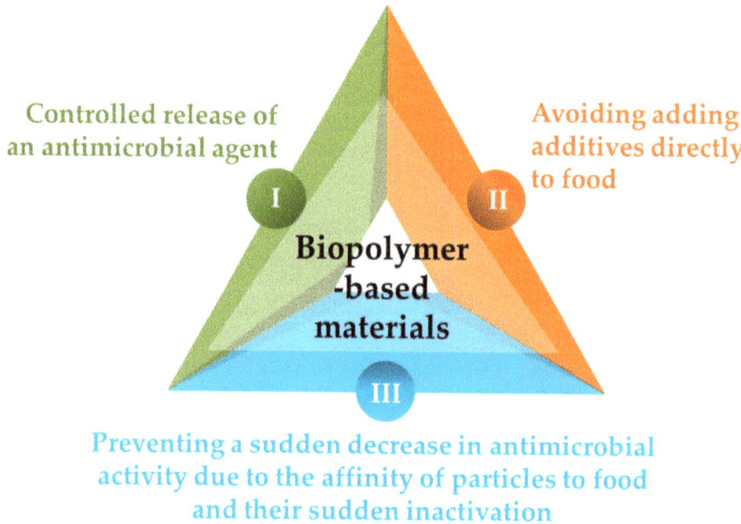

Figure 3. The requirements of biopolymer-based materials as a carrier for antimicrobials.

According to Radusin et al. [121], antimicrobial substances incorporated into packaging systems have one of three types of mechanisms of action on microorganism cells: destruction of the cell wall and/or membrane, inhibition of enzymes in the cell, or destruction of genetic material. Antimicrobial substances include inorganic metal compounds (silver, titanium dioxide, zinc oxide, magnesium oxide, etc.), organic acids (sorbic, citric, propanoic, etc.), enzymes (lysozyme, lactoferrin, etc.), bacteriocins (nisin, pediocin, etc.), fungicides (benomyl, imazalil, etc.), poymers (chitosan), natural extracts (bay leaf, oregano, lemon grass, etc.), antibiotics (natamycin), surfactants (lauric arginate), and other compounds (phenolic, Maillard reaction products, etc.). Regardless of which substance it is, the selection of suitable packaging material should be based on its spectrum and mode of action, chemical composition, and speed of action [122,123].

It most often happens that a certain antimicrobial substance is effective only on one group of microorganisms. That is why silver ions are often used due to the wide spectrum of antimicrobial activity against gram-negative and gram-positive bacteria, fungi, protozoa, and certain viruses [122,124]. In addition to silver, metal oxides such as TiO_2, ZnO, and MgO have antibacterial activity attributed to their effect on the cell's respiratory system (creating reactive oxygen). Titanium dioxide is non-toxic and has been approved by the FDA for use in food, drugs, and food contact materials [125]. On the other hand, ZnO particles in contact with microbial cells can act bacteriostatically or bacteriocidally depending on the concentration of the compound, but they act equally well on gram-positive and -negative bacteria [122]. For now, the only assumed bactericidal mechanism of MgO is related to the production of high concentrations of superoxide anions on its surface, which react with the carboxyl groups of peptide bonds in bacterial cells, thereby destroying them [122]. Antimicrobial activity has been observed with other metals, semimetals, and alkaline earth metals, especially in the form of nanoparticles (CdSe, CdTe, Au, Al_2O_3, and iron oxides) [117].

In recent years, the use of inorganic nanoparticles as antimicrobial substances in packaging materials has particularly intensified. This is attributed to the good stability of these materials and their ability to withstand process conditions such as high pressures and temperatures in plastic manufacturing processes [126]. In addition, organic acids have a long history as food preservatives with GRAS status, most of which do not have an acceptable daily intake limit for humans. As for enzymes as antimicrobial agents, lysozyme is the most widely used. It is often incorporated into packaging films, where, in contact with the microbial cell, it hydrolyzes or dissolves the cell wall [127]. Also, recent scientific works suggest that the effect of lysozyme is enhanced in the presence of detergents and chelates, or that the enzymatic effect of this substance can be enhanced by the addition of lactoferrin [117]. As a bacteriogenic product, bacteriocins have gained GRAS status and are used as natural antimicrobial substances. For example, nisin, which is produced by Lactococcus lactis, can protect this bacterium against Listeria, Staphylococcus, Bacillus, and Clostridium. Nisin is an interesting choice for incorporation into antimicrobial packaging on an industrial level, as it interacts with the microbial surface and does not need to be incorporated into the matrix to exert its effect [128]. Natamycin is a natural antifungal agent produced by the bacterium Streptomyces natelensis during fermentation. It is widely used in the food industry to prevent fungal contamination in meat, cheese, and fruit. It is approved as a food additive (E235) in over 40 countries, carrying GRAS status. Natamycin is an effective compound that acts specifically by binding to ergosterol, thereby inhibiting vacuolar fusion. Due to this mechanism of action, it is active against molds and yeasts but not against bacteria and viruses [129]. Natamycin has an advantage over other preservatives because it does not affect the taste and the appearance of the final product [130].

A wide variety of natural extracts, such as pigments, garlic, lemongrass, cinnamon, cloves, and oregano, have shown antimicrobial activity in packaging material against a large number of bacterial pathogens [131]. The most common mechanism of action of these substances is disruption of the cell and mitochondrial membrane, which leads to disruption of the cell membrane, cytoplasmic leakage, cell lysis, and, finally, death. However, the negative side of adding plant extracts is the possibility of adding them in low concentrations due to their effect on the smell and taste of food. In addition, these extracts are susceptible to lipid oxidation [132].

Finally, it should be emphasized that the direct addition of an antimicrobial substance to food can reduce food quality, changing the organoleptic and textural qualities of food [117]. Consequently, packaging with an antimicrobial effect will play a very important role in inhibiting the growth of targeted microorganisms on/in food while simultaneously improving food safety and extending shelf life without loss of quality.

8. Proposal for Comprehensive Determination of Antimicrobial Potential of Biopolymer-Based Active Packaging with Incorporated Essential Oils

While in vitro studies provide valuable insights into the antimicrobial properties of biopolymer-based active packaging, they have limitations and should be complemented with in vivo experiments on the specific food products the packaging is designed for. Generally, when it comes to testing the antimicrobial potential of newly designed biopolymer-based active packaging with incorporated essential oils, researchers should follow these steps:

1. Preliminary antimicrobial analysis of the selected essential oils by disc-diffusion method;
2. Determination of the minimal inhibition concentration (MIC) of the selected essential oils;
3. In vitro assessment of the antimicrobial activity of active packaging systems;
4. In vivo assessment of the antimicrobial activity of active packaging systems;
5. Sensory analysis.

As presented in Figure 4, the first mandatory step in testing the antimicrobial potential of active packaging prepared with various essential oils should be the examination of the antimicrobial activity of the essential oils themselves. The most common approach when testing the antimicrobial activity of the essential oils is to first examine them using the disc-diffusion method. This method is relatively cheap and easy to perform, so it is a choice of many authors [133–136]. The method consists of several steps: (i) activation of the chosen microorganisms on a suitable culture medium; (ii) preparation of cell suspension with an approximate concentration of 10^6 CFU/mL; (iii) homogenization of 1 mL of cell suspension with 9 mL of melted and tempered culture medium, which should be poured into Petri dishes; (iv) after the solidification, the sterile discs (6 mm in diameter) should be placed onto the inoculated medium; (v) on each disc, an aliquot of 15 μL of the tested essential oil and suitable positive and negative controls is applied; and (vi) after the incubation period, the diameter of the halo zone can be measured for each disc and expressed in mm [134].

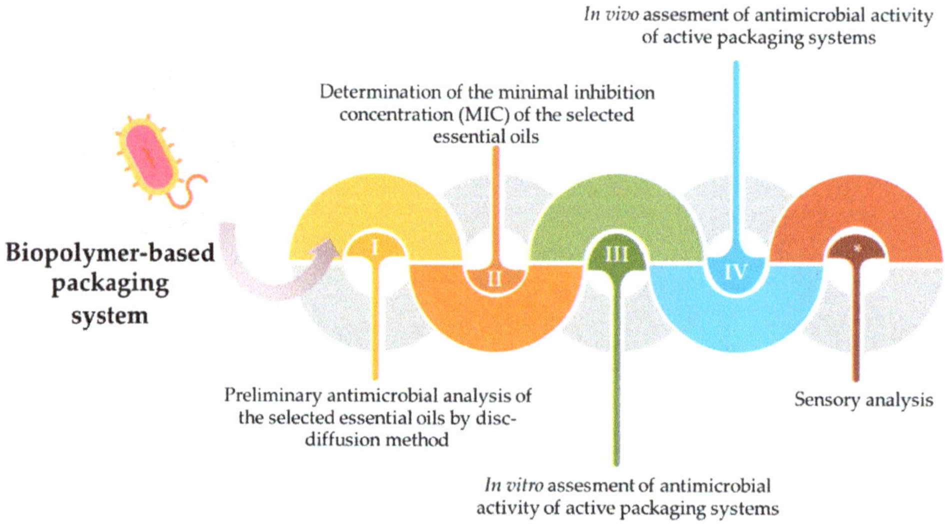

Figure 4. Traceability of steps in antimicrobial potential and sensory testing of packaging systems that involves biopolimer-based carrier and essential oil(s).

In order to obtain the minimal inhibitory concentration (MIC) of the selected essential oil capable of inhibiting microbial growth up to 90%, the microdilution method is usually employed. The preparation of cell suspension is performed in the same manner as the previously described disc diffusion method. Afterwards, the serial dilutions of the tested essential oil were prepared, and equal volumes (100 μL) of each dilution and inoculated media were transferred to a sterile flat-bottom, 96-well microtiter plates. After the period of incubation, 100 μL of mixture from each well was poured into Petri dishes and homogenized with suitable culture media. Petri dishes are commonly incubated under the same conditions as microtiter plates, and the grown colonies are enumerated by viable count. The final results of the MIC determination are calculated as follows:

$$100 \times \frac{(N_c - N_t)}{N_c} \ (\%)$$

where N_c is a number of cells in a positive control and N_t is a number of cells after the contact of essential oil dilution and microbial cells. This method seems to be indispensable when testing compounds with promising antimicrobial effects [137–139].

In vitro assesment of antimicrobial activity of active packaging systems involves conducting laboratory experiments to evaluate the effectiveness of each packaging layer in inhibiting the growth of microorganisms that can spoil or contaminate food products. In this step, it is very important to test each layer individually and their combinations to ensure their activity against the selected microorganisms [70]. Also, the choice of relevant microorganisms that are commonly associated with food spoilage or contamination is crucial. When the packaging materials and microorganisms are chosen, the disc diffusion method and the determination of minimal inhibitory concentration should be performed as previously described. It should be pointed out that control experiments must always be an integral part of the experiments related to the evaluation of antimicrobial activity. When testing active packaging systems, control experiments refer to the use of packaging materials without antimicrobial agents to establish a baseline for microbial growth inhibition. Also, the testing is completed using positive controls by using known antimicrobial substances (antibiotics, antimycotics, etc.) to validate the experimental setup. Finally, it is important to perform multiple replicates of the experiments to ensure the reliability and statistical significance of the results. Some authors suggest that when preparing the active packaging systems with two or more antimicrobial agents, their synergistic effects have to be examined [140,141]. By mixing various antimicrobial agents and through their synergistic activity, many advantages can be expected: (i) induction of stronger antimicrobial activity; (ii) the extension of the spectrum of antimicrobial action; and (iii) the prevention and suppression of the regrowth of undesirable microorganisms [141]. However, further analysis, including in vivo trials, are essential to validate the exact effectiveness of active packaging systems under practical conditions.

In vivo assessment of the antimicrobial activity of active packaging systems involves conducting experiments in real-life conditions to evaluate the effectiveness of packaging materials in inhibiting the growth of microorganisms and preserving the quality and safety of food products. Unlike in vitro assessments, which are conducted in controlled laboratory settings, in vivo assessments provide a more realistic understanding of how active packaging systems perform in practical situations. After choosing the relevant microorganisms or pathogens that are likely to affect the quality and safety of the specific food being packaged, their suspension should be made, and the selected food should be artificially contaminated with them. Afterwards, the active packaging materials with antimicrobial agents can be placed on the selected food, ensuring direct contact with it. The packaged food is then stored under the conditions that simulate the intended storage environment (temperature, humidity, etc.), and periodically, the samples of the packaged food are performed to assess microbial populations over time. The common microbial analyses that are conducted for this purpose are colony counting by using standardized methods [142], PCR (polymerase chain reaction), or some statistical analysis to avoid more complex destructive methods of analysis [70]. Also, in this type of analysis, comparative studies should be incorporated. Comparative studies are related to testing the same food product using traditional or non-active packaging systems at the same time and under the same conditions as the active packaging systems. This allows a direct comparison of the antimicrobial effects of the newly designed active packaging system with the old-fashioned one. Since essential oils, hydrolates, or some plant extracts are commonly used as active ingredients in active packaging, sensory analysis must be conducted when such a packaging system comes into direct contact with food.

Sensory analysis of active packaging systems involves evaluating how the packaging materials affect the sensory attributes (taste, smell, appearance, and texture) of the packaged food products. This type of analysis helps determine whether the active packaging materials introduce any changes in the sensory qualities of the food, which can influence consumer perception and acceptance. In order to perform sensory tests, a panel of trained sensory analysts or consumers who are skilled in evaluating food products should be recruited [143]. The sensory analysts should consume food products prepared with and without an active packaging system. It is very important to ensure that the packaging is consistent and that any differences are solely due to the active packaging system. Also, to prevent bias, the samples should be coded or numbered and randomized during the presentation to the sensory panel. For this purpose, different sensory tests can be used [144]:

1. Difference Test—determine if there are detectable differences between food samples packaged with and without active ingredients;
2. Descriptive Analysis—evaluate specific sensory attributes (e.g., taste, odor, texture) and quantify the intensity of these attributes using a trained panel;
3. Consumer Acceptance Test—Assess consumer preferences and overall acceptance of the food products with active packaging systems compared to controls.

The results obtained by the sensory panel should be interpreted and analyzed to determine if there are any noticeable sensory changes introduced by the active packaging system, taking into account whether these changes are acceptable to consumers or if they may impact the marketability of the product. Moreover, the results of sensory analysis can be compared with the data obtained during microbial analysis in order to understand if any changes in sensory attributes correspond to changes in microbial populations.

Sensory analysis of active packaging systems is crucial for ensuring that the packaging materials do not adversely affect the sensory characteristics of the food products. This information is essential for product development, quality control, and consumer acceptance.

9. Conclusions and Future Perspectives for Real Application

The incorporation of essential oils as antimicrobial substances within biopolymer-based active packaging has demonstrated the packaging material's antimicrobial efficacy. The bioactive compounds inherent in essential oils exhibit pronounced inhibitory effects against a spectrum of pathogenic and spoilage microorganisms, thereby manifesting a tangible extension of the shelf life of packaged commodities. This innovative approach offers a more sustainable alternative by mitigating reliance on conventional synthetic antimicrobial additives, thereby aligning with the contemporary drive for sustainable packaging modalities. The strategic incorporation of essential oils into biopolymeric matrices constitutes a propitious intervention, effectively attenuating the reliance on chemical preservatives and satisfying the increasing demand for environmentally based packaging solutions. The consequential elongation of product shelf life is a noteworthy outcome of this integration, notably benefiting perishable commodities encompassing many food items. The noticeable inhibition effect on spoilage microorganism proliferation is crucial in solving the perishability predicament that compromises product quality. Moreover, the incorporation of essential oils can offer ancillary advantages, particularly in the realm of flavor preservation. The aromatic origin of essential oils imparts a natural flavor profile to packaged foods, thereby augmenting their sensorial allure.

By addressing these critical fronts, the integration of essential oils within biopolymer-based active packaging is poised to substantiate its role as a pivotal stride towards efficacious and sustainable food preservation patterns. However, the journey is not without challenges, especially concerning essential oil volatility and compatibility within diverse biopolymer matrices. The vulnerability of essential oils to gradual volatilization underscores the need for meticulous considerations to ensure sustained antimicrobial efficacy. Furthermore, the homogenous dispersion or encapsulation of essential oils within packaging materials necessitates precise techniques due to the intricate nature of the process. The regulatory landscape also requires attention, as the utilization of essential oils in active packaging calls for adherence to rigorous safety and food contact standards. The variability in permissible concentrations across jurisdictions accentuates the need for strict regulatory compliance. The exploration of synergistic interactions among essential oils and other antimicrobial agents offers a promising avenue to enhance antimicrobial potency further. Understanding the mechanistic nuances underlying these interactions opens novel avenues to fortify the antimicrobial efficacy of active packaging materials. Moving forward, research endeavors should focus on optimizing formulation techniques, refining processing methodologies, and elucidating the long-term stability and controlled release kinetics of essential oil-infused packaging materials under varying storage conditions. Addressing these critical aspects will underpin the integration of essential oils within biopolymer-based active packaging as a pivotal step toward effective and sustainable food preservation strategies. The symbiotic alliance between essential oils and biopolymers holds immense potential for redefining packaging's role in ensuring food safety and longevity while aligning with evolving environmental paradigms. Sensory evaluations discerning alterations in sensory attributes and preferences are imperative in refining the formulation of biopolymer-based packaging fortified with essential oils. Prospective research trajectories should endeavor to optimize formulation methodologies, augment processing techniques, and illuminate the long-term stability and controlled release kinetics of essential oil-infused packaging across varying storage conditions.

In conclusion, the integration of essential oils as potent antimicrobial agents within biopolymer-based active packaging materials represents a transformative advancement in the realm of food preservation and packaging. The incorporation of essential oils and biopolymers synergistically marries the innate antimicrobial attributes of the former with the structural advantages and eco-friendliness of the latter. This convergence not only bolsters packaging's role in safeguarding product quality and shelf life but also resonates with the global call for sustainable packaging solutions. Crucially, the selection of appropriate biopolymers is an essential determinant of the success of active packaging systems. Different biopolymers bring distinct mechanical, barrier, and compatibility properties to the table, influencing the overall performance and practicality of the packaging. The adaptability of essential oils to diverse biopolymers is a testament to their versatility, with each combination offering a unique and tailored approach to combating microbial proliferation. Furthermore, the dynamic landscape of consumer preferences underscores the need for a holistic evaluation of the sensory attributes imparted by essential oils in packaged products. As consumers increasingly seek natural and minimally processed alternatives, the interplay between essential oils, flavors, and product quality gains paramount significance. Looking ahead, continued research is indispensable in fine-tuning the formulation and processing techniques of essential oil-infused packaging materials. The optimization of factors like essential oil concentrations, release kinetics, and shelf stability will pave the way for robust and scalable applications. Collaboration across multidisciplinary domains, encompassing chemistry, packaging engineering, microbiology, and consumer studies, holds the potential to yield comprehensive solutions that address both technical and consumer-driven challenges. The alignment of industry efforts and academic exploration will drive innovation in antimicrobial active packaging, propelling it from a nascent concept to a standard practice in ensuring food safety and extending shelf life. In summary, the integration of essential oils within biopolymer-based active packaging encapsulates a dynamic convergence of science, sustainability, and sensory appeal. By harnessing the power of nature's antimicrobial arsenal and the ingenuity of biopolymers, this interdisciplinary approach forges a path toward safer, longer-lasting, and more environmentally conscious food products. The journey is ongoing, but the strides made so far signify a promising future where essential oil-infused packaging stands as a cornerstone in the modern food packaging landscape.

Author Contributions: Conceptualization, O.Š. and T.E.; investigation, A.T.; resources, O.Š. and T.E.; writing—original draft preparation, O.Š. and T.E.; writing—review and editing, A.T.; visualization, O.Š. All authors have read and agreed to the published version of the manuscript.

Funding: This research was funded by the Ministry of Education, Science, and Technological Development of the Republic of Serbia (grant no. 451-03-68/2023-14/200134) and Provincial Secretariat for Higher Education and Scientific Research of AP Vojvodina (grants no. 142-451-3106/2022-01 and 142-451-2657/2021-01).

Institutional Review Board Statement: Not applicable.

Informed Consent Statement: Not applicable.

Data Availability Statement: Not applicable.

Conflicts of Interest: The authors declare no conflict of interest.

References

1. Kumar, R.; Verma, A.; Shome, A.; Sinha, R.; Sinha, S.; Jha, P.K.; Kumar, R.; Kumar, P.; Shubham; Das, S.; et al. Impacts of Plastic Pollution on Ecosystem Services, Sustainable Development Goals, and Need to Focus on Circular Economy and Policy Interventions. *Sustainability* **2021**, *13*, 9963. [CrossRef]
2. Nielsen, T.D.; Hasselbalch, J.; Holmberg, K.; Stripple, J. Politics and the plastic crisis: A review throughout the plastic life cycle. *Wiley Interdiscip. Rev. Energy Environ.* **2020**, *9*, e360. [CrossRef]
3. Mangaraj, S.; Yadav, A.; Bal, L.M.; Dash, S.K.; Mahanti, N.K. Application of Biodegradable Polymers in Food Packaging Industry: A Comprehensive Review. *J. Package Technol. Res.* **2019**, *3*, 77–96. [CrossRef]

4. Alizadeh-Sani, M.; Khezerlou, A.; Ehsani, A. Fabrication and characterization of the bionanocomposite film based on whey protein biopolymer loaded with TiO_2 nanoparticles, cellulose nanofibers and rosemary essential oil. *Ind. Crop. Prod.* **2018**, *124*, 300–315. [CrossRef]
5. Ishangulyyev, R.; Kim, S.; Lee, S.H. Understanding Food Loss and Waste—Why Are We Losing and Wasting Food? *Foods* **2019**, *8*, 297. [CrossRef] [PubMed]
6. Li, X.; Yang, X.; Deng, H.; Guo, Y.; Xue, J. Gelatin films incorporated with thymol nanoemulsions: Physical properties and an-timicrobial activities. *Int. J. Biol. Macromol.* **2020**, *150*, 161–168. [CrossRef]
7. Zubair, M.; Shahzad, S.; Hussain, A.; Pradhan, R.A.; Arshad, M.; Ullah, A. Current Trends in the Utilization of Essential Oils for Polysaccharide- and Protein-Derived Food Packaging Materials. *Polymers* **2022**, *14*, 1146. [CrossRef]
8. Newell, D.G.; Koopmans, M.; Verhoef, L.; Duizer, E.; Aidara-Kane, A.; Sprong, H.; Opsteegh, M.; Langelaar, M.; Threfall, J.; Scheutz, F.; et al. Food-borne diseases—The challenges of 20 years ago still persist while new ones continue to emerge. *Int. J. Food Microbiol.* **2010**, *139*, S3–S15. [CrossRef]
9. Cantas, L.; Suer, K. The Important Bacterial Zoonoses in "One Health" Concept. *Front. Public Health* **2014**, *2*, 144. [CrossRef]
10. Rahman, M.T.; Sobur, M.A.; Islam, M.S.; Ievy, S.; Hossain, M.J.; El Zowalaty, M.E.; Rahman, A.T.; Ashour, H.M. Zoonotic Diseases: Etiology, Impact, and Control. *Microorganisms* **2020**, *8*, 1405. [CrossRef]
11. Dowling, A.; O'Dwyer, J.; Adler, C. Alternatives to antibiotics-future trends. In *Microbial Pathogens and Strategies for Combating then: Science, Technology and Education*; Microbiology Book Series; Formatex Research Center: Badajoz, Spain, 2013; pp. 216–226.
12. Bazy, M.B.; Hoffmann, S.; Moris, J.G. Ranking the Disease Burden of 14 Pathogens in Food Sources in the United States Using Attribution Data from Outbreak Investigations and Expert Elicitation. *J. Food Prot.* **2012**, *75*, 1278–1291.
13. Johnson, N.B.; Hayes, L.D.; Brown, K.; Hoo, E.C.; Ethier, K.A. *CDC National Health Report: Leading Causes of Morbidity and Mortality and Associated Behavioral Risk and Protective Factors—United States, 2005–2013*; MMWR Suppl.; Centers for Disease Control and Prevention (CDC): Atlanta, GA, USA, 2014; Volume 63, pp. 3–27.
14. FDA. Foodborne Illness-Causing Organisms in the U.S. Factsheet. 2015. Available online: http://www.fda.gov/downloads/Food/FoodborneIllnessContaminants/UCM187482.pdf (accessed on 25 December 2022).
15. Karl, R.; Matthews, K.E.; Montville, T.J. *Food Microbiology: An Introduction*, 4th ed.; John Wiley & Sons: Hoboken, NJ, USA, 2017.
16. Cvetković, D.; Markov, S.; Ranitović, A. *Mikrobiološka Kontrola Bioprocesa, Praktikum ZA Studente Tehnološkog Fakulteta Novi Sad*; Tehnološki fakultet Novi Sad, Univerzitet u Novom Sadu: Novi Sad, Srbija, 2017.
17. Markov, S. *Mikrobiologija, Udžbenik ZA Studente Tehnološkog Fakulteta Novi Sad*; Tehnološki fakultet Novi Sad, Univerzitet u Novom Sadu: Novi Sad, Srbija, 2012.
18. Caya, J.G. Clostridium botulinum and the Ophthalmologist: A Review of Botulism, Including Biological Warfare Ramifications of Botulinum Toxin. *Surv. Ophthalmol.* **2001**, *46*, 25–34. [CrossRef]
19. Meloni, D.; Consolati, S.G.; Mazza, R.; Mureddu, A.; Fois, F.; Piras, F.; Mazzette, R. Presence and molecular characterization of the major serovars of Listeria monocytogenes in ten Sardinian fermented sausage processing plants. *Meat Sci.* **2014**, *97*, 443–450. [CrossRef] [PubMed]
20. Deacon, J. *Fungal Biology*, 4th ed.; Blackwell Publishing: Malden, MA, USA, 2006; ISBN 10:1-4051-3066-0.
21. Pitt, J.I.; Hocking, A.D. *Fungi and Food Spoilage*, 3rd ed.; Springer: Boston, MA, USA, 2009; ISBN 978-0-387-92206-5.
22. Wyatt, T.T.; Wösten, H.A.; Dijksterhuis, J. Fungal Spores for Dispersion in Space and Time. *Adv. Appl. Microbiol.* **2013**, *85*, 43–91. [CrossRef] [PubMed]
23. Sofi, S.; Singh, J.; Rafiq, S.; Ashraf, U.; Dar, B.; Nayik, G.A. A Comprehensive Review on Antimicrobial Packaging and its Use in Food Packaging. *Curr. Nutr. Food Sci.* **2018**, *14*, 305–312. [CrossRef]
24. White, D.G.; Zhao, S.; Simjee, S.; Wagner, D.D.; McDermott, P.F. Antimicrobial resistance of foodborne pathogens. *Microbes Infect.* **2002**, *4*, 405–412. [CrossRef] [PubMed]
25. Lynch, M.F.; Tauxe, R.V.; Hedberg, C.W. The growing burden of foodborne outbreaks due to contaminated fresh produce: Risks and opportunities. *Epidemiol. Infect.* **2009**, *137*, 307–315. [CrossRef] [PubMed]
26. Karaman, R.; Jubeh, B.; Breijyeh, Z. Resistance of Gram-Positive Bacteria to Current Antibacterial Agents and Overcoming Approaches. *Molecules* **2020**, *25*, 2888. [CrossRef]
27. Contreras, C.B.; Charles, G.; Toselli, R.; Strumia, M.C. Antimicrobial Active Packaging. In *Biopackaging*; CRC Press: Boca Raton, FL, USA, 2009; ISBN 9781315152349.
28. Dybka-Stępień, K.; Antolak, H.; Kmiotek, M.; Piechota, D.; Koziróg, A. Disposable Food Packaging and Serving Materials—Trends and Biodegradability. *Polymers* **2021**, *13*, 3606. [CrossRef]
29. Wang, X.; Ma, L.; Yan, S.; Chen, X.; Growe, A. Trade for Food Security: The Stability of Global Agricultural Trade Networks. *Foods* **2023**, *12*, 271. [CrossRef]
30. Suvarna, V.; Nair, A.; Mallya, R.; Khan, T.; Omri, A. Antimicrobial Nanomaterials for Food Packaging. *Antibiotics* **2022**, *11*, 729. [CrossRef] [PubMed]
31. Travičić, V.; Cvanić, T.; Cetković, G. Plant-Based Nano-Emulsions as Edible Coatings in the Extension of Fruits and Vegetables Shelf Life: A Patent Review. *Foods* **2023**, *12*, 2535. [CrossRef] [PubMed]
32. Xiao, Z.; Liu, W.; Zhu, G.; Zhou, R.; Niu, Y. Production and characterization of multinuclear microcapsules encapsulating lavender oil by complex coacervation. *Flavour. Fragr. J.* **2014**, *29*, 166–172. [CrossRef]

33. Chen, M.; Hu, Y.; Zhou, J.; Xie, Y.; Wu, H.; Yuan, T.; Yang, Z. Facile fabrication of tea tree oil-loaded antibacterial microcapsules by complex coacervation of sodium alginate/quaternary ammonium salt of chitosan. *RSC Adv.* **2016**, *6*, 13032–13039. [CrossRef]
34. de Matos, E.F.; Scopel, B.S.; Dettmer, A. Citronella essential oil microencapsulation by complex coacervation with leather waste gelatin and sodium alginate. *J. Environ. Chem. Eng.* **2018**, *6*, 1989–1994. [CrossRef]
35. Koupantsis, T.; Paraskevopoulou, A. Flavor retention in sodium caseinate—Carboxymethylcellulose complex coacervates as a function of storage conditions. *Food Hydrocoll.* **2017**, *69*, 459–465. [CrossRef]
36. Rojas-Moreno, S.; Osorio-Revilla, G.; Gallardo-Velázquez, T.; Cárdenas-Bailón, F.; Meza-Márquez, G. Effect of the cross-linking agent and drying method on encapsulation efficiency of orange essential oil by complex coacervation using whey protein isolate with different polysaccharides. *J. Microencapsul.* **2018**, *35*, 165–180. [CrossRef]
37. Rojas-Moreno, S.; Cardenas-Bailon, F.; Osorio-Revilla, G.; Gallardo Velazquez, T.; Proal-Najera, J. Effects of complex coacer-vation-spray drying and conventional spray drying on the quality of microencapsulated orange essential oil. *J. Food Meas. Charact.* **2018**, *12*, 650–660. [CrossRef]
38. Dima, C.; Cotârlet, M.; Alexe, P.; Dima, S. Microencapsulation of essential oil of pimento [*Pimenta dioica* (L.) *Merr.*] by chitosan/k-carrageenan complex coacervation method. *Innov. Food Sci. Emerg. Technol.* **2014**, *22*, 203–211. [CrossRef]
39. Shen, L.; Chen, J.; Bai, Y.; Ma, Z.; Huang, J.; Feng, W. Physical Properties and Stabilization of Microcapsules Containing Thyme Oil by Complex Coacervation. *J. Food Sci.* **2016**, *81*, N2258–N2262. [CrossRef]
40. Ban, Z.; Zhang, J.; Li, L.; Luo, Z.; Wang, Y.; Yuan, Q.; Zhou, B.; Liu, H. Ginger essential oil-based microencapsulation as an efficient delivery system for the improvement of Jujube (*Ziziphus jujuba* Mill.) fruit quality. *Food Chem.* **2020**, *306*, 125628. [CrossRef] [PubMed]
41. Yang, Z.; Peng, Z.; Li, J.; Li, S.; Kong, L.; Li, P.; Wang, Q. Development and evaluation of novel flavor microcapsules containing vanilla oil using a complex coacervation approach. *Food Chem.* **2014**, *145*, 272–277. [CrossRef]
42. Lin, L.; Gu, Y.; Cui, H. Moringa oil/chitosan nanoparticles embedded gelatin nanofibers for food packaging against Listeria monocytogenes and Staphylococcus aureus on cheese. *Food Packag. Shelf Life* **2019**, *19*, 86–93. [CrossRef]
43. Lin, L.; Mao, X.; Sun, Y.; Rajivgandhi, G.; Cui, H. Antibacterial properties of nanofibers containing chrysanthemum essential oil and their application as beef packaging. *Int. J. Food Microbiol.* **2019**, *292*, 21–30. [CrossRef] [PubMed]
44. Vafania, B.; Fathi, M.; Soleimanian-Zad, S. Nanoencapsulation of thyme essential oil in chitosan-gelatin nanofibers by noz-zle-less electrospinning and their application to reduce nitrite in sausages. *Food Bioprod. Process* **2019**, *116*, 240–248. [CrossRef]
45. Göksen, G.; Fabra, M.J.; Ekiz, H.I.; López-Rubio, A. Phytochemical-loaded electrospun nanofibers as novel active edible films: Characterization and antibacterial efficiency in cheese slices. *Food Control.* **2020**, *112*, 107133. [CrossRef]
46. Ghayempour, S.; Montazer, M. A novel controlled release system based on Tragacanth nanofibers loaded Peppermint oil. *Carbohydr. Polym.* **2019**, *205*, 589–595. [CrossRef]
47. Rafiq, M.; Hussain, T.; Abid, S.; Nazir, A.; Masood, R. Development of sodium alginate/PVA antibacterial nanofibers by the incorporation of essential oils. *Mater. Res. Express* **2018**, *5*, 035007. [CrossRef]
48. Jafari, S.M. *Nanoencapsulation Technologies for the Food and Nutraceutical Industries*; Academic Press: Cambridge, MA, USA, 2017; pp. 1–34.
49. Rajaei, A.; Hadian, M.; Mohsenifar, A.; Rahmani-Cherati, T.; Tabatabaei, M. A coating based on clove essential oils encapsulated by chitosan-myristic acid nanogel efficiently enhanced the shelf-life of beef cutlets. *Food Packag. Shelf Life* **2017**, *14*, 137–145. [CrossRef]
50. Medeiros, J.; Blick, A.; Galindo, M.; Alvim, I.; Yamashita, F.; Ueno, C.; Shirai, M.; Grosso, C.; Corradini, E.; Sakanaka, L. Incorporation of Oregano Essential Oil Microcapsules in Starch-Poly (Butylene Adipate Co-Terephthalate) (PBAT) Films. *Mac-Romol Symp.* **2019**, *383*, 1800052. [CrossRef]
51. Parris, N.; Cooke, P.H.; Hicks, K.B. Encapsulation of Essential Oils in Zein Nanospherical Particles. *J. Agric. Food Chem.* **2005**, *53*, 4788–4792. [CrossRef] [PubMed]
52. Aguiar, M.C.S.; das Gracas Fernandes da Silva, M.F.; Fernandes, J.B.; Forim, M.R. Evaluation of the microencapsulation of orange essential oil in biopolymers by using a spray-drying process. *Sci. Rep.* **2020**, *10*, 11799. [CrossRef] [PubMed]
53. Cui, H.; Xu, R.; Hu, W.; Li, C.; Abdel-Samie, M.A.; Lin, L. Effect of soy protein isolate nanoparticles loaded with litsea cubeba essential oil on performance of lentinan edible films. *Int. J. Biol. Macromol.* **2023**, *242*, 124686. [CrossRef] [PubMed]
54. Kord Heydari, M.; Assadpour, E.; Jafari, S.M.; Javadian, H. Encapsulation of rose essential oil using whey protein concen-trate-pectin nanocomplexes: Optimization of the effective parameters. *Food Chem.* **2021**, *356*, 129731. [CrossRef] [PubMed]
55. Sharma, S.; Mulrey, L.; Byrne, M.; Jaiswal, A.K.; Jaiswal, S. Encapsulation of Essential Oils in Nanocarriers for Active Food Packaging. *Foods* **2022**, *11*, 2337. [CrossRef]
56. de Oliveira, E.F.; Paula, H.C.; de Paula, R.C. Alginate/cashew gum nanoparticles for essential oil encapsulation. *Colloids Surf. B* **2014**, *113*, 146–151. [CrossRef]
57. Ozdemir, N.; Bayrak, A.; Tat, T.; Altay, F.; Kiralan, M.; Kurt, A. Microencapsulation of basil essential oil: Utilization of gum arabic/whey protein iso-late/maltodextrin combinations for encapsulation efficiency and in vitro release. *Food Meas.* **2021**, *15*, 1865–1876. [CrossRef]
58. Hilmaier-Delgadillo, F.; Lara-Espinoza, C.L.; Félix-Arias, K.G.; Gomeztagle-Romero, M.Z.; Gomez-Rodriguez, G.H.; Sánchez-Villegas, J.A.; Rascón-Chu, A. Pectin nanoparticles: Fabrication and uses 2022. In *Polysaccharide Nanoparticles*; Venkatesan, J., Kim, S.-K., Anil, S., Sukumaran Anil, R.P.D., Eds.; Elsevier: Amsterdam, The Netherlands, 2022; pp. 163–201.
59. Negi, A.; Kesari, K.K. Chitosan Nanoparticle Encapsulation of Antibacterial Essential Oils. *Micromachines* **2022**, *13*, 1265. [CrossRef]

60. Morsy, M.K.; Khalaf, H.H.; Sharoba, A.M.; El-Tanahi, H.H.; Cutter, C.N. Incorporation of Essential Oils and Nanoparticles in Pullulan Films to Control Foodborne Pathogens on Meat and Poultry Products. *J. Food Sci.* **2014**, *79*, M675–M684. [CrossRef]
61. Qiu, C.; Chang, R.; Yang, J.; Ge, S.; Xiong, L.; Zhao, M.; Li, M.; Sun, Q. Preparation and characterization of essential oil-loaded starch nanoparticles formed by short glucan chains. *Food Chem.* **2017**, *221*, 1426–1433. [CrossRef]
62. Fathi, M.; Karim, M.; Ahmadi, N. Nanostructures of cellulose for encapsulation of food ingredients. In *Nanoencapsulation in the Food Industry: Biopolymer Nanostructures for Food Encapsulation Purposes*; Jafari, S.M., Ed.; Academic Press: Cambridge, MA, USA, 2019; pp. 493–519.
63. Zhang, X.; Liu, D.; Jin, T.Z.; Chen, W.; He, Q.; Zou, Z.; Zhao, H.; Ye, X.; Guo, M. Preparation and characterization of gellan gum-chitosan polyelectrolyte complex films with the incorporation of thyme essential oil nanoemulsion. *Food Hydrocoll.* **2021**, *114*, 106570. [CrossRef]
64. Fernandes, R.V.d.B.; Silva, E.K.; Borges, S.V.; de Oliveira, C.R.; Yoshida, M.I.; da Silva, Y.F.; do Carmo, E.L.; Azevedo, V.M.; Botrel, D.A. Proposing Novel Encapsulating Matrices for Spray-Dried Ginger Essential Oil from the Whey Protein Isolate-Inulin/Maltodextrin Blends. *Food Bioprocess. Technol.* **2017**, *10*, 115–130. [CrossRef]
65. Pessoa Silva, M.; Fabi, J.P. Food biopolymers-derived nanogels for encapsulation and delivery of biologically active compounds: A perspective review. *Food Hydrocoll. Health* **2022**, *2*, 100079. [CrossRef]
66. Gao, X.; Han, S.; Zhang, R.; Liu, G.; Wu, J. Progress in electrospun composite nanofibers: Composition, performance and applications for tissue engineering. *J. Mater. Chem. B* **2019**, *7*, 7075–7089. [CrossRef]
67. Min, T.; Zhou, L.; Sun, X.; Du, H.; Zhu, Z.; Wen, Y. Electrospun functional polymeric nanofibers for active food packaging: A review. *Food Chem.* **2022**, *391*, 133239. [CrossRef]
68. Nath, D.; Santhosh, R.; Pal, K.; Sarkar, P. Nanoclay-based active food packaging systems: A review. *Food Packag. Shelf Life* **2022**, *31*, 100803. [CrossRef]
69. Bahrami, A.; Delshadi, R.; Assadpour, E.; Jafari, S.M.; Williams, L. Antimicrobial-loaded nanocarriers for food packaging applications. *Adv. Colloid. Interface Sci.* **2020**, *278*, 102140. [CrossRef]
70. Adel, A.M.; Ibrahim, A.A.; El-Shafei, A.M.; Al-Shemy, M.T. Inclusion complex of clove oil with chitosan/β-cyclodextrin citrate/oxidized nanocellulose biocomposite for active food packaging. *Food Packag. Shelf Life* **2019**, *20*, 100307. [CrossRef]
71. Erceg, T.; Šovljanski, O.; Stupar, A.; Ugarković, J.; Aćimović, M.; Pezo, L.; Tomić, A.; Todosijević, M. A comprehensive approach to chitosan-gelatine edible coating with β-cyclodextrin/lemongrass essential oil inclusion complex—Characterization and food application. *Int. J. Biol. Macromol.* **2022**, *228*, 400–410. [CrossRef]
72. Celebioglu, A.; Yildiz, Z.I.; Uyar, T. Thymol/cyclodextrin inclusion complex nanofibrous webs: Enhanced water solubility, high thermal stability and antioxidant property of thymol. *Food Res. Int.* **2018**, *106*, 280–290. [CrossRef]
73. Duda-Chodak, A.; Tarko, T.; Petka-Poniatowska, K. Antimicrobial Compounds in Food Packaging. *Int J Mol Sci.* **2023**, *24*, 2457. [CrossRef]
74. Sung, S.-Y.; Sin, L.T.; Tee, T.-T.; Bee, S.-T.; Rahmat, A.; Rahman, W.; Tan, A.-C.; Vikhraman, M. Antimicrobial agents for food packaging applications. *Trends Food Sci. Technol.* **2013**, *33*, 110–123. [CrossRef]
75. Siracusa, V. Packaging Material in the Food Industry. In *Antimicrobial Food Packaging*; Academic Press: Cambridge, MA, USA, 2016; pp. 95–106. [CrossRef]
76. Tongnuanchan, P.; Benjakul, S. Essential Oils: Extraction, Bioactivities, and Their Uses for Food Preservation. *J. Food Sci.* **2014**, *79*, R1231–R1249. [CrossRef] [PubMed]
77. Masango, P. Cleaner production of essential oils by steam distillation. *J. Clean. Prod.* **2005**, *13*, 833–839. [CrossRef]
78. Dhifi, W.; Bellili, S.; Jazi, S.; Bahloul, N.; Mnif, W. Essential Oils' Chemical Characterization and Investigation of Some Biological Activities: A Critical Review. *Medicines* **2016**, *3*, 25. [CrossRef]
79. Krepker, M.; Shemesh, R.; Poleg, Y.D.; Kashi, Y.; Vaxman, A.; Segal, E. Active food packaging films with synergistic antimi-crobial activity. *Food Control* **2017**, *76*, 117–126. [CrossRef]
80. Erceg, T.; Vukić, N.; Teofilović, V.; Baloš, S.; Stupar, A.; Šovljanski, O. Optimisation of the applicative properties of biodegradable cellulose acetate-based films using the principles of green chemistry. In Proceedings of the STED Conference, Trebinje, Bosnia and Herzegovina, 2–5 June 2022.
81. Da Silva Dannenberg, G.; Funck, G.D.; dos Santos Cruxen, C.; Marques, J.D.L.; da Silva, W.P.; Fiorentini, M. Essential oil from pink pepper as an antimicrobial component in cellulose acetate film: Potential for application as active packaging for sliced cheese. *LWT Food Sci. Technol.* **2017**, *81*, 314–318. [CrossRef]
82. Erceg, T.; Vukić, N.; Šovljanski, O.; Stupar, A.; Šergelj, V.; Aćimović, M.; Baloš, S.; Ugarković, J.; Šuput, D.; Popović, S.; et al. Characterization of Films Based on Cellulose Acetate/Poly(caprolactone diol) Intended for Active Packaging Prepared by Green Chemistry Principles. *ACS Sustain. Chem. Eng.* **2022**, *10*, 9141–9154. [CrossRef]
83. Qin, Y.; Li, W.; Liu, D.; Yuan, M.; Li, L. Development of active packaging film made from poly (lactic acid) incorporated es-sential oil. *Prog. Org. Coat.* **2016**, *103*, 76–82. [CrossRef]
84. Silveira, M.P.; Silva, H.C.; Pimentel, I.C.; Poitevin, C.G.; Stuart, A.K.d.C.; Carpiné, D.; Jorge, L.M.d.M.; Jorge, R.M.M. Development of active cassava starch cellulose nanofiber-based films incorporated with natural antimicrobial tea tree essential oil. *J. Appl. Polym. Sci.* **2020**, *137*, 48726. [CrossRef]
85. Arezooa, E.; Mohammadrezaa, E.; Maryama, M.; Nafchi Abdorreza, M. The synergistic effects of cinnamon essential oil and nano TiO_2 on antimicrobial and functional properties of sago starch films. *Int. J. Biol. Macromol.* **2020**, *157*, 743–751. [CrossRef] [PubMed]

86. Perdana, M.I.; Ruamcharoen, J.; Panphon, S.; Leelakriangsak, M. Antimicrobial activity and physical properties of starch/chitosan film incorporated with lemongrass essential oil and its application. *LWT* **2021**, *141*, 110934. [CrossRef]
87. Handayasari, F.; Suyatma, N.E.; Nurjanah, S. Physiochemical and antibacterial analysis of gelatin–chitosan edible film with the addition of nitrite and garlic essential oil by response surface methodology. *J. Food Process. Preserv.* **2019**, *43*, e14265. [CrossRef]
88. Saavedra, S.C.; Ventura-Aguilar, R.I.; Bautista-Baños, S.; Barrera-Necha, L.L. Biodegradable chitosan coating for improving quality and controlling Alternaria alternata growth in figs. *World J. Adv. Res. Rev.* **2020**, *7*, 115–125. [CrossRef]
89. Socaciu, M.-I.; Fogarasi, M.; Semeniuc, C.A.; Socaci, S.A.; Rotar, M.A.; Mureşan, V.; Pop, O.L.; Vodnar, D.C. Formulation and Characterization of Antimicrobial Edible Films Based on Whey Protein Isolate and Tarragon Essential Oil. *Polymers* **2020**, *12*, 1748. [CrossRef]
90. Donsì, F.; Ferrari, G. Essential oil nanoemulsions as antimicrobial agents in food. *J. Biotechnol.* **2016**, *233*, 106–120. [CrossRef] [PubMed]
91. Ejaz, M.; Arfat, Y.A.; Mulla, M.; Ahmed, J. Zinc oxide nanorods/clove essential oil incorporated Type B gelatin composite films and its applicability for shrimp packaging. *Food Packag. Shelf Life* **2018**, *15*, 113–121. [CrossRef]
92. Tongnuanchan, P.; Benjakul, S.; Prodpran, T. Structural, morphological and thermal behaviour characterisations of fish gelatin film incorporated with basil and citronella essential oils as affected by surfactants. *Food Hydrocoll.* **2014**, *41*, 33–43. [CrossRef]
93. Wu, J.; Ge, S.; Liu, H.; Wang, S.; Chen, S.; Wang, J.; Li, J.; Zhang, Q. Properties and antimicrobial activity of silver carp (*Hypophthalmichthys molitrix*) skin gelatin-chitosan films incorporated with oregano essential oil for fish preservation. *Food Packag. Shelf Life* **2014**, *2*, 7–16. [CrossRef]
94. Peng, Y.; Yin, L.; Li, Y. Combined effects of lemon essential oil and surfactants on physical and structural properties of chitosan films. *Int. J. Food Sci. Technol.* **2013**, *48*, 44–50. [CrossRef]
95. Noshirvani, N.; Ghanbarzadeh, B.; Gardrat, C.; Rezaei, M.R.; Hashemi, M.; Le Coz, C.; Coma, V. Cinnamon and ginger essential oils to improve antifungal, physical and mechanical properties of chitosan-carboxymethyl cellulose films. *Food Hydrocoll.* **2017**, *70*, 36–45. [CrossRef]
96. Biswas, A.; Furtado, R.F.; Bastos, M.d.S.R.; Benevides, S.D.; Oliveira, M.; Boddu, V.; Cheng, H. Preparation and characteri-zation of carboxymethyl cellulose films with embedded essential oils. *J. Mater. Sci. Res.* **2018**, *7*, 16–25.
97. Han, Y.; Yu, M.; Wang, L. Physical and antimicrobial properties of sodium alginate/carboxymethyl cellulose films incorporated with cinnamon essential oil. *Food Packag. Shelf Life* **2018**, *15*, 35–42. [CrossRef]
98. Otoni, C.G.; Pontes, S.F.O.; Medeiros, E.A.A.; Soares, N.d.F.F. Edible Films from Methylcellulose and Nanoemulsions of Clove Bud (*Syzygium aromaticum*) and Oregano (*Origanum vulgare*) Essential Oils as Shelf Life Extenders for Sliced Bread. *J. Agric. Food Chem.* **2014**, *62*, 5214–5219. [CrossRef]
99. Kouravand, F.; Jooyandeh, H.; Barzegar, H.; Hojjati, M. Characterization of cross-linked whey protein isolate-based films containing *Satureja Khuzistanica* Jamzad essential oil. *J. Food Process. Preserv.* **2018**, *42*, e13557. [CrossRef]
100. Mohammadi, M.; Mirabzadeh, S.; Shahvalizadeh, R.; Hamishehkar, H. Development of novel active packaging films based on whey protein isolate incorporated with chitosan nanofiber and nano-formulated cinnamon oil. *Int. J. Biol. Macromol.* **2020**, *149*, 11–20. [CrossRef]
101. Sani, I.K.; Geshlaghi, S.P.; Pirsa, S.; Asdagh, A. Composite film based on potato starch/apple peel pectin/ZrO_2 nanoparticles/microencapsulated Zataria multiflora essential oil; investigation of physicochemical properties and use in quail meat packaging. *Food Hydrocoll.* **2021**, *117*, 106719. [CrossRef]
102. Fenga, X.; Wanga, W.; Chua, Y.; Gao, C.; Liu, Q.; Tang, X. Effect of cinnamon essential oil nanoemulsion emulsified by OSA modified starch on the structure and properties of pullulan based films. *LWT* **2020**, *134*, 110123. [CrossRef]
103. Sherry, M.; Charcosset, C.; Fessi, H.; Greige-Gerges, H. Essential oils encapsulated in liposomes: A review. *J. Liposome Res.* **2013**, *23*, 268–275. [CrossRef]
104. Al-Moghazy, M.; El-Sayed, H.S.; Salama, H.H.; Nada, A.A. Edible packaging coating of encapsulated thyme essential oil in liposomal chitosan emulsions to improve the shelf life of Karish cheese. *Food Biosci.* **2021**, *43*, 101230. [CrossRef]
105. Bastarrachea, L.; Dhawan, S.; Sablani, S.S. Engineering Properties of Polymeric-Based Antimicrobial Films for Food Packaging: A Review. *Food Eng. Rev.* **2011**, *3*, 79–93. [CrossRef]
106. Quintavalla, S.; Vicini, L. Antimicrobial food packaging in meat industry. *Meat Sci.* **2002**, *62*, 373–380. [CrossRef] [PubMed]
107. Arvanitoyannis, I.S.; Kotsanopoulos, K.V. Migration Phenomenon in Food Packaging. Food–Package Interactions, Mecha-nisms, Types of Migrants, Testing and Relative Legislation—A Review. *Food Bioproc Techn* **2013**, *7*, 21–36. [CrossRef]
108. Motelica, L.; Ficai, D.; Ficai, A.; Oprea, O.C.; Kaya, D.A.; Andronescu, E. Biodegradable Antimicrobial Food Packaging: Trends and Perspectives. *Foods* **2020**, *9*, 1438. [CrossRef]
109. Bhunia, K.; Sablani, S.S.; Tang, J.; Rasco, B. Migration of Chemical Compounds from Packaging Polymers during Microwave, Conventional Heat Treatment, and Storage. *Compr. Rev. Food Sci. Food Saf.* **2013**, *12*, 523–545. [CrossRef]
110. Becerril, R.; Nerín, C.; Silva, F. Encapsulation Systems for Antimicrobial Food Packaging Components: An Update. *Molecules* **2020**, *25*, 1134. [CrossRef]
111. Irkin, R.; Esmer, O.K. Novel food packaging systems with natural antimicrobial agents. *J. Food Sci. Technol.* **2015**, *52*, 6095–6111. [CrossRef]
112. Cerisuelo, J.; Muriel-Galet, V.; Bermúdez, J.M.; Aucejo, S.; Catalá, R.; Gavara, R.; Hernández-Muñoz, P. Mathematical model to describe the release of an antimicrobial agent from an active package constituted by carvacrol in a hydrophilic EVOH coating on a PP film. *J. Food Eng.* **2012**, *110*, 26–37. [CrossRef]

113. Balaguer, M.P.; Lopez-Carballo, G.; Catala, R.; Gavara, R.; Hernandez-Munoz, P. Antifungal properties of gliadin films incorporating cinnamaldehyde and application in active food packaging of bread and cheese spread foodstuffs. *Int. J. Food Microbiol.* **2013**, *166*, 369–377. [CrossRef]
114. Robertson, G. *Food Packaging—Principles and Practice*, 3rd ed.; CRC Press: Boca Raton, FL, USA, 2006; ISBN 978-1-4398-6242-1.
115. Feigenbaum, A.E.; Riquet, A.M.; Scholler, D. Fatty Food Simulants: Solvents to Mimic the Behavior of Fats in Contact with Packaging Plastics. In *Food Packaging Testing Methods and Applications*; Sara, J.R., Ed.; American Chemical Society: Washington, DC, USA, 2000.
116. Appendini, P.; Hotchkiss, J.H. Review of antimicrobial food packaging. *Innov. Food Sci. Emerg. Technol.* **2002**, *3*, 113–126. [CrossRef]
117. Miranda, J.M.; Jorge, F.; Dominguez, L.; Cepeda, A.; Franco, C.M. In vitro Growth Inhibition of Food-borne Pathogens and Food Spoilage Microorganism by Vitamin K5. *Food Bioprocess. Technol.* **2010**, *4*, 1060–1065. [CrossRef]
118. Muriel-Galet, V.; Cerisuelo, J.P.; López-Carballo, G.; Lara, M.; Gavara, R.; Hernández-Muñoz, P. Development of antimicrobial films for microbiological control of packaged salad. *Int. J. Food Microbiol.* **2012**, *157*, 195–201. [CrossRef] [PubMed]
119. Radusin, T.; Ristic, I.; Pilic, B.; Novakovic, A. Antimicrobial nanomaterials for food packaging applications. *Food Feed. Res.* **2013**, *43*, 119–126. [CrossRef]
120. de Azeredo, H.M.C. Antimicrobial nanostructures in food packaging. *Trends Food Sci. Technol.* **2013**, *30*, 56–69. [CrossRef]
121. Malhotra, B.; Keshwani, A.; Kharkwal, H. Antimicrobial food packaging: Potential and pitfalls. *Front. Microbiol.* **2015**, *6*, 611. [CrossRef] [PubMed]
122. Zahra, S.A.; Butt, Y.N.; Nasar, S.; Akram, S.; Fatima, Q.; Ikram, J. Food Packaging in Perspective of Microbial Activity: A Review. *J. Microbiol. Biotechnol. Food Sci.* **2016**, *6*, 752–757. [CrossRef]
123. Li, M.; Noriega-Trevino, M.E.; Nino-Martinez, N.; Marambio-Jones, C.; Wang, J.; Damoiseaux, R.; Ruiz, F.; Hoek, E.M. Synergistic Bactericidal Activity of Ag-TiO_2 Nanoparticles in Both Light and Dark Conditions. *Environ. Sci. Technol.* **2011**, *45*, 8989–8995. [CrossRef]
124. Rhim, J.-W.; Park, H.-M.; Ha, C.-S. Bio-nanocomposites for food packaging applications. *Prog. Polym. Sci.* **2013**, *38*, 1629–1652. [CrossRef]
125. Aminlari, L.; Hashemi, M.M.; Aminlari, M. Modified Lysozymes as Novel Broad Spectrum Natural Antimicrobial Agents in Foods. *J. Food Sci.* **2014**, *79*, R1077–R1090. [CrossRef]
126. Meira, S.M.M.; Zehetmeyer, G.; Jardim, A.I.; Scheibel, J.M.; de Oliveira, R.V.B.; Brandelli, A. Polypropylene/Montmorillonite Nanocomposites Containing Nisin as Antimicrobial Food Packaging. *Food Bioprocess. Technol.* **2014**, *7*, 3349–3357. [CrossRef]
127. Resa, C.P.O.; Gerschenson, L.N.; Jagus, R.J. Natamycin and nisin supported on starch edible films for controlling mixed culture growth on model systems and Port Salut cheese. *Food Control* **2014**, *44*, 146–151. [CrossRef]
128. Lantano, C.; Alfieri, I.; Cavazza, A.; Corradini, C.; Lorenzi, A.; Zucchetto, N.; Montenero, A. Natamycin based sol–gel antimicrobial coatings on polylactic acid films for food packaging. *Food Chem.* **2014**, *165*, 342–347. [CrossRef] [PubMed]
129. Otoni, C.G.; de Moura, M.R.; Aouada, F.A.; Camilloto, G.P.; Cruz, R.S.; Lorevice, M.V.; de, F.F. Soares, N.; Mattoso, L.H.C. Antimicrobial and physical-mechanical properties of pectin/papaya puree/cinnamaldehyde nanoemulsion edible composite films. *Food Hydrocoll.* **2014**, *41*, 188–194. [CrossRef]
130. Hill, L.E.; Gomes, C.; Taylor, T.M. Characterization of beta-cyclodextrin inclusion complexes containing essential oils (trans-cinnamaldehyde, eugenol, cinnamon bark, and clove bud extracts) for antimicrobial delivery applications. *LWT* **2013**, *51*, 86–93. [CrossRef]
131. Mith, H.; Duré, R.; Delcenserie, V.; Zhiri, A.; Daube, G.; Clinquart, A. Antimicrobial activities of commercial essential oils and their components against food-borne pathogens and food spoilage bacteria. *Food Sci. Nutr.* **2014**, *2*, 403–416. [CrossRef]
132. Micić, D.; Đurović, S.; Riabov, P.; Tomić, A.; Šovljanski, O.; Filip, S.; Tosti, T.; Dojčinović, B.; Božović, R.; Jovanović, D.; et al. Rosemary essential oils as a promising source of bioactive compounds: Chemical composition, thermal properties, biological activity and gastronomical perspectives. *Foods* **2021**, *10*, 2734. [CrossRef]
133. Aćimović, M.; Šovljanski, O.; Šeregelj, V.; Pezo, L.; Zheljazkov, V.D.; Ljujić, J.; Tomić, A.; Ćetković, G.; Čanadanović-Brunet, J.; Miljković, A.; et al. Chemical composition, antioxidant and antimicrobial activity of *Dracocephalum moldavica* L. essential oil and hydrolate. *Plants* **2022**, *11*, 941. [CrossRef]
134. Šovljanski, O.; Saveljić, A.; Aćimović, M.; Šeregelj, V.; Pezo, L.; Tomić, A.; Ćetković, G.; Tešević, V. Biological profiling of essential oils and hydrolates of *Ocimum basilicum* var. *genovese* and var. *minimum* originated from Serbia. *Processes* **2022**, *10*, 1893. [CrossRef]
135. Pavlić, B.; Teslić, N.; Vidaković, A.; Vidović, S.; Velićanski, A.; Versari, A.; Radosavljević, R.; Zeković, Z. Sage processing from by-product to high quality powder: I. *Bioact. Potential. Ind. Crop. Prod.* **2017**, *107*, 81–89. [CrossRef]
136. Riabov, P.A.; Micić, D.; Božović, R.B.; Jovanović, D.V.; Tomić, A.; Šovljanski, O.; Filip, S.; Tosti, T.; Ostojić, S.; Blagojević, S.; et al. The chemical, biological and thermal characteristics and gastronomical perspectives of *Laurus nobilis* essential oil from different geograohical origin. *Ind. Crop Prod.* **2020**, *151*, 112498. [CrossRef]
137. Hulankova, R. The Influence of Liquid Medium Choice in Determination of Minimum Inhibitory Concentration of Essential Oils against Pathogenic Bacteria. *Antibiotics* **2022**, *11*, 150. [CrossRef] [PubMed]
138. Havelt, T.; Brettschneider, S.; Schmitz, M. Evaluation of practical applicability and synergistic effects of bio-based food pack-aging materials combined with plant-based stabilisers. *Processes* **2021**, *9*, 1838. [CrossRef]
139. Karbowiak, M.; Szymanski, P.; Zielinska, D. Synergistic effect of combination of various microbial hurdles in the biopreserva-tion of meat and meat products—Systematic review. *Foods* **2023**, *12*, 1430. [CrossRef] [PubMed]

140. Nur Hanani, Z.A.; Reich, F.; Tolksdorf, T.; Siemen, H.; Bandick, N. Monitoring the effect of active packaging films with sil-ver-kaolinite using different packaging systems on the quality of the beef meat. *Heliyon* **2022**, *8*, e11019. [CrossRef]
141. Vizzini, P.; Beltrame, E.; Zanet, V.; Vidić, J.; Manzano, M. Development and evaluation of qPCR detection method and Zn-MgO/alginate active packaging for controlling Listeria monocytogenes contamination in cold-smoked salmon. *Foods* **2020**, *9*, 1353. [CrossRef]
142. Pateiro, M.; Domínguez, R.; Bermúdez, R.; Munekata, P.E.; Zhang, W.; Gagaoua, M.; Lorenzo, J.M. Antioxidant active packaging systems to extend the shelf life of sliced cooked ham. *Curr. Res. Food Sci.* **2019**, *1*, 24–30. [CrossRef]
143. Ruskova, M.; Šiškova, A.O.; Mosnackova, K.; Gago, C.; Guerreiro, A.; Bučkova, M.; Puškarova, A.; Pangallo, D.; Antunes, M.D. Biodegradable active packaging enriched with essential oils for enhacing the shelf life of strawberries. *Antioxidants* **2023**, *12*, 755. [CrossRef]
144. Sipos, L.; Nyitrai, A.; Hitka, G.; Friedrich, L.F.; Kokai, Z. Sensory Panel Performance Evaluation—Comprehensive Review of Practical Approaches. *Appl. Sci.* **2021**, *11*, 11977. [CrossRef]

antibiotics

MDPI

Review

Bacillus VOCs in the Context of Biological Control

Jovana Grahovac *, Ivana Pajčin * and Vanja Vlajkov

Faculty of Technology Novi Sad, University of Novi Sad, Bulevar cara Lazara 1, 21000 Novi Sad, Serbia
* Correspondence: johana@uns.ac.rs (J.G.); ivana.pajcin@uns.ac.rs (I.P.)

Abstract: A contemporary agricultural production system relying on heavy usage of agrochemicals represents a questionable outlook for sustainable food supply in the future. The visible negative environmental impacts and unforeseen consequences to human and animal health have been requiring a shift towards the novel eco-friendly alternatives for chemical pesticides for a while now. Microbial-based biocontrol agents have shown a promising potential for plant disease management. The bacteria of the genus *Bacillus* have been among the most exploited microbial active components due to several highly efficient mechanisms of action against plant pathogens, as well as a palette of additional plant-beneficial mechanisms, together with their suitable properties for microbial biopesticide formulations. Among other bioactive metabolites, volatile organic compounds (VOCs) have been investigated for their biocontrol applications, exhibiting the main advantage of long-distance effect without the necessity for direct contact with plants or pathogens. The aim of this study is to give an overview of the state-of-the-art in the field of *Bacillus*-based VOCs, especially in terms of their antibacterial, antifungal, and nematicidal action as the main segments determining their potential for biocontrol applications in sustainable agriculture.

Keywords: antibacterial; antifungal; biocontrol agent; mechanism of action; microbial biopesticides; nematicidal; plant disease; plant pathogen; sustainable agriculture

1. Introduction

Microbial volatile organic compounds (mVOCs) represent a diverse group of molecules synthesized through different metabolic pathways by microorganisms, predominantly bacteria and fungi [1,2]. The role of mVOCs was explained through microorganisms' evolution in the context of microbial communities due to their ability to mediate interactions with certain VOCs acting like infochemicals [1,3]. Bacteria use a cell-to-cell communication system (quorum sensing) as a method for monitoring the population density [3,4] relying on the synthesis, release, and subsequent detection of small diffusible signal molecules known as autoinducers [4]. Quorum sensing is variable depending on the bacteria type, allowing both intra- and inter-species communication. The chemical communication enabled by diffusible autoinducers is possible at short distances between cells, also requiring a high concentration of signaling molecules. Recent research, on the other hand, showed that microorganisms also produce different inorganic and organic volatile compounds that can be used as signals in intra- and inter-kingdom interactions, even at lower concentrations and over long distances [2]. This kind of communication system enables the coordinated behavior of a group of organisms to achieve process regulation leading to virulence, biofilm formation, and other developmental processes. The important finding in this matter was that microorganisms employ volatiles during interactions with plants, fungi, nematodes, and bacteria [4].

The beneficial effect of VOCs is additionally supported by several environmentally friendly properties, including biodegradability, meaning they do not leave toxic residues on plant surfaces, low molecular weight (100–500 Da), the lipophilic character with a low boiling point, and high vapor pressure (0.01 kPa), making them easily evaporative at normal temperature and pressure and enabling diffusion through the atmosphere and soil over different distances [2,5–7]. These characteristics enable them to fulfill their roles in plant growth and protection via pores in soil and rhizosphere environments. Additionally, mVOCs act as ideal signal/messenger molecules for mediating interactions at both short and long distances in microbes and plants [2,7]. One key characteristic suggested as the main difference compared to soluble compounds lies in the independence from solvents. Due to the restricted number of functional groups, many volatiles are defined as non-polar, showing low solubility in water that is sufficient to allow dissemination into the water phase. However, volatiles spread fast in both the gas and water phases. Through the gaseous phase, volatiles can spread in highly complex ecosystems such as soil, insect, and spider nests. This allows them to achieve functions such as communication and antimicrobial defense, which, on the other hand, cannot be performed by solvents due to the lack of effective spreading [8].

Based on chemical structure, mVOCs can be divided into different classes, including alkenes, alcohols, ketones, benzenoids, pyrazines, sulfides, and terpenes. The first systematic review on bacterial volatiles was published by Schulz and Dickschat in 2007 [9], describing in detail the biosynthesis of common volatiles such as fatty acids or sulfur compounds, which are predominantly produced by bacteria, as well as some not-so-common VOCs such as halogenated compounds. The research addressing the occurrence of volatiles in bacteria indicated that the compounds can be classified into three different groups: common, group, and specific compounds. Common compounds are being produced by different strains throughout the bacterial kingdom, and include basic fermentation products and primary metabolism-derived compounds. The typical representatives of the described group are dimethyl disulfide, 2-phenylethanol, aliphatic methyl ketones, and indole. The group compounds are mostly produced within certain genera or species. However, different mixtures made of the aforementioned compounds can be strain- or species-specific, resulting in specific biological effects [8,10,11]. The studies also confirmed that environmental parameters, including the medium composition in the first place but also temperature, humidity, pH, and oxygen levels, influence the composition of volatiles produced by microorganisms. The effects of the parameters can be direct, in terms of their physical properties (temperature and humidity will clearly affect molecule volatility), or indirect, by influencing the growth rate and metabolic activity. The presence or absence of oxygen has a strong impact on the production of volatile compounds, taking into account the mode of metabolism preferred by the particular producing strain, whether it is respiration or fermentation. Additionally, it is to be expected that volatiles' production rate changes depending on the growth stage. Aside from abiotic factors, recent studies have shown that biotic factors, such as interactions between microorganisms of different species, can also cause or stop the release of volatiles [10]. This explains that volatiles are considered chemical signals that can be released specifically when needed and as results of complex two-way directed interactions existing between other members of the microbial community. Microorganisms can respond to a range of volatile compounds, which are diverse in terms of their structural and functional properties. However, a better understanding of how exactly cells perceive microbial volatiles is still limited and necessary due to the lack of information regarding the volatile-specific receptors in microorganisms. At this moment, it is confirmed that the physico-chemical properties of microbial volatiles make possible a passive diffusion through the cell wall or membrane. This implies that the target could be all cell components, including nucleoids, resulting in gene expression control. Taking into account the existing differences in volatile profiles among microorganisms, the relationship between them varies, and they are recognized within each other as friends, foes, or prey, consequently adjusting the behavior—persist, invade, escape, or defend. In microbial interactions, bacteria–bacteria, fungi–fungi, fungi–bacteria, or bacteria–protists relations, the response directly depends on the interacting partner; a volatile compound can have an opposite effect on different organisms [2,10,11].

The increased interest in microbial volatiles and a growing number of studies have been noticed in the last two decades, addressing their beneficial and environmentally friendly roles in the form of beneficial interactions among producing strains and plants. This results in the induction of systemic resistance against biotic and abiotic elements, plant growth promotion, and inhibition of plant fungal and bacterial pathogens [10,12]. The action mode of VOCs has an additional advantage over other biocontrol and growth-regulating mechanisms since the VOCs do not require any physical contact with pathogens or plant parts, in contrast with most of the other processes involved in controlling phytopathogens and promoting plant growth. In the scientific literature, it was reported that 300 bacteria and fungi are recognized as VOC producers. A total of 671 VOCs belong to 212 bacterial species, while 335 belong to 96 species of fungi, as recorded in the database of volatiles emitted by microorganisms [13]. The most common representatives also recognized based on beneficial activity that includes the influence on plant growth promotion and induction of systemic resistance are members of the *Bacillus, Pseudomonas, Stenotrophomonas, Serratia,* and *Arthrobacter* genus [12]. In recent years, the production of mVOCs has been considered a promising biocontrol method that enables short- and long-distance pathogen control [14]. The capability of volatiles to act as suppressive agents on neighboring pathogens and signal to plants confirms their potential role as sustainable alternatives to chemical fertilizers and pesticides [2]. The specificity of mVOCs in terms of target pathogens explains that the inhibitory effects of VOCs can mediate virulence factor expression of target pathogens, but also suppress metabolic processes, such as toxins biosynthesis [2,14]. Several recent studies are focused on a better understanding of possible modes of action in pathogens suppression, on the necessity to widen the investigation, and on addressing questions regarding clarifying the molecular targets of mVOCs across a broader range of pathogens. The studies also reported that the suppressing effects of mVOCs produced by bacterial mixtures in co-culturing methods can be significantly different from those produced by single species. In this kind of competitive interaction, mVOCs themselves can serve as signals to trigger or reduce the production of other mVOCs, with the additional possibility that some volatiles can be produced by precursors synthesized by different strains [7].

The potential of VOCs as biocontrol agents and eco-friendly alternatives to the chemical products conventionally used in agricultural practices for pest management is topic of a great scientific and practical interest recognized by many research groups worldwide. The present study is focused on an overview of the state-of-the-art in the field of *Bacillus*-based VOCs in terms of their antibacterial, antifungal, and nematicidal activity as the main factors determining their potential for biocontrol applications in sustainable agriculture. This study has summarized available scientific data regarding the Bacillus strains as VOC producers, focusing on clarifying the mechanisms of action and describing potential application routes, giving insights into the direction of the subsequent research steps and scientific questions addressed in the future.

2. Antibacterial *Bacillus*-Based VOCs and Their Mechanisms of Action

Biocontrol activity of *Bacillus*-emitted VOCs against different plant pathogenic bacteria was previously reported in numerous studies (Table 1). Different mechanisms of antibacterial action against plant pathogens exhibited by the *Bacillus*-based VOCs are discussed below and summarized in Figure 1, while the most abundant antibacterial VOCs are presented in Figure 2.

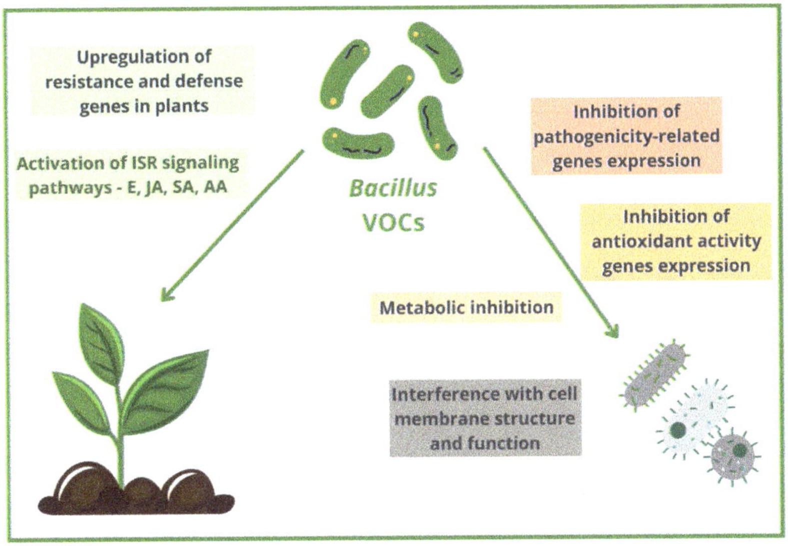

Figure 1. Mechanisms of antibacterial activity of *Bacillus*-based VOCs (ISR—induced systemic resistance; E—ethylene; JA—jasmonic acid; SA—salycilic acid; AA—abscisic acid).

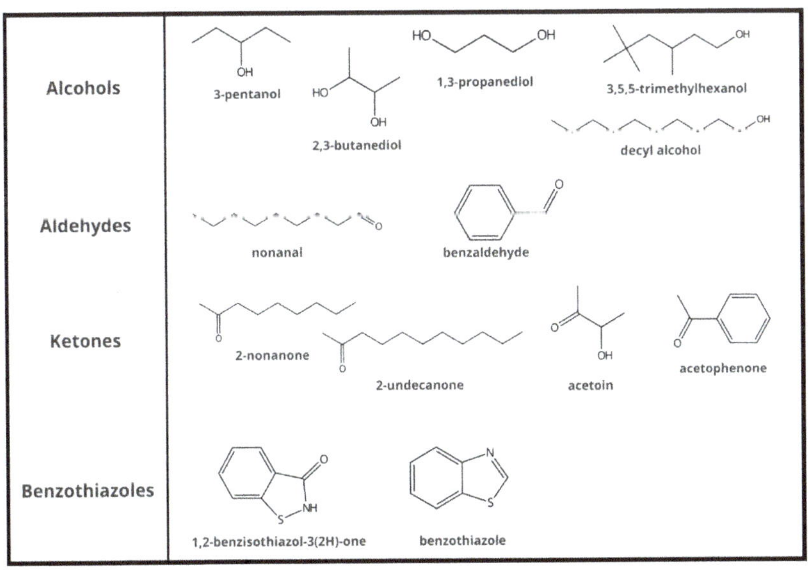

Figure 2. The most common antibacterial *Bacillus*-based VOCs.

2.1. ISR (Induced Systemic Resistance) Induction via Different Signaling Pathways as the Mechanism of Antibacterial Activity of Bacillus VOCs

Among the pioneers in this field, Ryu et al. [15] have proven the antibacterial effect of 2,3-butanediol produced by *Bacillus subtilis* GB03 and *B. amyloliquefaciens* IN937a against *Pectobacterium carotovorum* subsp. *carotovorum* (syn. *Erwinia carotovora* subsp. *carotovora*). The main mechanism of antibacterial action in the aforementioned study was ISR (induced systemic resistance) in *Arabidopsis thaliana* after 4 days of exposure to *Bacillus* VOCs, which was mediated through the ethylene-dependent signaling pathways, while the ISR was independent of the salicylic acid or jasmonic acid signaling pathways. VOCs produced by *B. subtilis* GB03 and *B. amyloliquefaciens* IN937a have shown a supreme biocontrol effect by reducing the number of symptomatic leaves to one in *Arabidopsis* plants, even in comparison to 2,3-butanediol applied as a pure compound (1–2 symptomatic leaves) as well as compared to water used as a control (4–5 symptomatic leaves) [15]. Acetoin (3-hydroxy-2-butanone) was found to be the main VOC produced by *B. subtilis* FB17 that triggers systemic resistance in *Arabidopsis thaliana* against *Pseudomonas syringae* pv. *tomato* DC3000 via induction of salicylic acid and ethylene signaling pathways, while the jasmonic acid signaling pathway was not essential for ISR. Plants treated with *B. subtilis* FB17 or acetoin as a pure compound have shown milder disease symptoms in terms of chlorosis, as well as a significant reduction of pathogen incidence measured as CFU/g of fresh weight (around 1 log unit) [16]. The antibacterial activity of 3-pentanol and 2-butanon supplied by the drench treatment in concentrations of 1 mM and 0.1 μM, respectively, was reported through the consistent triggering of systemic resistance in cucumber against *Pseudomonas syringae* pv. *lachrymans*, causing bacterial angular leaf spots, whereas 2,3-butanediol had been ineffective in eliciting induced resistance in cucumber plants in the aforementioned concentrations [17]. Later, it was reported that ten Petri dishes containing 10 μM 2,3-butanediol (the main VOC produced by *B. subtilis* GB03) were utilized in the miniature greenhouse system to successfully induce systemic resistance against *Pseudomonas syringae* pv. *lachrymans* on cucumber plants, which was mediated via the jasmonic acid signaling pathway. The disease severity score of cucumber angular leaf spot was reduced to 2.7 for *B. subtilis* GB03 VOCs treatment, compared to 4.2 for plants without VOCs treatment (on the scale in the range 0–5) [18]. The subsequent study revealed that 3-pentanol primes salicylic acid and jasmonic acid signaling pathways responsible for ISR towards *Pseudomonas syringae* pv. *tomato* in *Arabidopsis* plants [19]. Similar results regarding the ISR mechanisms were reported by Choi et al. [20], in which 3-pentanol from *B. amyloliquefaciens* IN937a has shown a significant reduction in pepper bacterial spots severity caused by *Xanthomonas axonopodis* pv. *vesicatoria* in field trials over two years. The disease index, measured 40 days after plant transplantation in the field, was reduced to 0.7 and 1.7 in 3-pentanol treatments, compared to 4.0 and 3.8 for water used as control (scale 0–5) in two subsequent years [20].

2.2. Modulation of Pathogens' Gene Expression by Antibacterial Bacillus-Based VOCs

Inhibition of virulence traits and metabolic activity by inhibition of the related genes' expression and modulating the metabolic pathways responsible for pathogenic behavior are among the most important mechanisms of action of *Bacillus*-generated VOCs in terms of their antibacterial activity. Furthermore, several studies have shown improved antibacterial activity achieved by the mixture of VOCs compared to separate compounds, thereby targeting the expression of different pathogenicity-related genes. The antibacterial activity of the VOC mixture produced by *B. amyloliquefaciens* SQR-9 was proven against *Ralstonia solanacearum* ZJ3721 (biovar 3), the causal agent of tomato bacterial wilt, with an efficiency of 70% in bacterial pathogen growth suppression when the VOC mixture was applied as a biocontrol agent, contrary to the 1–11% growth inhibition achieved by the individual VOCs [21]. The underlying mechanisms of antibacterial activity included inhibition of motility, biofilm formation, and root colonization by *Ralstonia solanacearum*, as well as inhibited production of antioxidant enzymes and exopolysaccharides, with significant down-regulation of genes involved in virulence traits, carbohydrate and amino acid metabolism, protein translation, and folding, as well as antioxidant activity [19]. Almost similar mechanisms of action were observed in the case of *B. amyloliquefaciens* T-5 VOCs antibacterial activity against the tomato bacterial wilt pathogen, where pathogen growth inhibition rates of 75%, 62%, and 85% were achieved using the mixture of VOCs produced by the *Bacillus* antagonist on the agar medium, in sterilized soil, and natural soil, respectively [22]. This study also reported down-regulation of several virulence- and metabolism-related genes of *Ralstonia solanacearum* in the range 27–54%, including transcriptional regulator (*phcA*), catalase (*katG*), and SOD (superoxide dismutase—*sobB*) genes motility-related genes (twitching motility (*pilT*) and flagellin (*fliC*)) as well as metabolism-related genes, DNA polymerase (*polA*) and pyruvate dehydrogenase (*aceE*) [22]. The same research group has also investigated induced VOC production in the presence of organic fertilizers prepared from different animal and plant organic waste materials [23], where the production of VOCs was significantly improved when combined with the application of organic fertilizers. This suggests a possible novel good agricultural practice in tomato bacterial wilt management. It was concluded that maximal production of 2-nonanone, nonanal, xylene, benzothiazole, and butylated hydroxy toluene was achieved by the strain *B. amyloliquefaciens* T-5 in the presence of organic fertilizer made of amino acid organic fertilizer (prepared from the microbially hydrolyzed oil rapeseed cake) and pig manure compost (1:1, *w*/*w*). On the other hand, maximal production of 2-nonanone, nonanal, xylene, and 2-undecanone was achieved by *B. amyloliquefaciens* SQR-9 in the presence of organic fertilizer composed of 41% vinegar-production residue, 20% rice straw, and 39% cattle dung [23].

The suppression of *Ralstonia solanacearum* as the causal agent of tobacco bacterial wilt was also investigated by Tahir et al. [12,24]. Albuterol and 1,3-propanediol produced by *B. subtilis* SYST2 were found to be responsible for ISR and growth promotion of tobacco plants at the level of inhibition of gene expression related to ethylene production, while on the other hand, genes related to expansin, wilt resistance, and plant defense were overexpressed. Moreover, the wilt index in tobacco plants was reduced from 90.66% to 33.00%, 19%, and 27% by applying inoculation with *B. subtilis* SYST2 or treatments with 1,3-propanediol (1 mM) and albuterol (0.1 mM) [12]. Benzaldehyde, 1,2-benzisothiazol-3(2H)-one, and 1,3-butadiene were found to be major VOCs produced by *B. amyloliquefaciens* FZB42 and *B. atrophaeus* LSSC22, which suppressed *Ralstonia solanacearum* in tobacco plants by reducing the colony size, pathogen cell viability, and motility, and negatively influencing chemotaxis. One of the major mechanisms of action was the induction of morphological and ultrastructural changes/abnormalities in *Ralstonia solanacearum* cells. Furthermore, expression of pathogenicity-related genes was significantly down-regulated, including *PhcA* (a global virulence regulator), type III secretion system (T3SS), type IV secretion system (T4SS), extracellular polysaccharides, and chemotaxis-related genes. On the other hand, genes related to pathogen resistance and defense were significantly overexpressed, where the salicylic acid pathway was found to be responsible for the induction of systemic resistance, with up-regulation of the *EDS1* and *NPR1* genes as its main components. All of the aforementioned mechanisms of action have resulted in the reduced tobacco wilt index during *in planta* experiments (28% for *B. amyloliquefaciens* FZB42 and 43.2% for *B. atrophaeus* LSSC22 VOCs compared to 98% for the non-exposed control) [24].

Growth inhibition of *Ralstonia solanacearum* was also achieved by 3,5,5-trimethylhexanol produced by *B. cereus* D13, which has also been successful in suppression of *Pseudomonas syringae* pv. *tomato* DC3000 and *Xanthomonas oryzae* pv. *Oryzicola*. This is while both 3,5,5-trimethylhexanol and decyl alcohol have shown antibacterial activity against *Xanthomonas oryzae* pv. *oryzae* with growth inhibition of 60.7% and 53.6% at minimum inhibitory amounts of 0.48 and 2.4 mg, respectively [25]. The same study has revealed several mechanisms of antibacterial activity against *Xanthomonas oryzae* pv. *oryzae* as the causal agent of bacterial leaf blight in rice. The first one was the inhibition of pathogen swimming and swarming motility after 3-day exposure to *B. cereus* D13 VOCs, with significant down-regulation of the genes *motA*, encoding flagellar motor component MotA, and *motC*, encoding the flagellar motor protein. Interestingly, while pathogen motility was restricted during the first 3 days of exposure, it took 6 days of exposure to observe a sharp decline in the number of viable pathogen cells, indicating that a certain period of time was required to achieve lethal VOCs concentration, while a certain extent of pathogen spreading inhibition could be achieved in earlier phases of antagonist-pathogen interaction at the sub-lethal level of VOCs concentration. Considering that the rhizosphere is a relatively closed environment, it is a favorable place for maximization of VOCs' antibacterial activity, considering the shorter time necessary to achieve a certain VOCs concentration threshold required for bactericidal effect. In the case of *Xanthomonas oryzae* pv. *oryzae*, rice rhizosphere is therefore a good place to apply antagonist or VOCs solely in order to prevent or inhibit infection via root wounds [25].

2.3. Structural and Functional Changes at Cell Level Caused by Antibacterial Bacillus VOCs

Another mechanism of antibacterial activity was observed in the case of *B. cereus* D13 VOCs, including alteration of *Xanthomonas oryzae* pv. *oryzae* cell membrane permeability resulting in changed cell morphology, which could be directed in two ways: (a) increased membrane permeability through membrane distortion, resulting in leakage of intracellular contents, and (b) decreased membrane permeability resulting in concentrated cytoplasm [25]. Hence, the action mode of 3,5,5-trimethylhexanol and decyl alcohol VOCs could be explained by their ability to cause leakage or impede the interchange of materials at the cell membrane surface [4].

On the other hand, one of the possible antibacterial activity mechanisms related to pathogen cells' morphological changes is also inducing several cell abnormalities at the ultrastructural level, as mentioned before [24]. The same was observed by Rajer et al. [5], where benzaldehyde, nonanal, benzothiozole, and acetophenone emitted by *B. subtilis* FA26 induced a wide range of abnormalities in cells of *Clavibacter michiganensis* ssp. *sepedonicus*, a causal agent of potato bacterial ring rot, including distorted colony morphology, misshapen cells and their disintegration, the formation of inclusions, movement of cytoplasmic content toward the ruptured cytoplasmic membrane, and lack of cytoplasmic content or fragmented cytoplasm due to intracellular content leakage. The same authors concluded that the production and activity of *B. subtilis* FA26 VOCs depend on cultivation conditions and that an increase in their biocontrol potential against *Clavibacter michiganensis* ssp. *sepedonicus* is related to the increased VOC concentrations [5].

2.4. Effects of Antibacterial Bacillus VOCs Concentration and Treatment Timing on Biocontrol Efficiency

Besides cultivation conditions, the other important variable determining the efficacy of the VOC treatment is the time of application, considering the current pathogen growth and development stage. Han et al. [25] have shown that the mixture of VOCs produced by *B. velezensis* strains JCK-1618 and JCK-1696 was more successful in suppressing *Xanthomonas arboricola* pv. *pruni* when *B. velezensis* strains were inoculated three days before pathogen inoculation, compared to a one-day window between the antagonist and pathogen inoculation, where the pathogen suppression efficacy ranged between 22.4% and 72.2%.

A mixture of *B. velezensis* X5-2, *B. megaterium* X6-3, and *Pseudomonas orientalis* X2-1P VOCs, including alkanes, alkenes, pyrazines, acids, alcohols, and indoles, was found to be effective during the in vitro and in vivo suppression of the winter oilseed rape black rot pathogen *Xanthomonas campestris* pv. *campestris*, with disease reductions of 82.37% and 72.47% in preventive and curative treatments, respectively [26]. Pyrazines (pyrazine, 2-ethyl-3-methyl, pyrazine, 2-ethyl-, pyrazine, 2, 5-dimethyl, and pyrazine, 2-methyl) were also found as active VOCs of *B. megaterium* BmBP17 against the bacterial wilt pathogen *Ralstonia solanacearum*, where pyrazine, 2-ethyl-3-methyl, was found to be the most effective compound with a required dosage of 672 μg/mL for complete inhibition of *Ralstonia solanacearum* [27]. This study also confirmed an increase in antibacterial activity with an increase in VOC concentrations.

Table 1. Literature overview concerning VOCs exhibiting antibacterial activity against plant pathogens produced by *Bacillus* spp.

***Bacillus* Strain**	**Plant Pathogen (Disease)**	**Antibacterial VOCs**	**Reference**
B. subtilis FB17	*Pseudomonas syringae* pv. *tomato*	acetoin	Rudrappa et al. [16]
B. subtilis FA26	*Clavibacter michiganensis* ssp. *sepedonicus* (potato bacterial ring rot)	benzaldehyde nonanal benzothiazole acetophenone	Rajer et al. [5]
B.s subtilis SYST2	*Ralstonia solanacearum* (tobacco bacterial wilt)	albuterol 1,3-propanediol	Tahir et al. [12]
B. subtilis GB03	*Pseudomonas syringae* pv. *lachrymans*	2,3-butanediol	Song et al. [18]
B. amyloliquefaciens IN937a	*Xanthomonas axonopodis* pv. *vesicatoria* (pepper bacterial spot)	3-pentanol	Choi et al. [20]
B. amyloliquefaciens T-5	*Ralstonia solanacearum* (tomato bacterial wilt)	mixture of VOCs	Raza et al. [22]
B. amyloliquefaciens SQR-9	*Ralstonia solanacearum* (tomato bacterial wilt)	mixture of VOCs	Raza et al. [21]
		2-nonanone 2-undecanone nonanal xylene benzothiazole butylated hydroxy toluene	Raza et al. [23]
B. megaterium BmBP17	*Ralstonia solanacearum*	pyrazine, 2-ethyl-3-methyl pyrazine, 2-ethyl- pyrazine, 2, 5-dimethyl pyrazine, 2-methyl	Munjal et al. [27]
B. cereus D13	*Xanthomonas oryzae pv. oryzae* (rice bacterial leaf blight) *Xanthomonas oryzae pv. oryzicola* *Pseudomonas syringae pv. tomato* *Ralstonia solanacearum*	decyl alcohol 3,5,5-trimethylhexanol	Xie et al. [25] Xie et al. [4]
B. atrophaeus JZB120050	*Ralstonia solanacearum* *Pseudomonas tolaasii* *Pseudomonas syringae pv. lachrymans*	mixture of VOCs	Ni et al. [28]
B. subtilis GB03 *B. amyloliquefaciens* IN937a	*Erwinia carotovora* subsp. *carotovora*	2,3-butanediol acetoin	Ryu et al. [15]
B. amyloliquefaciens FZB42 *B. atrophaeus* LSSC22	*Ralstonia solanacearum* (tobacco bacterial wilt)	benzaldehyde 1,2-benzisothiazol-3(2H)-one 1,3-butadiene	Tahir et al. [24]
B. velezensis X5-2 *B. megaterium* X6-3 *Pseudomonas orientalis* X2-1P	*Xanthomonas campestris* pv. *campestris* (black rot of winter oilseed rape)	mixture of VOCs	Jelušić et al. [26]
B. velezensis JCK-1618 *B. velezensis* JCK-1696	*Xanthomonas arboricola* pv. *pruni*	mixture of VOCs	Han et al. [25]

3. Mechanisms of Action of Antifungal *Bacillus*-Based VOCs

The overview of published literature data investigating the antifungal activity of *Bacillus*-based VOCs shows a supreme number of studies compared to literature investigating antibacterial and nematicidal effects. Hence, a general overview of the mechanisms involved in the suppression of plant-pathogenic fungi by the *Bacillus* VOCs will be given here (summarized in Figure 3), emphasizing the most abundant and effective VOCs in terms of antifungal activity. A more detailed overview of the published data regarding the antifungal activity of VOCs produced by different strains of the genus *Bacillus* can be found in Table 2, while the most abundant *Bacillus*-based VOCs with antifungal activity towards plant pathogens are presented in Figure 4.

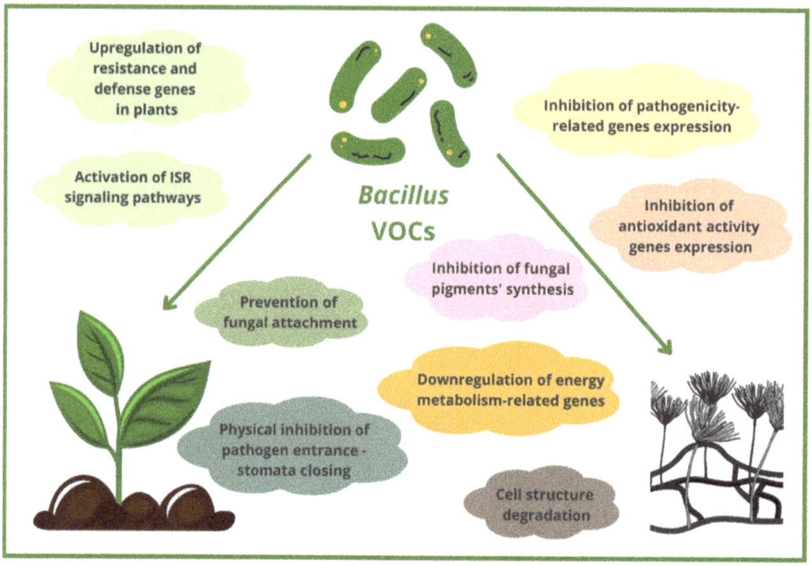

Figure 3. Antifungal mechanisms of action of *Bacillus*-based VOCs (ISR—induced systemic resistance).

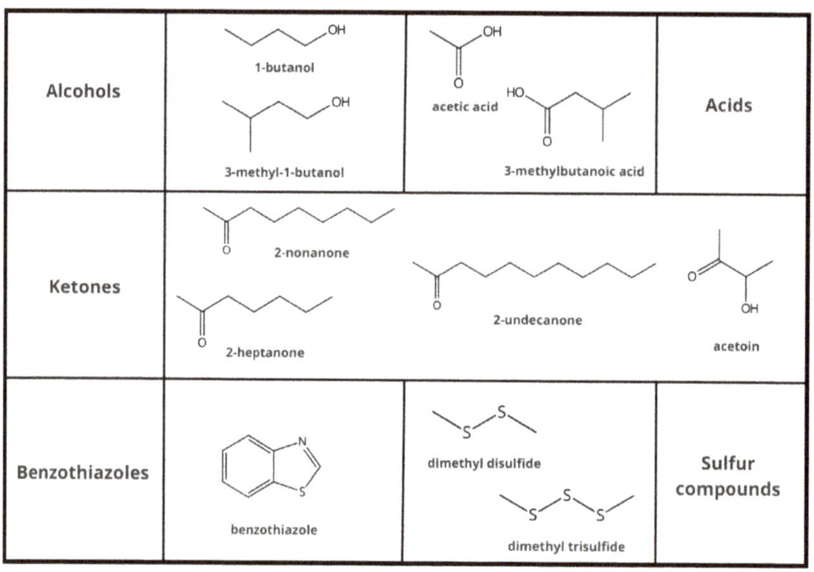

Figure 4. The most common antifungal VOCs produced by *Bacillus* spp.

3.1. *Cultivation and Treatment Variables Affecting Antifungal Efficiency of Bacillus VOCs*

The effect of the growth medium on VOCs production and antibacterial activity was reported by Huang et al. [29], where 90% growth inhibition of *Rhizoctonia solani* and *Pythium aphanidermatum* (Edson) was achieved using *B. mycoides* grown on TSA (tryptic soy agar) or SPMA (soy powder milk agar). This is while the application of KBA (King's B agar) and LBA (Luria-Bertani agar) resulted in moderate pathogen growth inhibition and NA (nutrient agar) and PDA (potato dextrose agar) showed almost no inhibitory activity against fungal pathogens. Similar results in terms of the suitability of TSA as a growth medium were obtained by Gotor-Vila et al. [30] for *B. amyloliquefaciens* CPA-8, whose antifungal activity was the highest compared to NYDA (nutrient yeast glucose agar) and NAglu20 (nutrient agar supplemented with glucose) in the cases of *Monilinia laxa* (>78.6%), *Botrytis cinerea* (86.8%), and *Monilinia fructicola* (68.6%) suppression. In the study by Fujimoto et al. [31], TSB (tryptone soya broth) and TSA favored the production of VOCs by *Bacillus* sp. ACB-65 and *Bacillus* sp. ACB-73, which exhibited antifungal activity against *Phyllosticta citricarpa*, the orange-black spot pathogen, over the NA, PDA, and King B media. Specific VOCs were produced by *B. amyloliquefaciens* strains UCMB5033, UCMB5036, UCMB5113, and FZB42 using different cultivation media: 2,3-butanedione and acetoin on M9A medium, while 5-methyl-heptanone, 2-methylpyridine, and 2-pentanone were produced on TSA and LBA media [32]. The highest production of antifungal VOCs (chloroacetic acid, tetradecyl ester, octadecane and hexadecanoic acid, and methyl ester) by *B. atrophaeus* HAB-5 in submerged cultivation was obtained in LB medium, followed by BPY (beef peptone yeast) and MH (Mueller Hinton) medium, inhibiting the growth of *Colletotrichum gloeosporioides* by 47.81, 45.51, and 44.55%, respectively [33]. Different types of growth media (NA, TSA, LBA, and TMEA (TM Enterprise agar) were investigated for their effect on VOCs production by *B. pumilus* TM-R and their antifungal activity against *Alternaria alternata, Aspergillus niger, Cladosporium cladosporioides, Curvularia lunata, Fusarium oxysporum, and Penicillium italicum* in both small- and large-scale tests (plate and 12L-tests, respectively). TMEA medium resulted in the strongest antifungal activity, supported by the production of methyl isobutyl ketone, ethanol, 5-methyl-2-heptanone, and S-()-2-methylbutylamine as the predominant antifungal VOCs [34]. MOLP medium (medium for optimum lipopetide production) used for the production of VOCs by *B.velezensis* BUZ-14 and *B. ginsengihumi* S38 resulted in 90% suppression of *Botrytis cinerea* in table grapes, while grape juice was the least favorable medium for VOC efficacy [35].

Furthermore, cultivation time also affects the type and content of the bacterial VOCs produced. The largest diversity of VOCs in the cultivation broth of *B. subtilis* CF-3 was detected after 48 hof cultivation, while the peak of the antifungal efficiency (73.46% on *Monilinia fructicola*, causing peach brown rot, and 63.63% on *Colletotrichum gloeosporioides*, causing litchi antrachnose), was achieved after 24 h of cultivation. Benzothiazole and 2,4-di-tert-butylphenol showed a strong inhibitory effect on both pathogens in vitro and vivo [36], with EC_{50} values of 9.90×10^{-4} mol/L for *Monilinia fructicola* and 1.26×10^{-2} mol/L for *Colletotrichum gloeosporioides* [37]. Similar results were obtained by Ni et al. [28], where *B. atrophaeus* JZB120050 produced 29 alkanes, three alkenes, four acids, one aldehyde, and one phenol after 24 h, while 41 compounds were detected via GC-MS analysis, including 34 alkanes, three alkenes, two acids, one benzene, and one phenol after 48 h of cultivation. Zheng et al. [38] investigated the mixture content of VOCs produced by *B. amyloliquefaciens* PP19 to suppress *Peronophythora litchi* and found significant differences in VOCs production over the course of the cultivation, where a total of 9, 33, 14, 28, and 17 compounds were detected at each of the five investigated time points (24, 36, 48, 60 and 72 h, respectively). However, only two compounds (2-nonanone and 6-methyl-2-heptanone) were common at all time points and constantly produced during the cultivation. Zhang et al. [39] have found that there was no significant difference in biocontrol activity regarding the in vivo suppression of raspberry postharvest diseases caused by *Botrytis cinerea* and *Rhizopus stolonifer* when VOCs produced by *B. siamensis* G-3 in NA medium and at pH 7.0 were applied for treatment after 72 h and 84 h of cultivation. This points out the necessity to optimize cultivation time in order to achieve maximal VOCs biocontrol efficacy while minimizing production operational costs.

The timing of inoculation/VOCs in correspondence with the pathogen infection time frame has been considered an important aspect affecting the efficiency of plant pathogen suppression, pointing out the importance of choosing between the preventive/curative plant disease management strategies. Previously mentioned molecular signaling between antagonists and plant pathogens and the related induction of VOC production in the pathogen's presence need to be understood in more detail to be able to define the appropriate timing of the treatment to maximize its efficiency. For example, Han et al. [25] have shown that the inoculation of antagonists *B. velezensis* JCK-1618 and JCK-1696 3 days before the fungal pathogen inoculation has significantly increased the treatment efficiency compared to a shorter time period (1 day) between the subsequent antagonist and pathogen inoculation. The efficiency of the VOCs produced by *B. velezensis* JCK-1696 was increased from 67% to 75.7% inhibition for *Mycosphaerella cerasella* and from 44.9% to 66.8% inhibition for *Epicoccum tobaicum*, taking into account a 1-day and 3-day inoculation interval [25]. These findings support several mechanisms of action described for *Bacillus* spp. biocontrol activity, including competition for growth space and nutrients with extra time given to establish antagonist populations at the target site of application as well as the longer time necessary to achieve a fungicidal level of VOC content. Jangir et al. [40] have reported an increase in the antifungal activity of *Bacillus* sp. B44 VOCs against *Fusarium oxysporum* f. sp. *lycopersici* from 20% on the 1st day of the in vitro experiment to 70% on the 7th day of incubation, while the in vivo test showed a 36% reduction in tomato disease incidence. An increase in the antifungal activity of VOCs produced by *B. amyloliquefaciens* ALB629 and UFLA285—including 3-methylbutanoic acid, 2-methylbutanoic acid, isovaleric acid, and 2- methyl butyric acid—was observed in the reduction of common bean antrachnose from 83% on the first day to 93% disease incidence reduction on the 11th day [41]. This was also shown by Arrebola et al. [42], where VOCs produced by *B. amyloliquefaciens* PPCB004 exhibited the highest inhibition of fungal radial growth of *Penicillium crustosum* (73.3%) in vitro after 10 days. This is while a significant in vivo decrease of decay incidence and severity in Valencia orange was observed after a 12-day treatment. Similar results were observed by Leelasuphakul et al. [43], where the disease incidence of green mold caused by *Penicillium digitatum* Sacc. in citrus fruit was decreased by 86.7% and disease symptoms were delayed by 6 days and decay symptoms to day 9 by the VOCs produced by the *B. subtilis* 155 suspensions, which was inoculated 24 h before pathogen inoculation. *B. amyloliquefaciens* NJN-6 inhibited the mycelial growth of *Fusarium oxysporum* f. sp. *cubense* by 30% to 40% compared with the control after 3 days of treatment, while in the soil test the number of *Fusarium oxysporum* f. sp. *cubense* was significantly reduced (10^2 spores/g compared to 10^4 spores/g in control samples) after 45 days of treatment [44]. The same study identified benzene (2,3,6-trimethyl-phenol) and ketone (2-undecanone, 2-dodecanon, and 2-tridecanone) compounds as the most effective in terms of antifungal activity, where the number of carbon atoms in ketones negatively correlated with their antifungal activity against *Fusarium oxysporum* f. sp. *cubense* [44]. *B. subtilis* Bs 8B-1 has produced a sufficient amount of antifungal VOCs after 5 days of incubation with *Phytophthora capsici*, causing cucumber damping-off, and *Rhizoctonia solani*, causing radish damping-off [45]. *B. velezensis* RDA1 VOCs inhibited the growth of *Rosellinia necatrix* by approximately 60–70% compared to control after 10 days of treatment [46].

3.2. Wide Spectrum of Bacillus VOCs Antifungal Activity

A wide spectrum of antifungal activity for the mixture of *Bacillus*-derived VOCs as well as for separate VOCs has been reported widely in the literature. For example, the soil isolate *B. subtilis* G_8 has inhibited mycelial growth and completely prevented the pigment production of different soil-borne pathogens, where inhibition rates of *Sclerotinia sclerotiorum, Botrytis cinerea,* and *Cercospora kikuchii* Chupp were over 75%, while inhibition rates were less than 46% for *Alternaria brassicae* and *Rhizoctonia solani* [47]. DG4 (an isomer of acetylbutanediol) produced by *B. subtilis* C9 has shown strong antifungal activity in terms of inhibition of mycelial growth against a wide range of fungal pathogens, including

Colletotrichum gloeosporioides (44.41%), *Chatomium globosum* (59.38%), *Glomerella cingulata* (73.40%), *Fusarium oxysporum* (93.61%), *Aspergillus niger* (78.97%), *Corynespora cassiicola* (44.37%) and *Rhizoctonia solani* (79.14%) [48]. Chaves-Lopez et al. [1] have ranked several fungal strains according to their sensitivity to the VOCs produced by *B. subtilis*, *B. amyloliquefaciens*, and *B. cereus* as follows: *Moniliophthora perniciosa* > *Aspergillus niger* > *Fusarium oxysporum* f.sp. *lactucae* and *Aspergillus flavus* > *Aspergillus clavatus* > *Aspergillus parasiticus*. For example, 1-butanol, 3-methyl-1-butanol, acetic acid, 2-methylpropanoic acid, carbon disulphide, 3-methylbutanoic acid, and ethyl acetate successfully inhibited the mycelial growth of *Moniliophthora perniciosa* by about 84% and that of *Fusarium oxysporum* f.sp. *lactucae* by about 50% [1]. *B. megaterium* USB2103 VOCs have also been shown to have antifungal activity against a wide range of fungi, including *Botrytis cinerea*, *Phytophthora nicotianae*, *Rhizoctonia solani*, *Sclerotinia sclerotiorum*, *Verticillium dahliae*, as well as *Fusarium oxysporum* and *Macrophomina phaseolina*, with acetic acid and 2-nonanone as dominant antifungal VOCs [49]. *B. velezensis* ZSY-1 isolated from Chinese cabbage has produced VOCs exhibiting significant antifungal activity against *Alternaria solani* (81.1%), *Botrytis cinerea* (93.8%), *Valsa mali* (83.2%), *Monilinia fructicola* (80.9%), *Fusarium oxysporum* f. sp. *capsicum* (76.7%), and *Colletotrichum lindemuthianum* (70.6%). Among the produced VOCs, pyrazine (2,5-dimethyl), benzothiazole, 4-chloro-3-methyl, and phenol-2,4-bis(1,1-dimethylethyl) had shown significant antifungal activity against *Alternaria solani* (87.5%, 100%, 100%, and 89.14%, respectively) and *Botrytis cinerea* (100%, 100%, 100%, and 91.19%, respectively) [50]. *B. amyloliquefaciens* DA12 VOCs inhibited the growth of six pathogens including *Botrytis cinerea* (cucumber grey mold), *Colletotrichum coccodes* (pepper anthracnose), *Endothia parasitica* (chestnut blight), *F. oxysporum* f. sp. *lycopersici* (tomato wilt), *Raffaelea quercus-mongolicae* (oak wilt), and *Rhizoctonia solani* (rice sheath blight), with inhibition rate in the range 31.6–95.5%, as well as mycelial growth and mycotoxin production by eight toxigenic *Fusarium* spp. (*Fusarium asiaticum*, *Fusarium graminearum*, *Fusarium proliferatum*, *Fusarium verticillioides*, and *Fusarium oxysporum*) producing nivalenol, deoxynivalenol (and its acetylated derivatives), and fumonisin, with an inhibition rate ranging from 57.1% to 74.0% [51]. Inhibition of mycotoxigenic fungi was also observed by the VOCs produced by *B. megaterium* KU143 and *Pseudomonas protegens* AS15 in the case of *Aspergillus flavus*, where the total aflatoxin production in rice grains was reduced by 90.4%, besides the reduced fungal population [52]. Hlebová et al. [53] have shown complete inhibition of ochratoxin synthesis in *Aspergillus ochraceus* and *Aspergillus westerdijkiae* by VOCs produced by *B. mycoides*, *B. subtilis*, and *B. thuringiensis*. Acetoin was found to be the major VOC produced by *B. velezensis* G341, inhibiting mycelial growth of *Sclerotinia sclerotiorum* (cucumber *Sclerotinia rot*), *Rhizoctonia solani* (rice sheath blight), and *Botrytis cinerea* (tomato grey mold) [54]. VOCs in a 24-h cultivation broth of *B. subtilis* CF-3 inhibited the mycelial growth of *Botrytis cinerea*, *Colletotrichum gloeosporioides*, *Penicillium expansum*, *Monilinia fructicola*, and *Alternaria alternata*, with a mean inhibition rate of 59.97% [35]. Biovolatiles produced by *B. velezensis* NKG-2 suppressed the mycelial growth of *Fusarium oxysporum* (57%), *Fusarium graminearum* (68%), *Botrytis cinerea* (57%), *Alternaria alternata* (46%), *Fulvia fulva* (65%), and *Ustilaginoidea virens* (51%) [55].

3.3. Morphological and Ultrastructural Abnormalities in Fungal Cells Caused by Bacillus VOCs

Mycelia morphological abnormalities were observed in *Sclerotinia sclerotiorum* by Liu et al. [56], together with spore cracking causing the brownish color of sporaceous inclusion and its effusion after 24–48 h of treatment using *Paenibacillus polymyxa* BMP-11, *B. subtilis* BL02, *B. pumilus* BSH-4, and *B. pumilus* ZB13 VOCs. Several VOCs from *B. megaterium* USB2103 have caused ultrastructural alterations at cell organelles, mostly membranes, mitochondria, and endoplasmic reticulum of *Sclerotinia sclerotiorum* [49]. Hemolytic activity of the majority of the pure VOCs confirmed that the membrane appeared to be one of the primary targets in terms of the antifungal mechanism of action since 2-nonanone caused damage to the cytoplasmic membrane, resulting in complete or partial hyphae emptying. Detachment of the membrane from the outer cell wall resulted in strong vacuolization with internal residues of membranes in the cytoplasm. DL-limonene treatment has also led to cytoplasmic membrane detachment from the cell wall, as well as cytoplasm granulation, the absence of organelles, multi-vesciculation, and the accumulation of protein and lipidic material in the cytoplasm. Dimethyl disulfide has shown strong ultrastructural modifications, including missing or altered cytoplasm, hyper-vesiculation, hypocrested and vesiculated mitochondria, and accumulation of protein and lipidic material in the cytoplasm [49]. Ultrastructural damage of *Sclerotinia sclerotiorum* hyphae due to the VOCs of *B. velezensis* VM11 included abnormalities on cell membranes, mitochondria, nucleus, multivesicular structures, and cytoplasm, together with increased vacuoles' size and disorganized cytoplasmic materials to the extent of non-descript cell organelles [57]. On the other hand, Monteiro et al. [58] have not observed any hyphae alteration in *Sclerotinia sclerotiorum* causing white mold in *Lactuca sativa* after contact with VOCs produced by *B. subtilis*, although the reduction of mycelial growth was 83.84%, indicating the fungistatic effect of the produced VOCs.

Abnormalities on conidiophores of *Penicillium crustosum* were observed in treatment with VOCs produced by *B. subtilis* PPCB001, while complete loss of conidiophore structures was detected in combined treatment with *B. amyloliquefaciens* PPCB004 VOCs, with the presumed dominant role of 3-hydroxy-2-butanone (acetoin), which has induced reduction of the multiple phialides at the end of each hyphae, as well as vacuolation and swelling in hyphae and sporangium [41]. Besides the reduced radial growth in vitro, dimethyl disulphide and ammonia as the main VOCs produced by *B. mycoides* had reduced the damping-off disease of cabbage seedlings caused by *Pythium aphanidermatum* Edson by 45% in greenhouse experiments, while the disease incidence caused by *Rhizoctonia solani* had not been reduced. The bacterial VOCs affected the morphology of fungal hyphae, causing poor rigidity, shrinkage, curling, swelling, and hyphal deformation, together with organelle degeneration [29]. Abnormal swelling and increased branching of the *Fusarium oxysporum* f. sp. *niveum* hyphae were induced by VOCs produced by *B. subtilis* IBFCBF-4 [59].

O-anisaldehyde produced by *B. atrophaeus* CAB-1 showed a higher in vitro inhibitory effect than L-alaninol on hyphal elongation of *Botrytis cinerea* when applied at the concentration of 80 μL/plate (70.2% growth inhibition). Interestingly, the individual VOCs produced by *B. atrophaeus* CAB-1 have not been successful in the biocontrol of cucumber powdery mildew (*Sphaerotheca fuliginea*), while the mixture of VOCs has shown supreme biocontrol efficacy (71.54%) under greenhouse conditions compared to the other bioactive compounds of the same strain, including lipopeptides (29.57%) and crude secreted proteins (41.94%) [60]. Several VOCs produced by *B. subtilis* M29, including 2,6-diisocyanato-1-methyl-benzene, 1-propoxy-2-propanol, and benzophenone, were reported to destroy normal hyphae morphology and induce mycelial fragmentation and crumpling in *Botrytis cinerea* [61]. *Botrytis cinerea* hyphae treated with *B. velezensis* XT1 and *B. atrophaeus* L193 volatiles produced in the MOLP medium showed severe cytoplasmic cavitation and vacuolation, and no organelles were identified, while the reduction of fungal growth was 27% and 46%, respectively [62].

Chaves-Lopez et al. [1] have reported changes in colony morphology, spore production, and microstructural changes of the hyphae in different fungal pathogens induced by the VOCs produced by *B. subtilis, B. amyloliquefaciens,* and *B. cereus*. The presence of VOCs from *B. subtilis* SV75-1 has significantly contributed to degenerative changes in the hyphal morphology of *Moniliophthora perniciosa*, including the observation of flaccid hyphae presenting retracted protoplasm and the formation of empty segments and a thinner wall. Retraction of protoplasm was also observed in *Aspergillus parasiticus* exposed to VOCs from *B. cereus* SV40, while exposure to *B. amyloliquefaciens* SV20-2 VOCs resulted in shortened and swollen somatic hyphae. *Fusarium oxysporum* f. sp. *lactucae* MA284 exposure to the VOCs of *B. subtilis* SV75-1 has resulted in a reduction in conidia number and granulation of the mycelia [1].

Malformations, vacuolations, and swellings were observed in hyphae of *Verticillium dahliae*, causing tomato *Verticillium* wilt as induced by *B. velezensis* C2 VOCs and resulting in an approximately 70% reduction in disease incidence [63]. The hyphae of *Verticillium dahliae* were completely lysed/dissolved after a 5-day treatment with styrene produced by *Bacillus* sp. T6 [64].

The VOCs produced by *B. vallismortis* 12a and *B. altitudinis* 14b seriously decomposed the cell walls and damaged the protoplast of *Monilinia fructicola*, causing peach brown rot, with a special emphasis on the outer cell walls, whose structure was thin or gapped, which might allow leaking out of the cell contents. Additionally, the result was 77.1% and 50% disease suppression in fumigation treatment with cultivation broth of these two strains, respectively [65]. Similar thin or gapped structures of the uneven cell wall surface presenting a retracted protoplasm were also observed in *B. cereus* CF4-51 VOCs-treated mycelia of *Sclerotinia sclerotiorum* [66]. Acetic acid (20.68%), propanoic acid (33.30%), butanoic acid (26.87%), valeric acid (43.71%), and isovaleric acid (53.10%) produced by *Bacillus* sp. LPPC170 significantly inhibited the mycelial growth of *Fusarium kalimantanense*, causing Panama disease of banana, by damaging the vegetative and reproductive structures of the fungus and causing a lower density of mycelium with dehydrated, considerably deformed, withered, and malnourished hyphae [67].

Hyphae with wrinkled surface cells, surface swelling, and thinner cell walls were observed as a consequence of 6-methyl-2-heptanone (emitted by *B. subtilis* ZD01) treatment in *Alternaria solani*. As a result, the cytoplasm was shrunken, with an increased number of inclusions and larger liquid droplets, together with cytoplasmic content movement toward the ruptured cell walls or cytoplasmic membranes [68]. Hyphae of *Alternaria alternata* (tobacco brown spot) without any attached conidia appeared ruptured, shrunken, and twisted after being treated with 2-methylbutanoic acid and 3-methylbutanoic acid produced by *B. siamensis* LZ88 [69]. The mycelium of *Alternaria solani*, the causal agent of tomato early blight, became thin, twisted, deformed, bifurcated, and fractured, with a wrinkled and cracked surface, followed by intracellular content leakage after the treatment with *B. velezensis* ZJ1 VOCs led by isooctanol and 2-nonanol as the major active compounds [70]. Similar results were found for *Alternaria solani* causing early potato blight when exposed to the VOCs produced by *B. subtilis* ZD01 [71], as well as for *Mucor circinelloides*, *Fusarium arcuatisporum*, *Alternaria iridiaustralis*, and *Colletotrichum fioriniae* due to 2,3-butanedione and 3-methylbutyric acid produced by *B. subtilis* CL2 [72]. Twisted, flattened, and enlarged hyphae that lost their linearity were observed in *Alternaria iridiaustralis*, caused by the VOCs produced by *B. velezensis* L1 with 2,3-butanedione as the leading VOC [73].

Twisted hyphae were also observed in Colletotrichum acutatum, Colletotrichum coccodes, Colletotrichum dematium, and Colletotrichum gloeosporioides after treatment with the VOC mixture produced by B. velezensis CE 100 [74]. VOCs of B. velezensis JRX-YG39 have caused hyphae abnormalities such as coiling and discoloration in Colletotrichum gloeosporioides (walnut and jujube anthracnose), while the pure compounds 5-nonylamine and 3-methylbutanoic acid have caused similar morphological changes followed by cell wall lysis and fracturing [75].

Hyphal swelling, cytoplasm and protoplasm aggregation, and distortion of large amounts of balloon-shaped cells were reported for *Fusarium verticillioides*, *Fusarium graminearum*, and *Rhizoctonia solani* after treatment with *B. mojavensis* I4, with mycelial growth inhibition in the range of 16–76% [76]. Hyphae of *Phyllosticta citricarpa* were fattened, twisted, and deformed, with a reduced amount of conidia at the lesion site on the surface of orange plants after treatment with the VOCs produced by *Bacillus* sp. ACB-65 and *Bacillus* sp. ACB-73 [31].

In *Monilinia laxa* and *Monilinia fructicola*, the hyphal membrane and cell walls were thinner and degraded, while the cytoplasmic content was completely coagulated and no organelles could be identified [62]. One of the main mechanisms of action related to the degradation of the structure of fungal cell walls and cell membrane relies on the modification of fatty acids and ergosterol content. Benzothiazole produced by *B. subtilis* CF-3 reduced the content of long-chain saturated fatty acids (trans-linoleic acid, oleic acid, and palmitic acid) in the *Monilinia fructicola* membrane, indicating decreased cell membrane unsaturation resulting in the gradual weakening of membrane fluidity and leakage of intracellular content. Furthermore, benzothiazole treatment also reduced ergosterol content in the cell wall of *Monilinia fructicola*, affecting the integrity of the fungal cell wall and thus weakening the cell membrane and material transport [77].

3.4. Inhibition of Different Fungal Growth Stages by Bacillus VOCs

The VOCs of *B. subtilis* G_8 have been shown to efficiently prevent the overwintered sclerotoid germination of *Sclerotinia sclerotiorum*, which is a major mechanism for disease suppression due to reduced apothecial formation and decimated ascospore infection [47]. Liu et al. [56] have observed significant morphological changes affecting sclerotia function, including odd shape and lack of plumpness, as well as reduced mean weight of sclerotia (44.2%, 48.0%, 29.1%, and 22.4%) in treatments with VOCs produced by *Paenibacillus polymyxa* BMP-11, *B. subtilis* BL02, *B. pumilus* BSH-4, and *B. pumilus* ZB13, respectively. A higher minimal inhibitory concentration of the VOCs produced by *B. megaterium* USB2103 was required to inhibit sclerotia germination compared to mycelial growth of *Sclerotinia sclerotiorum*, except in the case of dimethyl trisulfide whose minimal inhibitory concentration has shown similar results either on mycelium growth or sclerotia germination [49]. *B. cereus* CF4-51 VOCs (2-pentadecanone, 6,10,14-trimethyl-, 1,2-benzenedicarboxylic acid bis(2-methylpropyl) ester, dibutyl phthalate, cyclododecane, and heptadecane) have shown supreme inhibition of *Sclerotinia sclerotiorum* (65.4%) in comparison with the cell free supernatant (18.2–42.4%) and lipopeptides (55.6%) by altering the expression of four genes related to sclerotia formation (*Ss-sl2, SOP1, SsAMS2,* and *SsSac1*) [66]. *B. velezensis* VM11, *B. velezensis* VM10, and *B. amyloliquefaciens* VM42 VOCs exhibited fungistatic effects toward *Sclerotinia sclerotiorum* by inhibiting sclerotia production by 62.9%, 54.7%, and 72.5%, respectively, while healthy harvested sclerotia lost their germination ability after being incubated together with 5 µL of *Bacillus* endophyte cultures [57].

B. subtilis PPCB001 and *B. amyloliquefaciens* PPCB004 VOCs affected the germination and germ tube elongation of *Penicillium crustosum* [42]. Inhibition of spore germination and germ tube elongation were also observed in *Penicillium digitatum* and *Penicillium italicum* in the presence of the VOCs produced by *B. amyloliquefaciens* JBC36, which resulted in 57.8% and 54.1% in vitro inhibition of mycelial growth of *Penicillium digitatum* and *Penicillium italicum*, respectively, as well as a reduced incidence of green and blue mold on wounded mandarin fruits with control efficacies of 88% and 80.2%, respectively [78]. Inhibition of conidial germination of *Thielaviopsis paradoxa* ranged from 12% to 68.8% during the 9-h exposure to the VOCs of *B. siamensis* N-1 [79].

Reduced sporification was observed in *Aspergillus flavus* in the presence of *B. cereus* SV40, *B. subtilis* SV36/2, and *B. coagulans* SV95 VOCs [1]. A significant decrease in spore density of *Fusarium verticillioides* and *Fusarium graminearum* was observed after treatment with *B. mojavensis* I4 VOCs [76]. The different concentrations of 1%, 3%, 5%, 7%, and 10% of the VOCs produced by *B. velezensis* CE 100 reduced the spore germination of *Colletotrichum gloeosporioides* (walnut and jujube antrachnose) by 15.4%, 18.9%, 25.4%, 30.0%, and 36.4%, respectively, with remarkably reduced germ tube elongation [75]. Incompact and irregular structures of spores of *Verticillium dahliae*, causing cotton *Verticilium* wilt, together with visible holes on the spores' surface, appeared after treatment using styrene produced by *Bacillus* sp. T6 [64]. *B. velezensis* SBB VOCs (2-nonanol—0.06 µL/mL, 2-heptanone—0.3 µL/mL, 6-methyl-2-heptanone—0.3 µL/mL, and 2-nonanone—0.6 µL/mL) completely inhibited *Verticillium dahliae* growth in vitro and inhibited production of conidia and microsclerotia [80]. Phenylacetic acid and methylphenyl acetate produced by *B. mycoides* BM02 suppressed spore germination but had no effects on the hyphal growth of *Fusarium oxysporum* f. sp. *lycopersici* in tomato [81]. Deformed and collapsed spores of *Alternaria alternata*, causing tobacco brown spot, resulted from treatment with 2-methylbutanoic acid and 3-methylbutanoic acid produced by *B. siamensis* LZ88, while inhibition of spore germination was achieved with EC_{50} values of 139.63 mg/mL and 88.07 mg/mL for the aforementioned VOCs, respectively [69].

Damaged conidial internal structures with collapsed and shrunken small vesicles, extracellular secretions around the conidial cell-wall surface, and larger lipid droplets within the conidia were observed in *Alternaria solani* after treatment with 6-methyl-2-heptanone (EC_{50} value of 10.88 μL) produced by *B. subtilis* ZD01 [68]. The germination rate of the morphologically disrupted conidia was lowered to 75%, and these conidia formed irregular (shorter) germ tubes that were not able to penetrate and invade host epidermal cell junctions. This was also confirmed by the down-regulation of the expression of two genes: the *slt2* gene, involved in mycelial growth, penetration, and pathogenicity [71], and the *wetA* gene, involved in sporulation and conidial wall formation [68]. *B. safensis* STJP VOCs (phenol, 2,4-bis (1,1-dimethylethyl)-, 3-hexadecanol, pyrrolo (1,2-a)pyrazine-1,4-dione, hexahydro-3-(2-methyl-propyl)-, 5,10-diethoxy-2,3,7,8-tetrahydro-1H,6H-dipyrrolo(1,2-a:10,20-d)pyrazine and hexadecanoic acid) have completely inhibited spore formation and conidia germination of *Alternaria alternata* [82]. The VOCs produced by *B. subtilis* ZD01 can inhibit the conidia germination (19.2%) and reduce the lesion areas and number of *Alternaria solani* in vivo significantly, which was further confirmed by the down-regulation of transcriptional expression of the *slt2* gene, a key gene that regulates the mycelial growth, penetration, sporulation, and virulence in vivo in *Alternaria solani* [71]. In the study by Xie et al. [83], 2-heptanone and isopentyl acetate produced by *B. subtilis* DZSY21 strongly inhibited the sporulation and germination of *Curvularia lunata* (maize leaf spot) conidia, while 2-methylbutyric acid inhibited sporulation, but did not affect germination. Furthermore, these VOCs repressed expression of the virulence-associated genes *clk1* and *clm1*, which encod mitogen-activated protein kinases required for conidia sporulation and pathogenicity in *Curvularia lunata* [83].

3.5. Prevention of Fungal Plant Attachment and Colonization by Bacillus VOCs

The VOCs of *B. subtilis* C9, with a special emphasis on DG4 (an isomer of acetyl butanediol) as an antifungal compound, have significantly reduced the incidence of stem-segment colonization by *Rhizoctonia solani* in Zoysia grass [48]. Sharifi and Ryu [84] have concluded that VOCs produced by *B. subtilis* GB03 might interfere with mycelial attachment to the hydrophobic cuticular surface of the *Arabidopsis* leaves, hence causing epiphytic mycelial growth of *Botrytis cinerea* and its inability to penetrate and colonize host tissue. Castro et al. [85] have made a relation between *B. velezensis* XT1 VOCs and the reduced number of *Verticillium dahliae* microsclerotia in the soil. *B. velezensis* OEE1 VOCs supported the reduction of *Verticillium dahliae* microsclerotia density in the naturally infested soil around olive trees [86]. The VOCs produced by *B. amyloliquefaciens* UQ154, *B. velezensis* UQ156, and *Acinetobacter* sp. UQ202 (isovaleraldehyde, 2-ethylhexanol, 2-heptanone, benzyl alcohol, and 3-methylbutanol) in a concentration of 10 μg/mL inhibited sporangia production and zoospore motility of *Phytophthora capsici* [87].

3.6. Altering the Expression of Genes Related to Pathogenicity, Metabolism and Antioxidant Activity of Fungal Pathogens

Zhang et al. [64] have reported the down-regulation of genes related to transport and catabolism, cell growth, and biosynthesis, especially peptidases, lipases, proteases, and chitinases, which act as plant cell wall-degrading enzymes, as well as methionyl-tRNA synthetases, in *Verticillium dahliae*, causing *Verticillium* cotton wilt, while the gene expression was modulated via styrene produced by *Bacillus* sp. T6.

Wang et al. [88] investigated differentially expressed genes and proteins in *Colletotrichum gloeosporioides* after treatment with *B. subtilis* CF-3 VOCs. The results revealed significant down-regulation of expression of genes related to cell membrane fluidity, cell wall integrity, energy metabolism, and production of cell wall-degrading enzymes, with a special emphasis on the biosynthesis of unsaturated fatty acids and ergosterol as the significant components of cell membranes, where 2,4-di-tert-butylphenol has been detected as the major antifungal VOC [88]. *B. subtilis* CF-3 VOC 2,4-di-tert-butylphenol can inhibit the activity of the pathogenic enzymes (pectinase and cellulase) secreted by *Colletotrichum gloeosporioides* to reduce the decomposition of plant tissues in litchi fruits [89], as well as benzothiazole with the same mechanism of antifungal activity against *Monilinia fructicola* in peaches [77]. The VOCs of *Bacillus* endophytes (*B. velezensis* VM11, *B. velezensis* VM10, and *B. amyloliquefaciens* VM42) induced strong ROS (reactive oxygen species) production in *Sclerotinia sclerotiorum* mycelial cells [57]. Down-regulation of the *SOD* gene, which plays a significant role in the SOD (superoxide dismutase) synthetic pathway in *Alternaria solani*, was found as a consequence of in vivo treatment by the VOCs produced by *B. subtilis* ZD01, suggesting the inhibition of the pathogen's antioxidant metabolism [71]. ROS can damage DNA replication and cell membranes, leading to cell death. In the study by Xie et al. [83], isopentyl acetate produced by *B. subtilis* DZSY21 caused ROS accumulation in the conidia of *Curvularia lunata* (maize leaf spot), while 2-methylbutyric acid and 2-heptanone did not affect ROS accumulation in conidia and mycelia. Here, it is suggested that these VOCs target different germination-related processes in *Curvularia lunata* conidia [83].

3.7. ISR Induced by Bacillus VOCs as Antifungal Mechanism of Action

One of the ways to induce resistance in plants against pathogens is physical inhibition of pathogen entrance to plant inner tissues by closing stomata. Acetoin and 2,3-butanediol as VOCs of *B. amyloliquefaciens* FZB42 modulated stomatal closure in *Arabidopsis thaliana* and *Nicotiana benthamiana*, where root absorption of VOCs was more effective than volatilization considering that VOC concentration of 250 μL was enough for stomata closure via root treatment, while 1 mM of VOCs was required for volatilization treatment. Furthermore, these VOCs have been successful in targeting pathogen entry points into hosts by triggering salicylic acid and abscisic acid signaling pathways and inducing the accumulation of hydrogen peroxide and nitric oxide, which are required for stomata closure [90]. Sharifi and Ryu [84] have found that the optimized concentration of *B. subtilis* GB03 that did not directly inhibit fungal growth of *Botrytis cinerea* successfully protected *Arabidopsis* from fungal infection, which indicates that ISR elicited by the bacterial VOCs has a more important role in biocontrol than direct inhibition of fungal growth on *Arabidopsis* plants. It was further confirmed that the ISR proportion was 90.63% and direct inhibition of fungi was 9.36% of the overall biocontrol activity, which means that ISR had the main role in suppressing *Botrytis cinerea* on *Arabidopsis* plants in conditions of low VOCs concentration. An almost three-fold increase in expression levels of plant defensin PDF1.2 indicated that the jasmonic acid signaling pathway had a key role in VOC-elicited plant defense responses, followed by the salicylic acid signaling pathway, as determined by the 2.8-fold increase in the expression level of PR1 (pathogenesis-related protein 1). On the other hand, the ethylene signaling pathway was not included in the *Arabidopsis* defense response since the expression level of the *ChiB* (basic endochitinase) gene did not display statistically significant differences between the VOCs-treated and control plants. This was also the first study to make a distinction between direct and indirect mechanisms of fungal pathogen suppression [84]. Pepper priming using the *B. velezensis* strains 5YN8 and DSN012 as VOC producers has resulted in more rapid transcription of the three pathogenicity-related genes (*NPR1*, *PR1*, and peroxidase gene), thus enhancing pepper resistance to *Botrytis cinerea* by activating the salicylic acid-mediated defense signaling pathway. In this way, gray mold biocontrol efficacy was above 50% in greenhouse experiments, with increased leaf number, stem diameter, and chlorophyll content in pepper seedlings [91]. Zheng et al. [38] have concluded that α-farnesene produced by several *Bacillus* isolates is probably related to ISR considering that it had not shown any antifungal activity in vitro against *Peronophythora litchi* while in vivo it had suppressed litchi downy blight with an efficacy of 52.34%.

B. siamensis LZ88 VOCs induced plant basal immunity through the induction of defense-related enzymes against *Alternaria alternata*, including peroxidase and polyphenol oxidase, thus contributing to the reduction of brown spots in tobacco leaves [92]. *B. velezensis* XT1 VOCs increased polyphenol oxidase activity by 395%, indicating induced resistance against *Verticillium* wilt of olive (*Verticillium dahliae*) in plant tissues, resulting in reduced disease severity in young olives by almost 80% [85]. Activation of antioxidant enzymes (peroxidase, polyphenol oxidase, catalase, and superoxide dismutase) in litchi fruit to eliminate excessive reactive oxygen species to reduce plant cell damage and activate disease resistance enzymes (phenylalanine ammonia-lyase, chitinases, β-1,3-glucanase) and enhance the resistance of litchi fruits to *Colletotrichum gloeosporioides* by inhibiting its growth was observed to be enhanced by 2,4-di-tert-butylphenol produced by *B. subtilis* CF-3 [89]. Similar mechanisms of action were observed for benzothiazole produced by the same *Bacillus* isolate in the suppression of *Monilinia fructicola* peach rot [77].

3.8. Inhibition of Fungal Pigments Production by Bacillus VOCs

Another interesting mechanism of action of *Bacillus*-produced VOCs is the inhibition of the production of different fungal pigments. Inhibition of pigment formation by the volatiles produced by *B. subtilis* G_8 [47], *Paenibacillus polymyxa* BMP-11, *B. subtilis* BL02, *B. pumilus* BSH-4, and *B. pumilus* ZB13 [56] was observed in *Ascochyta citrullina, Alternaria solani,* and *Alternaria brassicae.* The VOCs *of B. amyloliquefaciens* M49 inhibited the production of pink pigment by *Fusarium oxysporum* f. sp. *lactucae* [1]. *B. velezensis* SBB VOCs (2-nonanol, 2-heptanone, 6-methyl-2-heptanone, and 2-nonanone) inhibited melanin production by *Verticillium dahliae* [80]. Melanin plays an important role in providing the mechanical strength required for germ tubes, obtained by conidia germination, to penetrate host tissues [93]. The VOCs produced by *B. subtilis* DZSY21 caused inhibition of the expression of *SCD* and *brn1* genes involved in the synthesis of melanin in *Curvularia lunata* (maize leaf spot), where the inhibitory effect of isopentyl acetate was higher than that of 2-heptanone [83].

3.9. In Vivo Application of Bacillus VOCs in Biocontrol of Fungal Diseases

3.9.1. Fungal Diseases Caused by *Colletotrichum gloeosporioides*

Zheng et al. [94] have reported successful inhibition of *Colletotrichum gloeosporioides,* the causal agent of mango anthracnose, in vitro (88.87% and 80.07%) and in vivo (94.28% and 87.06%) using the VOCs produced by *B. pumilus* TB09 *and B. thuringiensis* TB72, respectively. The main identified bioactive VOCs and their minimal inhibitory concentrations for mycelial growth inhibition were 2-nonanone, b-benzeneethanamine, 2-decanone, and 2-methylpyrazine in a concentration of 100 μL/L and thymol in a concentration of 50 μL/L. The disease incidence of mango fruit anthracnose, caused by *Colletotrichum gloeosporioides* and treated by *B. siamensis* N-1, was reduced by 44.6%, while the litchi fruit disease index and browning index were reduced by 57.8% and 82.3% through mediation by the VOCs [73].

3.9.2. Fungal Diseases Caused by *Fusarium* spp.

Different *Bacillus* strains produced VOCs that inhibited *Fusarium solani,* including *B. amyloliquefaciens* subsp. *plantarum* YAU B9601-Y2, *Bacillus* spp. 041, 285, 033, 355 and *B. subtilis* XF-1, which had shown exceptionally strong inhibitory activities (75–82% inhibition), as well as *B. velezensis* FZB42 and *B. subtilis* 168, whose VOCs demonstrated 67% and 56% inhibition, respectively [95]. *B. subtilis* IBFCBF-4 VOCs successfully inhibited the mycelial growth of *Fusarium oxysporum* f. sp. *niveum* in vitro by 47.9%, while the reduction of *Fusarium* wilt in watermelon in greenhouse experiments was 51.1% [59]. *B. amyloliquefaciens* L3 VOCs (2-nonanone and 2-heptanone) were found to suppress *Fusarium* wilt of watermelon (*Fusarium oxysporum* f. sp. *niveum*) in greenhouse pot experiments, while acetoin and 2,3-butanediol were responsible for watermelon plant growth promotion [96]. Greenhouse experiments confirmed the efficacy of *B. mojavensis* I4 VOCs in the suppression of *Fusarium verticillioides, Fusarium graminearum,* and *Rhizoctonia solani* in *Arabidopsis thaliana* plants, with significant improvements in plant growth, biomass production, and chlorophyll content [76]. The VOCs of *B. cereus* MH778713 (hentriacontane and 2,4-di-tert-butylphenol) reduced the disease severity of tomato *Fusarium* wilt (*Fusarium oxysporum*) from 88.1 ± 4.1% to only 23 ± 8.2%, followed by a several-fold increase in tomato root and shoot length as well as in the fresh and dry weight of plants in treatment with 50 μg of the bioactive VOCs [97]. *In-planta* assays showed that *B. mycoides* BM02 treatment mediated by phenylacetic acid and methylphenyl acetate reduced spore attachment and germination of *Fusarium oxysporum* f. sp. *lycopersici* and increased the formation of swollen hyphae, thus protecting tomato seedlings against *Fusarium* wilt [81].

3.9.3. Fungal Diseases Caused by *Sclerotinia* spp.

Shifa et al. [98] were the first to report the production of tridecane by *B. subtilis* G-1, which participated in the suppression of *Sclerotium rolfsii*, which causes stem rot or white mold of groundnut. Wu et al. [99] have identified toluene, phenol, and benzothiazole as the main VOCs produced by *B. amyloliquefaciens* NJZJSB3, which have shown comparable effects to chemical fungicides in terms of reduction of canola stem rot incidence (by 83.3%), caused by *Sclerotinia sclerotiorum*, in pot experiments. Southern blight of *Aconitum carmichaelii* Debx., caused by *Sclerotium rolfsii*, was successfully inhibited (30% with a long-acting duration of up to 62 days) in a field trial by fermentation culture VOCs of *B. subtilis* JY-7-2L [100].

3.9.4. Fungal Diseases Caused by *Monilinia* spp.

Gotor-Vila et al. [30] have identified 1,3 pentadiene, acetoin (3-hydroxy-2-butanone), and thiophene as the main VOCs produced by *B. amyloliquefaciens* CPA-8, whereas thiophene was the most effective VOC in the suppression of *Monilinia laxa*, *Monilinia fructicola*, and *Botrytis cinerea* in vitro. On the other hand, during in vivo tests, it has not shown a biocontrol effect as a pure compound, while the mixture of VOCs decreased the disease incidence of cherry decay to 25% (compared to 65% in the control). The efficacy of VOCs produced by *B. amyloliquefaciens* SF14, *B. amyloliquefaciens* SP10, *Alcaligenes faecalis* ACBC1, and *Pantoea agglomerans* ACBP1 against *Monilinia fructigena* and *Monilinia laxa* causing apple brown spot was confirmed in a semi-commercial large-scale trial, with efficacy comparable to the commercial biocontrol agents (*B. subtilis* Y1336 and *Pantoea agglomerans* P10c) [101]. *B. subtilis* CF-3 VOCs combined with heat treatment could significantly reduce the rot index of peach and litchi fruit caused by *Monilinia fructicola* and *Colletotrichum gloeosporioides*, respectively, and effectively maintained fruit firmness and soluble solids content, reducing the fruit weight loss [102].

3.9.5. Fungal Diseases Caused by *Alternaria* spp.

B. velezensis ZJ1 VOCs 2-nonanol and isooctanol showed well in vitro antifungal activity and in vivo biocontrol effect against the two pathogens causing tomato early blight and gray mold, with 40.58% and 50.90% for *Alternaria solani* and *Botrytis cinerea*, respectively, while the highest decrease in disease incidence (74.16%) was observed in 2-nonanol treatment (25 μL/mL) [70]. The VOCs produced by *B. velezensis* L1 considerably decreased the wolfberry's disease index and decay incidence *in vivo*, caused by *Alternaria iridiaustralis*, where no mycelial growth was observed on the wolfberry fruits after exposure to the 8 LB (Luria-Bertrani) plates. The leading VOC with the strongest antifungal effect was 2,3-butanedione, which totally inhibited *Alternaria iridiaustralis* in wolfberry fruit at a concentration of 60 μL/L [73]. The VOCs produced by *B. subtilis* ZD01 significantly reduced lesion diameter in potato leaves, as well as the population density of *Alternaria solani* (early blight pathogen), with acetophenone, 2-nonanone, *m*-tolunitrile, 2-ethylhexanol, 2-heptanone, benzylacetone, 6-methyl-2-heptanone, benzothiazole, 5-methyl-2-hexanone, aniline, 4-methylanisole, benzoxazole, valerophenone, and 2,5-dimethylpyrazine as the major antifungal VOCs [68].

3.9.6. Fungal Diseases Caused by *Botrytis cinerea*

Dibutyl phthalate produced by *B. velezensis* JRX-YG39 has significantly reduced disease incidence in *Arabidopsis thaliana* caused by *Botrytis cinerea* up to 19.38% [103]. Zhang et al. [41] have reported 2,6-di-tert-butyl-4-methylphenol (BHT) and 2,4-di-tert-butylphenol (2,4-DTBP) produced by *B. siamensis* G-3 as biofumigants for controlling raspberry postharvest diseases caused by *Botrytis cinerea* and *Rhizopus stolonifer* in vivo, with biocontrol efficacy of 52.38% and 93.33%, respectively. This results in the possibility of storing raspberries for 20 days at 0 °C with the disease rate maintained at ~10% after the 2,4-DTBP treatment. Diacetyl and benzaldehyde produced by *B. velezensis* strains BUZ-14, I3, and I5 have been reported as promising VOCs for active packaging during the postharvest commercialization of fruit. Furthermore, VOCs of *B. velezensis* I3 suppressed gray mold (*Botrytis cinerea*) in grapes by 50%, while the VOCs of *B. velezensis* BUZ-14 decreased brown rot severity in apricots (*Monilinia fructicola*) from 60 to 4 mm. Diacetyl was shown as suitable for biocontrol of gray mold with a concentration of only 0.02 mL/L and blue rot in mandarins at the same dose up to 60% [35].

3.9.7. Suppression of Mycotoxigenic Fungi by *Bacillus*-Based VOCs

B. megaterium BM344-1 VOCs (hexadecanoic acid methyl ester (palmitic acid) and tetracosane) have caused 51% inhibition of *Aspergillus flavus* growth in in vivo experiments on maize kernels, as well as a reduction in aflatoxin synthesis from 91.81 ± 29.10 μg/kg to 25.34 ± 6.72 μg/kg. On the other hand, in vitro experiments have resulted in significant growth inhibition of mycotoxigenic fungi *Penicillium verrucosum* (66.7%), *Aspergillus flavus* (29.4%), and *Fusarium verticillioides* (18.2%), as well as in complete inhibition of aflatoxins (AFB1, AFG1, and AFG2), ochratoxin A, and fumonisin B1 (FB1) synthesis on artificial media [104]. In vivo assays on maize ears resulted in an 88% reduction in *Aspergillus flavus* growth and complete inhibition of fungal sporulation and aflatoxin accumulation by the VOCs produced by *B. licheniformis* BL350-2, dominated by 3-methyl-1-butanol [105].

3.9.8. Suppression of Other Fungal Diseases by *Bacillus*-Based VOCs

VOCs emitted by bacterial antagonists *B. amyloliquefaciens* UQ154, *B. velezensis* UQ156, and *Acinetobacter* sp. UQ202 negatively influenced the mycelial growth of the soil-borne phytopathogenic oomycete *Phytophthora capsici* by 35%, with significant positive effects on the increase in chili biomass (shoot and root fresh weights) and the primary root length, as well as the promotion of both root hair growth and lateral root development. The most important VOCs with antifungal activity were isovaleraldehyde, 2-ethylhexanol, 2-heptanone, benzyl alcohol, and 3-methylbutanol [87]. The leaf spot disease indexes of maize leaves sprayed with conidia of *Curvularia lunata* treated with the VOCs produced by *B. subtilis* DZSY21 were reduced from 60.52 to 26.64% [83]. In vivo application of 2,3-butanedione and 3-methylbutyric acid produced by *B. subtilis* CL2 significantly reduced the weight loss rate of wolfberry fruits caused by the pathogenic fungus *Mucor circinelloides*, as well as the decay incidence rate caused by *Fusarium arcuatisporum*, *Alternaria iridiaustralis*, and *Colletotrichum fioriniae* [72]. The VOCs produced by *B. methylotrophicus* BCN2 and *B. thuringiensis* BCN10 played complementary roles in controlling *Fusarium oxysporum*, *Botryosphaeria* sp., *Trichoderma atroviride*, *Colletotrichum gloeosporioides*, and *Penicillium expansum*, providing freshness to loquat fruits for ten days with a disease incidence of 20.19% compared to 54.17% in the control group [106]. The VOCs produced *Bacillus* sp. ACB-65 and *Bacillus* sp. ACB-73 cultured in TSB culture medium provided 86% inhibition of freckles that evolved into hard spots, with more superficial citrus black spot (*Phyllosticta citricarpa*) lesions in oranges [31]. The importance of the applied VOC concentration was pointed out by Zheng et al. [38], who discovered that 1-(2-aminophenyl)ethanone, benzothiazole, and α-farnesene had shown the highest efficacy in suppression of litchi downy blight (*Peronophythora litchi*) when applied in the lowest concentration (100 mg/L) from the examined concentration range (100–1000 mg/L). It suggested that VOCs in small concentrations could achieve the priming effect in plants, thus sensitizing plants for faster and/or stronger responses to successive pathogen attacks by acting as signaling molecules for environmental stresses.

Table 2. Literature overview concerning antifungal VOCs produced by *Bacillus* spp.

Bacillus Strain	Plant Pathogen (Disease)	Antifungal VOCs	Reference
B. subtilis 155	*Penicillium digitatum* Sacc. (green mold of citrus fruit)	mixture of VOCs	Leelasuphakul et al. [43]
B. subtilis G_8	*Sclerotinia sclerotiorum* *Botrytis cinerea* *Alternaria brassicae* *Alternaria solani* *Alternaria citrulina* *Fusarium oxysporum* *Cercospora kikuchii Chupp* *Rhizoctonia solani*	mixture of VOCs	Liu et al. [47]
B. subtilis	*Sclerotinia sclerotiorum* (white mold of *Lactuca sativa*)	mixture of VOCs	Monteiro et al. [58]
B. subtilis GB03	*Botrytis cinerea*	mixture of VOCs	Sharifi and Ryu [84]
B. subtilis ACB-AP3 *B. subtilis* ACB-83	*Phyllosticta citricarpa* (orange black spot)	mixture of VOCs	Kupper et al. [107]
B. subtilis IBFCBF-4	*Fusarium oxysporum* f. sp. *niveum* (watermellon Fusarium wilt)	mixture of VOCs	Zhu et al. [59]
B. subtilis JY-7-2L	*Sclerotium rolfsii* (southern blight of *Aconitum carmichaelii* Debx.)	mixture of VOCs	Zou et al. [100]
B. subtilis C9	*Rhizoctonia solani*	acetylbutanediol	Islam et al. [48]
B. subtilis G-1	*Sclerotium rolfsii* (stem rot or white mould of groundnut)	tridecane	Shifa et al. [98]
B. subtilis M29	*Botrytis cinerea*	1-butanol acetic acid butyl ester 1-heptylene-4-alcohol 3-methyl-3-hexanol furan-tetrahydro-2,5-dimethyl 2,6-diisocyanato-1-methyl-benzene 1-propoxy-2-propanol benzophenone	Mu et al. [61]
B. subtilis CF-3	*Monilinia fructicola* *Colletotrichum gloeosporioides*	1-octanol 2,4-di-tert-butylthiophenol	Gao et al., 2017 [37]
	Botrytis cinerea (strawberry gray mold) *Colletotrichum gloeosporioides* (litchi antrachnose) *Penicillium expansum* (blue mold of apple) *Monilinia fructicola* (peach brown rot) *Alternaria alternata* (Alternaria rot and black spot of jujube)	2,4-di-tert-butylthiophenol benzothiazole 1-octanol benzoic acid benzaldehyde 3-methylbutanal	Gao et al., 2018 [36]
	Monilinia fructicola *Colletotrichum gloeosporioides*	mixture of VOCs	Wu et al. [102]
	Monilinia fructicola	benzothiazole	Zhou et al. [77]
	Colletotrichum gloeosporioides	2,4-di-tert-butylphenol	Zhao et al. [89] Wang et al. [88]
B. subtilis CL2	*Mucor circinelloides* *Fusarium arcuatisporum* *Alternaria iridiaustralis* *Colletotrichum fioriniae*	2,3-butanedione 3-methylbutyric acid	Ling et al. [72]
B. subtilis BTK1	*Sarocladium oryzae* (rice sheath rot)	3-heptanone, 5-ethyl-4-methyl- butanoic acid, 2-methyl 1-propanol 2,2-dimethyl acetate	Surya et al. [108]
B. subtilis DZSY21	*Curvularia lunata* (maize leaf spot)	2-methylbutyric acid 2-heptanone isopentyl acetate	Xie et al. [83]

Table 2. *Cont.*

Bacillus Strain	Plant Pathogen (Disease)	Antifungal VOCs	Reference
B. subtilis ZD01	*Alternaria solani* (potato early blight)	acetophenone 2-nonanone m-tolunitrile 2-ethylhexanol 2-heptanone benzylacetone 6-methyl-2-heptanone benzothiazole 5-methyl-2-hexanone	Zhang et al. [71]
		6-methyl-2-heptanone	Zhang et al., [68]
B. subtilis BS-01	*Alternaria solani* (tomato Alternaria blight)	triphenylphosphine oxide pyrrolo[1,2-a] pyrazine-1,4-dione, hexahydro-3-(2-methylpropyl) pyrrolo[1,2-a] pyrazine-1,4-dione, hexahydro-3-(phenylmethyl) n-hexadecanoic acid n-tridecan-1-ol octadecane octadecanoic acid eicosane dodecyl acrylate	Awan et al. [109]
B. amyloliquefaciens JBC36	*Penicillium digitatum* (green mold of citrus fruit) *Penicillium italicum* (blue mold of citrus fruit)	mixture of VOCs	Yu et al. [78]
B. amyloliquefaciens NJN-6	*Fusarium oxysporum* f. sp. *cubense*	phenol 2,3,6-trimethyl-phenol 2-undecanone 2-dodecanone 2-tridecanone	Yuan et al., 2012 [44]
		mixture of VOCs	Yuan et al. [110]
B. amyloliquefaciens W19	*Fusarium oxysporum* f. sp. *cubense* (bannana *Fusarium* wilt)	o-xylene 2-heptanone benzene, 2-propenyl benzene,1,4-dichloro undecane, 1,2-methyl acetophenone 2-nonanone nonanane 1-(4-methylphenyl)ethanone 2- decanone naphthalene 2-undecanone tridecane 2- dodecanone tetradecane 2-tridecanone pentadecane hexadecane tetradecane	Wang et al. [111]
B. amyloliquefaciens NJZJSB3	*Sclerotinia sclerotiorum* (canola stem rot)	toluene phenol benzothiazole	Wu et al. [99]
B. amyloliquefaciens CPA-8	*Monilinia laxa* *Monilinia fructicola* *Botrytis cinera* (sweet cherry decay)	1,3-pentadiene acetoin thiophene	Gotor-Vila et al. [30]

Table 2. *Cont.*

Bacillus Strain	Plant Pathogen (Disease)	Antifungal VOCs	Reference
B. amyloliquefaciens DA12	*Fusarium asiaticum* *Fusarium graminearum* *Fusarium proliferatum* *Fusarium verticillioides* *Fusarium oxysporum* f. sp. *lycopersici* (tomato wilt) *Botrytis cinerea* (cucumber grey mould) *Colletotrichum coccodes* (pepper anthracnose) *Endothia parasitica* (chestnut blight) *Raffaelea quercus-mongolicae* (oak wilt) *Rhizoctonia solani* (rice sheath blight)	2-heptanone 5-methyl heptanone 6-methyl heptanone	Lee et al. [51]
B. amyloliquefaciens L3	*Fusarium oxysporum* f. sp. *niveum* (watermellon Fusarium wilt)	2-nonanone 2-heptanone	Wu et al. [96]
B. amylolicefaciens ALB629 *B. amylolicefaciens* UFLA285	*Colletotrichum lindemuthianum* (common bean antrachnose)	3-methylbutanoic 2-methylbutanoic acid	Martins et al. [41]
B. amyloliquefaciens BsA3MX *B. amyloliquefaciens* BsC11MX	*Macrophomina phaseolina* (cowpea charcoal rot)	mixture of VOCs	Rangel- Montoya et al. [112]
B. amyloliquefaciens D747 (Amylo-X®) *B. amyloliquefaciens* FZB24 (Taegro®) *B. amyloliquefaciens* MBI600 (Serifel®) *B. amyloliquefaciens* QST713 (Serenade®Aso)	*Plenodomus tracheiphilus* (Mal Secco disease of *Citrus volkameriana*)	mixture of VOCs	Aiello et al. [113]
B. velezensis 5YN8 *B. velezensis* DSN012	*Botrytis cinerea* (pepper gray mold)	mixture of VOCs	Jiang et al. [91]
B. velezensis NKG-2	*Fusarium oxysporum* *Fusarium graminearum* *Botrytis cinerea* *Alternaria alternata* *Fulvia fulva* *Ustilaginoidea virens*	mixture of VOCs	Myo et al. [55]
B. velezensis C2	*Verticillium dahliae* (tomato wilt disease)	mixture of VOCs	Dhouib et al. [63]
B. velezensis OEE1	*Fusarium solani*	mixture of VOCs	Cheffi et al. [114]
	Verticillium dahliae	cyclo (Leu-Pro)	Cheffi Azabou et al. [86]
B. velezensis XT1	*Verticillium dahliae* (Verticillium wilt of olive tree)	mixture of VOCs	Castro et al. [85]
B. velezensis RDA1	*Rosellinia necatrix*	mixture of VOCs	Sawant et al. [46]
B. velezensis JCK-1618 *B. velezensis* JCK-1696	*Epicoccum tobaicum* *Mycosphaerella cerasella*	mixture of VOCs	Han et al. [25]
B. velezensis ZSY-1	*Alternaria solani* *Botrytis cinerea* *Valsa mali* *Monilinia fructicola* *Fusarium oxysporum* f. sp. *capsicum* *Colletotrichum lindemuthianum*	pyrazine (2,5-dimethyl) benzothiazole 4-chloro-3-methyl phenol-2,4-bis (1,1-dimethylethyl)	Gao et al. [50]
B. velezensis G341	*Alternaria panax* (ginseng blight) *Botrytis cinerea* (tomato gray mold) *Colletotrichum coccodes* (red pepper antrachnose) *Fusarium oxysporum* f. sp. *lycopersici* (tomato *Fusarium* wilt) *Magnaporthe oryzae* (rice blast) *Phytophthora capsici* *Pythium infestans* (tomato late blight) *Pythium ultimum* (cucumber damping-off) *Rhizoctonia solani* (rice sheath blight) *Sclerotinia sclerotiorum* (cucumber Sclerotinia rot)	dimethylsulfoxide 1-butanol acetoin	Lim et al. [54]

Table 2. *Cont.*

Bacillus Strain	Plant Pathogen (Disease)	Antifungal VOCs	Reference
B. velezensis BUZ-14 *B. velezensis* I3 *B. velezensis* I5	*Monilinia fructicola* *Monilinia laxa* *Penicillium italicum* *Botrytis cinerea*	benzaldehyde diacetyl	Calvo et al. [115]
B. velezensis CT32	*Verticillium dahliae* *Glomerella cingulata* *Thanatephorus cucumeris* *F. oxysporum* f. sp. *cucumerinum* *F. oxysporum* f. sp. *fragariae* *F. oxysporum* f. sp. *niveum* *Botryosphaeria dothidea* *Botrytis cinerea*	decanal benzothiazole 3-undecanone 2-undecanone 2-undecanol undecanal 2,4-dimethyl-6-tert-butylphenol	Li et al. [116]
B. velezensis CE 100	*Colletotrichum gloeosporioides* (walnut and jujube antrachnose)	5-nonylamine 3-methylbutanoic acid	Choub et al. [75]
	Colletotrichum acutatum *Colletotrichum coccodes* *Colletotrichum dematium* *Colletotrichum gloeosporioides*	mixture of VOCs	Kim et al. [74]
B. velezensis JRX-YG39	*Botrytis cinerea* *Fusarium pernambucanum* *Alternaria alternata* *Colletotrichum gloeosporioides*	dibutyl phthalate	Feng et al. [103]
B. velezensis L1	*Alternaria iridiaustralis* *Phytophthora capsici* *Colletotrichum capsici* *Fusarium oxysporum* *Fusarium graminearum* *Fusarium annulatum* *Fusarium arcuatisporum* *Botrytis cinerea* *Rhizoctonia solani* *Talaromyces tumuli* *Colletotrichum fioriniae*	2,3-butanedione	Ling et al. [73]
B. velezensis ZJ1	*Alternaria solani* (tomato early blight) *Botrytis cinerea* (tomato gray mold)	isooctanol 2-nonanol	Ren et al. [70]
B. velezensis HY-3479	*Colletotrichum acutatum* (pepper ripe rot) *Cylindrocarpon destructans* (ginseng root rot) *Rhizoctonia solani* (pepper damping-off) *Sclerotinia sclerotiorum* (pepper white mold)	3-methyl-1-butanol (R, R)-2,3-butanediol acetoin benzoic acid	Song et al. [117]
B. velezensis SBB	*Verticillium dahliae*	2-nonanol 2-heptanone 6-methyl-2-heptanone 2-nonanone	Wang et al. [80]
B. licheniformis BL350-2	*Aspergillus westerdijkiae* *Aspergillus carbonarius* *Aspergillus niger* *Aspergillus flavus* *Aspergillus parasiticus* *Aspergillus ochraceus* *Penicillium verrucosum*	3-methyl-1-butanol	Ul Hassan et al. [105]
B. pumilus TM-R	*Alternaria alternata* *Cladosporium cladosporioides* *Curvularia lunata* *Fusarium oxysporum* *Penicillium italicum*	methyl isobutyl ketone ethanol 5-methyl-2-heptanone S-()-2-methylbutylamine	Morita et al. [34]
B. megaterium BmBP17	*Phytophthora capsici* *Magnaporthe oryzae*	pyrazine, 2-ethyl-3-methyl pyrazine, 2-ethyl- pyrazine, 2,5-dimethyl pyrazine, 2-methyl	Munjal et al. [27]

Table 2. *Cont.*

Bacillus Strain	Plant Pathogen (Disease)	Antifungal VOCs	Reference
B. megaterium BM344-1	*Aspergillus flavus* *Aspergillus carbonarius* *Penicillium verrucosum* *Fusarium verticillioides*	hexadecanoic acid methyl ester (palmitic acid) tetracosane	Saleh et al. [104]
B. mycoides	*Rhizoctonia solani* Kühn *Pythium aphanidermatum* Edson (cabbage damping-off)	dimethyl disulphide ammonia	Huang et al. [29]
B. mycoides BM02	*Fusarium oxysporum* f. sp. *lycopersici* (tomato *Fusarium* wilt)	phenylacetic acid methylphenyl acetate	Wu et al. [81]
B. atrophaeus CAB-1	*Botrytis cinerea* (tomato gray mold) *Sphaerotheca fuliginea* (cucumber powdery mildew)	O-anisaldehyde	Zhang et al. [60]
B. atrophaeus JZB120050	Botrytis cinerea *Fusarium oxysporum* f. sp. *conglutinans* *Fusarium oxysporum* f. sp. *niveum* *Fusarium oxysporum* f. sp. *vasinfectum* *Fusarium solani* f. sp. *pisi* *Fusarium oxysporum Schlecht* *Fusarium graminearum* *Rhizoctonia cereal* *Gaeumannomyces graminis* *Monilinia fructicola* *Botryosphaeria dothidea* *Colletotrichum gloeosporioides*	mixture of VOCs	Ni et al. [28]
B. atrophaeus HAB-5	*Colletotrichum gloeosporioides*	chloroacetic acid tetradecyl esters octadecane hexadecanoic acid, methyl ester	Rajaofera et al. [32]
B. cereus MH778713	*Fusarium oxysporum* (tomato *Fusarium* wilt)	hentriacontane 2,4-di-tert-butylphenol	Ramírez et al. [97]
B. cereus CF4-51	*Sclerotinia sclerotiorum*	2-pentadecanone, 6,10,14-trimethyl- 1,2-benzenedicarboxylic acid bis(2-methylpropyl) ester dibutyl phthalate cyclododecane heptadecane	Hu et al. [66]
B. mojavensis I4	*Fusarium verticillioides* *Fusarium graminearum* *Rhizoctonia solani*	mixture of VOCs	Ghazala et al. [76]
B. siamensis G-3	*Botrytis cinerea* *Rhizopus stolonifer*	2,6-di-tert-butyl-4-methylphenol 2,4-di-tert-butylphenol	Zhang et al. [39]
B. siamensis N-1	*Colletotrichum gloeosporioides* *Glomerella sp.* *Pestalotiopsis microspora* *Diaporthe phaseolorum* *Phomopsis sp.* *Diaporthe phaseolorum* *Geotrichum candidum* *Fusarium lateritium* *Fusarium oxysporm* *Fusarium equiseti* *Fusarium incarnatum* *Fusarium* sp. *Lasiodiplodia theobromae* *Phomopsis caricae-papayae* *Thielaviopsis paradoxa*	1-undecene 3-methyl-1-butanol 2-nonanone 1,3,5,7-cyclooctatetraene phenol	You et al. [79]

Table 2. *Cont.*

Bacillus Strain	Plant Pathogen (Disease)	Antifungal VOCs	Reference
B. siamensis LZ88	*Alternaria alternata* (tobacco brown spot)	mixture of VOCs	Xie et al. [92]
		2-methylbutanoic acid 3-methylbutanoic acid	Wang et al. [69]
B. safensis STJP	*Alternaria alternata*	phenol, 2,4-bis (1,1-dimethylethyl)-3-hexadecanol pyrrolo (1,2-a)pyrazine-1,4-dione hexahydro-3-(2-methyl-propyl)- 5,10-diethoxy-2,3,7,8-tetrahydro-1H,6H-dipyrrolo(1,2-a:10,20-d)pyrazine hexadecanoic acid	Prakash and Arora [82]
Bacillus sp. B44	*Fusarium oxysporum* f. sp. *lycopersici*	mixture of VOCs	Jangir et al. [40]
Bacillus sp. ACB-65 *Bacillus* sp. ACB-73	*Phyllosticta citricarpa* (orange black spot)	mixture of VOCs	Fujimoto et al. [31]
Bacillus sp. T6	*Verticillium dahliae* (cotton *Verticillium* wilt)	styrene	Zhang et al. [64]
Bacillus sp. LPPC170	*Fusarium kalimantanense* (Panama disease of bannana)	acetic acid propanoic acid butanoic acid valeric acid isovaleric acid	de Ávila Santos et al. [67]
B. subtilis XF-1 *B. amyloliquefaciens* subsp. *plantarum* FZB42 *B. amyloliquefaciens* subsp. *plantarum* YAU B9601-Y2 *B. subtilis* 168 *Bacillus* spp. strains 033, 041, 355 and 285	*Fusarium solani*	mixture of VOCs	Li et al. [97]
B. cereus KY094642 *B. safensis* KY094643	*Alternaria* sp. (leaf spot and blight disease of lentils)	mixture of VOCs	Roy et al. [118]
B. amyloliquefaciens RS-25 *B. licheniformis* MG-4 *B. subtilis* Z-14 *B. subtilis* Pnf-4	*Botrytis cinerea* (tomato, strawberry, and grapefruit gray mold)	mixture of VOCs	Chen et al. [119]
B. methylotrophicus BCN2 *B. thuringiensis* BCN10	*Fusarium oxysporum* *Botryosphaeria sp.* *Trichoderma atroviride* *Colletotrichum gloeosporioides* *Penicillium expansum*	mixture of VOCs	He et al. [106]
B. velezensis BUZ-14 *B. ginsengihumi* S38	*Botrytis cinerea*	mixture of VOCs	Calvo et al. [35]
B. mycoides *B. subtilis* *B. thuringiensis*	*Aspergillus ochraceus* *Aspergillus westerdijkiae* *Aspergillus flavus* *Aspergillus parasiticus*	mixture of VOCs	Hlebová et al. [53]
B. safensis RGM 2450 *B. siamensis* RGM	*Botrytis cinerea* *Colletotrichum acutatum* *Fusarium oxysporum* *Phytophtora cinnamomi*	mixture of VOCs	Altimira et al. [120]
B. subtilis PPCB001 *B. amyloliquefaciens* PPCB004	*Penicillium digitatum* Sacc. *Penicillium italicum* Wehmer *Penicillium crustosum* Thom	acetoin	Arrebola et al. [42]
B. pumilus TB09 *B. thuringiensis* TB72	*Colletotrichum gloeosporioides* (mango antrachnose)	2-nonanone b-benzeneethanamine 2-decanone thymol 2-methylpyrazine	Zheng et al. [94]

Table 2. *Cont.*

Bacillus Strain	Plant Pathogen (Disease)	Antifungal VOCs	Reference
B. subtilis *B. amyloliquefaciens* *B. cereus*	*Aspergillus niger* *Aspergillus flavus* *Aspergillus parasiticus* *Aspergillus clavatus* *Fusarium oxysporum* f.sp. *lactucae Moniliophthora perniciosa*	propanone 1-butanol 3-methyl-1-butanol acetic acid 2-methylpropanoic acid carbon disulphide 3-methylbutanoic acid ethyl acetate	Chaves-Lopez et al. [1]
B. vallismortis 12a *B. altitudinis* 14b	*Monilinia fructicola* (peach brown rot)	6-methyl-2-heptanone 2-pentylfuran cedrol isodecyl methacrylate	Liu et al. [65]
B. velezensis VM11 *B. velezensis* VM10 *B. amyloliquefaciens* VM42	*Sclerotinia sclerotiorum*	2-undecanone 1,3-butadiene benzothiazole N,N-dimethyldodecylamine	Massawe et al. [57]
B. amyloliquefaciens HA *B. stratosphericus* SO *B. acidiceler* SJJ *B. mycoides* HB	*Fusarium solani* *Fusarium* sp. *Colletotrichum gloeosporioides* *Phytophthora cinnamomi*	2,3,5-trimethylpyrazine 2-nonanone 2-decanone 2-dodecanone dimethyl disulfide dimethyl trisulfide	Guevara-Avendaño et al. [121]
B. nakamurai *B. pseudomycoides* *B. proteolyticus* *B. thuringiensis*	*Botrytis cinerea*	2-heptanone dodecanal dimethyl disulfide dimethyl trisulfide 3-methylbutan-1-ol	Chaouachi et al. [122]
Paenibacillus polymyxa BMP-11 *B. subtilis* BL02 *B. pumilus* BSH-4 *B. pumilus* ZB13	*Sclerotinia sclerotiorum* *Botrytis cinerea* *Alternaria brassicae* *Alternaria solani* *Ascochyta citrullina* *Fusarium oxysporum* *Cercospora kikuchii Chupp* *Rhizoctonia solani* *Phoma arachnidicola* *Verticillium dahiae* *Fusarium graminerum*	mixture of VOCs	Liu et al. [56]
Pseudomonas fluorescens Pf 9A-14 *Pseudomonas sp.* Psp. 8D-45 *B. subtilis* Bs 8B-1	*Pythium capsici* (cucumber damping-off) *Phytophthora capsici* (cucumber root rot) *Rhizoctonia solani* (radish damping-off)	mixture of VOCs	Khabbaz et al. [45]
B. megaterium KU143 *Pseudomonas protegens* AS15	*Aspergillus flavus*	mixture of VOCs	Mannaa et al. [52]
Pichia kudriavzevii *Candida labiduridarum* *B. acidiceler* *B. macauenses* *B. amyloliquefaciens* *B. pumilus*	*Sclerotinia sclerotiorum*	mixture of VOCs	Cavalcanti et al. [123]
B. amyloliquefaciens SF14 *B. amyloliquefaciens* SP10 *Alcaligenes faecalis* ACBC1 *Pantoea agglomerans* ACBP1	*Monilinia fructigena* *Monilinia laxa* (apple brown rot)	mixture of VOCs	Lahlali et al. [101]

Table 2. *Cont.*

Bacillus Strain	Plant Pathogen (Disease)	Antifungal VOCs	Reference
Pseudomonas brassicacearum *Pseudomonas putida* *B. megaterium*	*Botrytis cinerea* *Phytophthora nicotianae* *Rhizoctonia solani* *Sclerotinia sclerotiorum* *Verticillium dahliae* *Fusarium oxysporum* *Macrophomina phaseolina*	acetic acid 2-nonanone dimethyl trisulfide	Giorgio et al. [49]
Bacillus spp. *Paenibacillus* spp.	*Rhizoctonia solani* *Fusarium graminearum* *Phytophthora capsici* *Pythium aphanidermatum* *Podosphaera fuliginea*	acetoin diacetyl	Khalaf and Raizada [124]
B. amyloliquefaciens LI24 *B. amyloliquefaciens* PP19 *B. licheniformis* HS10 *B. pumilus* PI26 *Exiguobacterium acetylicum* SI17	*Peronophythora litchii* (litchi downy blight)	1-(2-aminophenyl)ethanone benzothiazole α-farnesene	Zheng et al. [38]
B. amyloliquefaciens UQ154 *B. velezensis* UQ156 *Acinetobacter sp.* UQ202	*Phytophthora capsici*	isovaleraldehyde 2-ethylhexanol 2-heptanone benzyl alcohol 3-methylbutanol	Syed-Ab-Rahman et al. [87]
B. atrophaeus L193 *B. velezensis* XT1 *Psychrobacillus vulpis* Z8	*Alternaria alternata* *Botrytis cinerea* *Fusarium oxysporum* *Fusarium solani* *Monilinia fructicola* *Monilinia laxa* *Sclerotinia sclerotiorum*	acetoin acetic acid 2,3-butanediol isopentanol dimethyl disulphide isopentyl isobutanoate	Toral et al. [62]

4. Nematicidal Action of *Bacillus*-Based VOCs

Besides the antimicrobial activity against bacterial and fungal pathogens, representatives of the *Bacillus* genus are recognized as potential biocontrol agents effective in the suppression of plant-parasitic nematodes. The overview of published literature data focused on the nematicidal activity of *Bacillus*-based VOCs is summarized and examples of active VOCs are given in Table 3. The mode of action of *Bacillus* strains is defined through several approaches, including regulation of nematode behavior, competition for nutrients, and interference with nematode-host recognition [125]. Some of the examples reported in the scientific literature include *B. firmus* YBf-10, which shows nematicidal activity against the root-knot nematode *Meloidogyne incognita*, *B. cereus* C1-7, which inhibits root gall formation and reduces egg production of the carrot and tomato parasite *Meloidogyne hapla* [126]; and *B. subtilis*, which is active even under high temperatures, making it applicable in greenhouses as a biocontrol agent of root-knot nematode [125]. The previous studies also reported that secondary metabolites produced by *Bacillus* strains including *B. megaterium*, *B. cereus*, *B. thuringiensis*, and *B. pumilus* are effective against *Meloidogyne exigua*, *Bursaphelenchus xylophilus*, and *Ditylenchus destructor*. The production of volatile metabolites was also recognized as a potential mechanism of action for nematode suppression. *B. nematocida* B16 was one of the examples reported in the literature, where it was explained that it lures nematodes by producing seven VOCs that attract worms and afterward enter the intestine of the nematodes [126].

4.1. *Styrene as the Nematicidal Bacillus-Based VOC*

In the study by Luo et al. [126], a total of 45 members of the *Bacillus* genus were isolated from the root-knot nematode-infested tomato rhizosphere soil, and 5 of them were positive in terms of nematicidal activity with a mortality rate over 60%. The strain exhibiting the highest potential of nematicidal activity, causing a 98.1% mortality rate, was identified as *B. mycoides* R2. Styrene was defined as the primary nematicidal substance produced by the investigated strain, expressing high nematicidal activity against both free-living nematodes (*Caenorhabditis elegans*) and the root-knot nematode *Meloidogyne incognita*. In comparison with other nematicides, for example, chloronicotinyl insecticide thiacloprid for the nematode *Meloidogyne incognita* J2, with the LC50 of 36.2 mg/L in tomato crops, this value for styrene was 4.55 μg/mL [126]. The additional unique advantage for the control of nematodes with this VOC in the field lies in the fact that it fully evaporates in the soil and quickly and efficiently repels nematodes from crops [126].

4.2. *Interference of Bacillus-Based VOCs with Nematodes' Chemotaxis*

In another study, the potential nematicidal strain, *B. subtilis* Bs-1, was isolated from tomato rhizosphere and tested for in vitro nematicidal and ovicidal activities against *Meloidogyne incognita*, but the study also included efficiency evaluation in the pot experiments and in the field [127]. The results indicated high nematicidal activity, with an egg mortality rate of 100%, and a positive outcome even in field conditions. *B. subtilis* Bs-1 successfully reduced the disease index and stimulated the growth and yield of cucumber. Previous studies also confirmed that the *B. subtilis* isolate repelled second-stage juveniles (J2s) and reduced nematode production in tomatoes [127]. The major VOC produced by *B. subtilis* Bs-1 was CO_2, and other identified active substances were acetic acid, 2-heptanone, pyrazine 2,5-dimethyl- and dimethyl disulfide, which were reported in previous studies as leading to chemotaxis in *Meloidogyne incognita* or *Caenorhabditis elegans* [128,129]. Considering the above-mentioned components' roles, it should be findings pointed out that *Meloidogyne incognita* was attracted by low concentrations of CO_2 and that acetic acid (0.1%) caused 100% mortality of *Meloidogyne incognita*. Organic sulfide also showed strong antimicrobial and insecticidal activities, and phenol, cyclohexanol, 2-octanol, and 2-undecanone expressed suppressive activity against nematodes [125]. The VOCs of another strain, *B. cereus* Bc-cm103, caused the mortality rates of *Meloidogyne incognita* J2s to be 90.8% and 97.2% after 24 h and 48 h of incubation, respectively. The identification of VOCs revealed the presence of 21 compounds, including alkanes, alkenes, esters, and sulfides, but the nematocidal activity was observed in the case of dimethyl disulfide (30.63%) and S-methyl ester butanethioic acid (30.29%) [130]. As it was suggested in previous studies, the mechanism of action included strong interference of VOCs with the chemotaxis of *Meloidogyne incognita* to cucumber roots.

4.3. *Interference of Bacillus-Based VOCs with Nematodes' Antioxidant Metabolism*

Ayaz et al. [131] conducted the experiments with *Bacillus* GBSC56 isolated from the Tibet region of China investigating the potential nematicidal activity against *Meloidogyne incognita*. The VOCs profile analysis revealed the presence of 10 compounds, while 3 of them, including dimethyl disulfide, methyl isovalerate, and 2-undecanone indicated strong nematicidal activity with mortality rates of 87%, 83%, and 80%, respectively. The activity of VOCs was based on severe oxidative stress caused by nematodes, resulting in rapid death. Additionally, the activity of antioxidant enzymes SOD, CAT, POD, and APX has enhanced in *Meloidogyne incognita*-infested roots in the presence of volatiles, which might reduce the adverse effect of oxidative stress induced after infection.

4.4. *Specific Bacillus-Based VOCs Exhibiting Nematicidal Action*

B. licheniformis JF-22 was another *Bacillus* strain recognized as a potential biocontrol agent active against *Meloidogyne incognita*. It was isolated from the tomato rhizosphere in the area where healthy plants were grown in the presence of the tomato root-knot nematode, and the study pointed out that acetoin, 2,3-butanediol, and hexamethylcyclotrisiloxane are the main components among the produced VOCs [132]. The VOCs produced by *B. altitudinis* AMCC 1040 were analyzed in the study by Ye et al. [133] and grouped into four major categories: ethers, alcohols, ketones, and organic acids. Out of eight compounds, six exhibited different levels of nematicidal activity, including 2,3-butanedione, acetic acid, 2-isopropoxy ethylamine, 3-methylbutyric acid, 2-methylbutyric acid, and octanoic acid. All four organic acids showed strong nematicidal activity, with octanoic acid showing the highest, followed by the activity of acetic acid as the second best, while two isomeric organic acids, 2-methyl-butanoic acid and 3-methyl-butanoic acid, had the same suppressive effect. Among the two ketones tested, only 2,3-butanedione showed activity [133].

Table 3. Literature overview—nematicidal VOCs produced by *Bacillus* spp.

Bacillus Strain	Plant Pathogen	Nematicidal VOCs	Reference
B. mycoides R2	*Caenorhabditis elegans* *Meloidogyne incognita*	styrene	Luo et al. [126]
B. subtilis Bs-1	*Meloidogyne incognita*	CO_2 acetic acid 2-heptanone pyrazine, 2,5-dimethyl- dimethyl disulfide	Cao et al. [125]
Bacillus sp. GBSC56	*Meloidogyne incognita*	dimethyl disulfide methyl isovalerate 2-undecanone	Ayaz et al. [131]
B. cereus Bc-cm103	*Meloidogyne incognita*	dimethyl disulfide S-methyl ester butanethioic acid	Yin et al. [130]
B. licheniformis JF-22	*Meloidogyne incognita*	acetoin 2,3-butanediol hexamethyl cyclotrisiloxane	Du et al. [132]
B. altitudinis AMCC 1040	*Meloidogyne incognita*	2,3-butanedione acetic acid 2-isopropoxy ethylamine 2-methyl-butyric acid 3-methylbutyric acid octanoic acid	Ye et al. [133]
Bacillus megaterium YMF3.25	*Meloidogyne incognita*	benzeneacetaldehyde decanal dimethyl disulfide 2-nonanone 2-undecanone	Huang et al. [129]
Bacillus aryabhattai MCCC 1K02966	*Meloidogyne incognita*	dimethyl disulfide methyl thioacetate	Chen et al. [134]

5. Future Outlook on *Bacillus*-Based VOCs Research and Application

As presented in the previous sections, recent research on *Bacillus*-based VOCs has provided useful results in terms of (a) screening of *Bacillus* strains producing VOCs exhibiting antibacterial, antifungal, and nematicidal activity; (b) identification of the VOCs present in the volatile mixtures emitted by *Bacillus* spp.; (c) targeting the specific VOCs responsible for the antibacterial, antifungal, and nematicidal effects, as well as evaluation of the bacteriostatic/bactericidal and fungistatic/fungicidal concentrations of the specific VOCs; (d) *in vitro*, *in vivo*, and field testing of the specific VOCs/VOCs mixtures on the suppression of bacterial, fungal, and nematode plant pathogens. While the first studies in this field focused on identifying *Bacillus* strains producing VOCs with possible biocontrol applications, the research was later directed towards the precise identification of the produced VOCs and promotion of the ones responsible for biocontrol activity. Recent and currently ongoing studies are mostly focused on understanding the underlying mechanisms of antibacterial, antifungal, and nematicidal activity, both at the levels of cell structure and metabolism. However, a more profound understanding of the aforementioned mechanisms is required to maximize the potential of *Bacillus*-based VOCs biocontrol applications, leaving a significant space for further research in this area. Furthermore, *in vivo* testing procedures have been mostly based on model plants so far, requiring the widening of the host palette to increase the applicability and test the VOCs' biocontrol potential in realistic application conditions, with more studies needed to be performed in greenhouses and in the field, followed by an investigation of the VOCs' possible negative effects to the environment, animal- and human health. One of the possible research directions is also related to the biotechnological production of VOCs, directly affecting the mode of their biocontrol applications. Specific remarks related to all of the aforementioned aspects are given in the following subsections.

5.1. The Necessity to Investigate the Effects of Microbial Communities on Bacillus-VOCs Synthesis and Vice-Versa

Considering the previously mentioned fact that VOCs serve as signaling molecules for intra- and interspecies interactions as well as communication mediators across the kingdoms, it is necessary to better understand the exact mechanisms of microbial VOCs-mediated communication, considering the complexity of microbial communities in different ecological niches. So far, it has been revealed that VOCs help microorganisms make distinctions between neighboring microorganisms (friend, foe, or prey) and adjust their behavior and performance (persist, invade, escape, or defend) accordingly [11,135]. Furthermore, it is necessary to understand the mechanisms underlying volatile emission and perception, since it has been very challenging to detect the signal senders, receivers, and putative eavesdroppers [10]. Biodiversity is a key driver of several ecosystem functions [136], hence the interactions among the ecosystem members affect the production and function of VOCs. Diverse examples of shifts in VOC production by bacteria in the presence of other organisms involved in different communication pathways could be found so far, although this field is still under-investigated. An increase or decrease of the produced VOCs' diversity and amount could be observed depending on the ecosystem community structure and the types of interactions, ranging from beneficial to antagonistic, resulting in the triggering/silencing of the VOCs' production (mostly mediated by quorum sensing). Beneficial interactions result in additive/complementary/facilitative effects on VOC production and could arise from the induction of certain VOC production in the presence of specific strains/their metabolites, possibly acting as molecular inducers or precursors for VOC synthesis. On the other hand, antagonistic interactions are usually related to direct antagonism as well as the necessity to provide a competitive advantage in terms of growth space and nutrients in a limited ecological niche [7]. The aforementioned interactions in complex microbial communities could result in the production of novel VOCs that were not detected in the respective monocultures, and consequently, in a higher diversity of VOCs with distinct biological functions observed separately and together. One of the reasons for that could be the horizontal acquisition of the genes for the synthesis of volatile secondary metabolites by bacteria [3], which should be further investigated. Hence, there is a necessity to increase the diversity of the investigated microbial communities and shift from pure monocultures to more complex systems that include (micro)organisms representative of certain applications of the investigated VOCs. Although the soil communities are the most complex in terms of diversity and the number of present species, it is also important to direct investigations to the plant phyllosphere as well as to endophytic microbial interactions resulting in VOC production.

5.2. The Necessity to Better Understand the VOCs' Mechanisms of Action against Broader Spectrum of Plant Pathogens and Hosts

Although a lot of literature data could be found regarding VOCs' effect in terms of antifungal activity, their effects against other types of plant pathogens are still not sufficiently investigated. Furthermore, the majority of the studies deal only with the confirmation of antifungal/antibacterial/nematicidal activity of the mixture of VOCs produced by the certain

Bacillus strain, while a minority of the studies involve a precise investigation of the activity of separate VOCs from the emitted mixture. There could be observed significant differences in terms of biocontrol efficacy between VOC blends (with specific concentrations and ratios or naturally produced) and single components, both in terms of general efficacy as well as in terms of the range of pathogenic targets. Currently, <10% of mVOCs have been assigned a function [13]. Taking into account overlaps in the biological roles of many VOCs as well as the raising evidence on different antimicrobial activities of chiral VOCs/enantiomers, there is a necessity for complete chemical characterization and molecular targets' profiling of the VOCs in future investigations [10]. Furthermore, limited knowledge about the perception of microbial volatiles by other (micro)organisms is currently available. Therefore, further research should focus on mechanisms of VOC cell entry and cell targets, and here microbial mutants could offer a useful toolbox to detect genes responsible for the perception of VOCs, as well as their cellular/molecular targets [11]. In general, a greater understanding of VOCs' mechanisms of action across a broader range of pathogenic microorganisms is required, besides the necessity to include a wider range of plant hosts going behind the model plant species, considering that most of the current research refers to *Arabidopsis thaliana* and *Nicotiana benthamiana* [13].

5.3. Research Directions Related to VOCs Production by Bacillus spp.

VOCs' potential application is directly related to the selected VOC source—pure compounds, *Bacillus*-based captured VOCs, or the use of viable cells for on-site VOC production and application. Some of the VOCs produced by *Bacillus* strains could be chemically synthesized and used as pure compounds in different modes of application. On the other hand, VOCs produced by *Bacillus* spp. could be captured in a closed system and used for plant pathogen suppression at the same or a different location. Moreover, simultaneous production and application of *Bacillus*-based VOCs could be achieved, either by direct inoculation of biocontrol strains to plants or the surrounding soil or by maintaining cultures producing VOCs in plants' close vicinity, which would be the suitable mode of application in closed and controlled systems, such as greenhouses. Independently of the application mode, it is necessary to consider the main bioprocess variables affecting VOC production by *Bacillus* strains. On the upstream side of the bioprocess, the main bioprocess development step is the selection of suitable nutrients to be included in the solid or liquid cultivation medium, depending on the metabolic pathways required for the production of targeted VOCs and the substrates required in these metabolic processes, as well as optimization of the medium pH value as one of the most important physiology-affecting parameters. The next step is to optimize nutrients' ratios and concentrations to maximize target VOC production, as well as to decide between the utilization of solid or liquid medium, which significantly affects other bioprocess variables, such as mass and oxygen transfer. This leads us to the cultivation step itself, where it is necessary to determine the production system design, significantly depending on the previous selection between solid and liquid cultivation medium, and to optimize the cultivation parameters (inoculum preparation and inoculation strategy, medium volume, T, mixing and aeration rate, duration) to minimize resource utilization and achieve cost-effectiveness in terms of energy consumption. Furthermore, downstream and analytical methods require constant advancements to collect and detect the produced volatiles correctly, especially in cases where the collected volatiles are further used as biocontrol agents. Most of the currently available studies deal with VOCs produced by a single strain cultivated on artificial nutrient-rich media [137], not taking into account the real conditions where the VOCs will be applied, both in terms of the previously mentioned problems related to the diversity of natural microbial communities and environmental conditions. Hence, future research should focus on the imitation of environmental conditions at the VOC application site in terms of nutrient supply, physico-chemical properties of the soil, and climate factors shaping the growth and development of the bacteria but also their volatile emission [3]. The factors that should be taken into account include soil aeration and limited oxygen availability in the rhizosphere, together with regional, seasonal, or climate dependencies and nutritional profiling in terms of the dependency of microbial growth and metabolism on root exudates. On the other hand, poor soil nutrient status is a raising trend in different geographic regions across the globe. Simulation of VOCs application environmental conditions should be implemented into the general bioprocessing strategy, starting from the cultivation medium whose composition strongly affects VOCs profile and amount and choice between solid and liquid media, mostly affecting oxygen availability [138]. Furthermore, different cultivation conditions (T, pH, mixing and aeration rates, duration) should be investigated to predict the VOC emission in a real-world application environment as well as to maximize their efficiency in terms of optimal diversity and concentration. Another important aspect for future investigations includes the monitoring and analysis of volatile secondary metabolites related to specific stages of bacterial growth and development, especially in terms of multicellular behaviors of *Bacillus* spp., including motility of freely available cells, sporulation, and biofilm formation [3].

5.4. VOCs Application-Related Remarks

Recent research of *Bacillus*-based VOCs has revealed varying differences in their effects from the lab to the field, mostly due to significant differences between in vitro production and testing conditions and real application conditions, including abiotic soil conditions (temperature, pH, moisture content, and soil texture), as well as the availability and quality of organic energy sources [137]. It points out the requirement for more field studies in terms of VOCs efficacy, which are currently scarce. Considering that the exact VOC concentration in the complex volatile mixture emitted by *Bacillus* spp. is usually not determined, it is very important to incorporate a wider concentration range in the testing protocols as many VOCs reveal dose-dependent biocontrol effects. The perception of a microbial VOC by other (micro)organisms could be related to its ratio/concentration in the complex volatile mixture, besides its presence. Therefore, this complex background should be incorporated as much as possible in the experimental setups designed to assess the biological activity of VOCs, facilitating the transition from laboratory research to real-life application conditions [10]. The incorporation of sensors for continuous monitoring of VOC concentration and big data computing analytics represent promising auxiliary tools for sustainable agricultural practice [2]. *Bacillus*-based VOCs could be applied, e.g., as repellents or biopesticides against plant diseases caused by microbial pathogens, soil fumigants, and fumigants in the management of post-harvest diseases. Their mode of use depends a lot on how far these VOCs travel before they cause a biological response in other organisms [11]. It opens a chapter of possibilities for VOCs delivery, including injection, dripping, drench versus spray application, companion cropping systems, etc. [13]. Utilization of different carriers for immobilization of *Bacillus*-producing VOCs, which could be supported by, e.g., 3D bioprinting, is worthy of investigation in future studies. One of the possible investigation routes includes the utilization of organic soil amendments that promote the production of VOCs during decomposition, where the necessity of the presence of VOC precursors in organic amendments should be further examined [137].

5.5. Possible Risks of Bacillus-Based VOCs Application in Biocontrol of Plant Diseases and Pathogens

Due to their biological origin, *Bacillus*- and other microbially-derived VOCs are usually perceived as safe for the environment, plants, animals, and humans due to their lower (eco)toxicity and biodegradability. Some studies have observed the phytotoxic effects of higher VOC concentrations at different plant growth stages. Hence, there is a necessity to optimize VOC dosage, delivery, and time of treatment. Furthermore, when applying a mixture of VOCs emitted by a certain *Bacillus* strain present directly on the plant or in its close vicinity, it is necessary to investigate the strain's overall capacity for VOC production depending on the growth conditions, i.e., to predict the strain's volatile profile expected under certain application conditions to prevent the emergence of (phyto)toxic volatiles.

Moreover, it is necessary to predict the strain's volatile profile independently of the growth conditions by knowing and understanding the strain's genetic basis for VOC production, where whole genome sequencing technology could be useful together with databases of genomic data on *Bacillus* strains capable of VOC production to provide the basis for the selection of safe strains in terms of possible VOC release risks. Due to high evaporation rates and a lack of stability, VOC application may require high initial concentrations, raising the risk of dose-dependent toxicity against plants and other non-target organisms [137]. Dimethyl disulfide, produced by many *Bacillus* strains, is commercialized as one of the most potent microbial VOCs, exhibiting antifungal and nematicidal action [139,140]. However, recent studies have reported possible toxicity-related issues, including potential eye- and skin-irritable properties during acute exposure, while exposure to large concentrations may cause nausea, headache, dizziness, and irritation of the upper respiratory tract [141]. Therefore, besides the utilization of VOCs as pure compounds, which have been previously proven to be safe for humans and animals, the toxicity and non-target effects of the VOCs need to be documented before any field application, including effects on mycorrhizal development, non-target beneficial soil organisms, and a possible increase in other harmful soil organisms, to overcome the translational gap related to *Bacillus*-VOCs unexpected effects [10,11,137].

Author Contributions: Conceptualization, I.P. and J.G.; methodology, I.P. and V.V.; software, I.P.; validation, J.G.; formal analysis, I.P. and V.V.; investigation, I.P. and V.V.; resources, J.G.; data curation, I.P. and V.V.; writing—original draft preparation, I.P. and V.V.; writing—review and editing, J.G.; visualization, I.P.; supervision, J.G.; project administration, I.P. and J.G.; funding acquisition, I.P. and J.G. All authors have read and agreed to the published version of the manuscript.

Funding: This research was funded by the program 451-03-47/2023-01/200134 of the Ministry of Science, Technological Development and Innovations of the Republic of Serbia, the project 142-451-3187/2022-01/01 financed by the Provincial Secretariat for Higher Education and Scientific Research of the Autonomous Province of Vojvodina, as well as the bilateral project between the Republic of Serbia and Hungary, financed by the Ministry of Education, Science and Technological development of the Republic of Serbia (project number 451-03-01345/2020-09/7) and by the Hungarian National Office for Research, Development and Innovation (NKFI, project number 2019-2.1.11-TÉT-2020-00249).

Institutional Review Board Statement: Not applicable.

Informed Consent Statement: Not applicable.

Conflicts of Interest: The authors declare no conflict of interest.

References

1. Chaves-López, C.; Serio, A.; Gianotti, A.; Sacchetti, G.; Ndagijimana, M.; Ciccarone, C.; Stellarini, A.; Corsetti, A.; Paparella, A. Diversity of food-borne *Bacillus* volatile compounds and influence on fungal growth. *J. Appl. Microbiol.* **2015**, *119*, 487–499. [CrossRef] [PubMed]
2. Chandrasekaran, M.; Paramasivan, M.; Sahayarayan, J.J. Microbial volatile organic compounds: An alternative for chemical fertilizers in sustainable agriculture development. *Microorganisms* **2023**, *11*, 42. [CrossRef] [PubMed]
3. Kai, M. Diversity and distribution of volatile secondary metabolites throughout *Bacillus subtilis* isolates. *Front. Microbiol.* **2020**, *11*, 559. [CrossRef] [PubMed]
4. Xie, S.; Zang, H.; Jun Wu, H.; Uddin Rajer, F.; Gao, X. Antibacterial effects of volatiles produced by *Bacillus* Strain D13 against *Xanthomonas oryzae* pv. *oryzae*. *Mol. Plant Pathol.* **2018**, *19*, 49–58. [CrossRef] [PubMed]
5. Rajer, F.U.; Wu, H.; Xie, Y.; Xie, S.; Raza, W.; Tahir, H.A.S.; Gao, X. Volatile organic compounds produced by a soil-isolate, *Bacillus subtilis* fa26 induce adverse ultra-structural changes to the cells of *Clavibacter michiganensis* ssp. *sepedonicus*, the causal agent of bacterial ring rot of potato. *Microbiology* **2017**, *163*, 523–530. [CrossRef]
6. Ajilogba, C.F.; Babalola, O.O. GC–MS analysis of volatile organic compounds from *Bambara groundnut* rhizobacteria and their antibacterial properties. *World J. Microbiol. Biotechnol.* **2019**, *35*, 83. [CrossRef]
7. Raza, W.; Wang, J.; Jousset, A.; Friman, V.P.; Mei, X.; Wang, S.; Wei, Z.; Shen, Q. Bacterial community richness shifts the balance between volatile organic compound-mediated microbe–pathogen and microbe–plant interactions. *Proc. R. Soc. B Biol. Sci.* **2020**, *287*, 20200403. [CrossRef]
8. Lammers, A.; Lalk, M.; Garbeva, P. Air ambulance: Antimicrobial power of bacterial volatiles. *Antibiotics* **2022**, *11*, 109. [CrossRef]
9. Schulz, S.; Dickschat, J.S. Bacterial volatiles: The smell of small organisms. *Nat. Prod. Rep.* **2007**, *24*, 814–842. [CrossRef]

10. Weisskopf, L.; Schulz, S.; Garbeva, P. Microbial volatile organic compounds in intra-kingdom and inter-kingdom interactions. *Nat. Rev. Microbiol.* **2021**, *19*, 391–404. [CrossRef]
11. Schulz-Bohm, K.; Martín-Sánchez, L.; Garbeva, P. Microbial volatiles: Small molecules with an important role in intra- and inter-kingdom interactions. *Front. Microbiol.* **2017**, *8*, 2484. [CrossRef]
12. Tahir, H.A.S.; Gu, Q.; Wu, H.; Raza, W.; Safdar, A.; Huang, Z.; Rajer, F.U.; Gao, X. Effect of volatile compounds produced by *Ralstonia solanacearum* on plant growth promoting and systemic resistance inducing potential of *Bacillus* volatiles. *BMC Plant Biol.* **2017**, *17*, 133. [CrossRef]
13. Lemfack, M.C.; Gohlke, B.O.; Toguem, S.M.T.; Preissner, S.; Piechulla, B.; Preissner, R. MVOC 2.0: A database of microbial volatiles. *Nucleic Acids Res.* **2018**, *46*, D1261–D1265. [CrossRef]
14. Thomas, G.; Withall, D.; Birkett, M. Harnessing microbial volatiles to replace pesticides and fertilizers. *Microb. Biotechnol.* **2020**, *13*, 1366–1376. [CrossRef]
15. Ryu, C.-M.; Farag, M.A.; Hu, C.-H.; Reddy, M.S.; Kloepper, J.W.; Paré, P.W. Bacterial volatiles induce systemic resistance in *Arabidopsis*. *Plant Physiol.* **2004**, *134*, 1017–1026. [CrossRef]
16. Rudrappa, T.; Biedrzycki, M.L.; Kunjeti, S.G.; Donofrio, N.M.; Czymmek, K.J.; Paré, P.W.; Bais, H.P. The rhizobacterial elicitor acetoin induces systemic resistance in *Arabidopsis thaliana*. *Commun. Integr. Biol.* **2010**, *3*, 130–138. [CrossRef]
17. Song, G.C.; Ryu, C.-M. Two volatile organic compounds trigger plant self-defense against a bacterial pathogen and a sucking insect in cucumber under open field conditions. *Int. J. Mol. Sci.* **2013**, *14*, 9803–9819. [CrossRef]
18. Song, G.C.; Riu, M.; Ryu, C.-M. Beyond the two compartments Petri-dish: Optimising growth promotion and induced resistance in cucumber exposed to gaseous bacterial volatiles in a miniature greenhouse system. *Plant Methods* **2019**, *15*, 9. [CrossRef]
19. Song, G.C.; Choi, H.K.; Ryu, C.-M. Gaseous 3-pentanol primes plant immunity against a bacterial speck pathogen, *Pseudomonas syringae* pv. *tomato* via salicylic acid and jasmonic acid-dependent signaling pathways in Arabidopsis. *Front. Plant Sci.* **2015**, *6*, 821. [CrossRef]
20. Choi, H.K.; Song, G.C.; Yi, H.-S.; Ryu, C.-M. Field evaluation of the bacterial volatile derivative 3-pentanol in priming for induced resistance in pepper. *J. Chem. Ecol.* **2014**, *40*, 882–892. [CrossRef]
21. Raza, W.; Ling, N.; Yang, L.; Huang, Q.; Shen, Q. Response of tomato wilt pathogen *Ralstonia solanacearum* to the volatile organic compounds produced by a biocontrol strain *Bacillus amyloliquefaciens* SQR-9. *Sci. Rep.* **2016**, *6*, 24856. [CrossRef] [PubMed]
22. Raza, W.; Wang, J.; Wu, Y.; Ling, N.; Wei, Z.; Huang, Q.; Shen, Q. Effects of volatile organic compounds produced by *Bacillus amyloliquefaciens* on the growth and virulence traits of tomato bacterial wilt pathogen *Ralstonia solanacearum*. *Appl. Microbiol. Biotechnol.* **2016**, *100*, 7639–7650. [CrossRef] [PubMed]
23. Raza, W.; Wei, Z.; Ling, N.; Huang, Q.; Shen, Q. Effect of organic fertilizers prepared from organic waste materials on the production of antibacterial volatile organic compounds by two biocontrol *Bacillus amyloliquefaciens* strains. *J. Biotechnol.* **2016**, *227*, 43–53. [CrossRef] [PubMed]
24. Tahir, H.A.S.; Gu, Q.; Wu, H.; Niu, Y.; Huo, R.; Gao, X. *Bacillus* volatiles adversely affect the physiology and ultra-structure of *Ralstonia solanacearum* and induce systemic resistance in tobacco against bacterial wilt. *Sci. Rep.* **2017**, *7*, 40481. [CrossRef] [PubMed]
25. Han, V.-C.; Yu, N.H.; Yoon, H.; Ahn, N.-H.; Son, Y.K.; Lee, B.-H.; Kim, J.-C. Identification, characterization, and efficacy evaluation of *Bacillus velezensis* for shot-hole disease biocontrol in flowering cherry. *Plant Pathol. J.* **2022**, *38*, 115–130. [CrossRef]
26. Jelušić, A.; Popović, T.; Dimkić, I.; Mitrović, P.; Peeters, K.; Miklavčić Višnjevec, A.; Tavzes, Č.; Stanković, S.; Berić, T. Changes in the winter oilseed rape microbiome affected by *Xanthomonas campestris* pv. *campestris* and biocontrol potential of the indigenous *Bacillus* and *Pseudomonas* isolates. *Biol. Control* **2021**, *160*, 104695. [CrossRef]
27. Munjal, V.; Nadakkakath, A.V.; Sheoran, N.; Kundu, A.; Venugopal, V.; Subaharan, K.; Rajamma, S.; Eapen, S.J.; Kumar, A. Genotyping and identification of broad spectrum antimicrobial volatiles in black pepper root endophytic biocontrol agent, *Bacillus megaterium* BP17. *Biol. Control* **2015**, *92*, 66–76. [CrossRef]
28. Ni, M.; Wu, Q.; Wang, J.; Liu, W.C.; Ren, J.H.; Zhang, D.P.; Zhao, J.; Liu, D.E.W.; Rao, Y.H.; Lu, C.G. Identification and comprehensive evaluation of a novel biocontrol agent *Bacillus atrophaeus*. *J. Environ. Sci. Health Part B* **2018**, *53*, 777–785. [CrossRef]
29. Huang, J.-S.; Peng, Y.-H.; Chung, K.-R.; Huang, J.-W. Suppressive efficacy of volatile compounds produced by *Bacillus mycoides* on damping-off pathogens of cabbage seedlings. *J. Agric. Sci.* **2018**, *156*, 795–809. [CrossRef]
30. Gotor-Vila, A.; Teixidó, N.; Di Francesco, A.; Usall, J.; Ugolini, L.; Torres, R.; Mari, M. Antifungal effect of volatile organic compounds produced by *Bacillus amyloliquefaciens* CPA-8 against fruit pathogen decays of cherry. *Food Microbiol.* **2017**, *64*, 219–225. [CrossRef]
31. Fujimoto, A.; Augusto, F.; Fill, T.P.; Moretto, R.K.; Kupper, K.C. Biocontrol of *Phyllosticta citricarpa* by *Bacillus* spp.: Biological and chemical aspects of the microbial interaction. *World J. Microbiol. Biotechnol.* **2022**, *38*, 53. [CrossRef]
32. Asari, S.; Matzén, S.; Petersen, M.A.; Bejai, S.; Meijer, J. Multiple effects *of Bacillus amyloliquefaciens* volatile compounds: Plant growth promotion and growth inhibition of phytopathogens. *FEMS Microbiol. Ecol.* **2016**, *92*, fiw070. [CrossRef]
33. Rajaofera, M.J.N.; Wang, Y.; Dahar, G.Y.; Jin, P.; Fan, L.; Xu, L.; Liu, W.; Miao, W. Volatile Organic compounds of *Bacillus atrophaeus* HAB-5 inhibit the growth of *Colletotrichum gloeosporioides*. *Pestic. Biochem. Physiol.* **2019**, *156*, 170–176. [CrossRef]
34. Morita, T.; Tanaka, I.; Ryuda, N.; Ikari, M.; Ueno, D.; Someya, T. Antifungal spectrum characterization and identification of strong volatile organic compounds produced by *Bacillus pumilus* TM-R. *Heliyon* **2019**, *5*, e01817. [CrossRef]

35. Calvo, H.; Roudet, J.; Gracia, A.P.; Venturini, M.E.; Fermaud, M. Comparison of efficacy and modes of action of two high-potential biocontrol *Bacillus* strains and commercial biocontrol products against *Botrytis cinerea* in table grapes. *OENO One* **2021**, *3*, 229–243. [CrossRef]
36. Gao, H.; Li, P.; Xu, X.; Zeng, Q.; Guan, W. Research on volatile organic compounds from *Bacillus subtilis* CF-3: Biocontrol effects on fruit fungal pathogens and dynamic changes during fermentation. *Front. Microbiol.* **2018**, *9*, 456. [CrossRef]
37. Gao, H.; Xu, X.; Zeng, Q.; Li, P. Optimization of headspace solid-phase microextraction for gc-ms analysis of volatile compounds produced by biocontrol strain *Bacillus subtilis* CF-3 using response surface methodology. *Food Sci. Technol. Res.* **2017**, *23*, 583–593. [CrossRef]
38. Zheng, L.; Situ, J.; Zhu, Q.; Xi, P.; Zheng, Y.; Liu, H.; Zhou, X.; Jiang, Z. Identification of volatile organic compounds for the biocontrol of postharvest litchi fruit pathogen *Peronophythora litchii*. *Postharvest Biol. Technol.* **2019**, *155*, 37–46. [CrossRef]
39. Zhang, X.; Gao, Z.; Zhang, X.; Bai, W.; Zhang, L.; Pei, H.; Zhang, Y. Control effects of *Bacillus siamensis* G-3 volatile compounds on raspberry postharvest diseases caused by *Botrytis cinerea* and *Rhizopus stolonifer*. *Biol. Control* **2020**, *141*, 104135. [CrossRef]
40. Jangir, M.; Pathak, R.; Sharma, S.; Sharma, S. Biocontrol mechanisms of *Bacillus* sp., isolated from tomato rhizosphere, against *Fusarium oxysporum* f. sp. *lycopersici*. *Biol. Control* **2018**, *123*, 60–70. [CrossRef]
41. Martins, S.J.; Faria, A.F.; Pedroso, M.P.; Cunha, M.G.; Rocha, M.R.; Medeiros, F.H.V. Microbial volatiles organic compounds control anthracnose (*Colletotrichum lindemuthianum*) in common bean (*Phaseolus vulgaris L.*). *Biol. Control* **2019**, *131*, 36–42. [CrossRef]
42. Arrebola, E.; Sivakumar, D.; Korsten, L. Effect of volatile compounds produced by *Bacillus* strains on postharvest decay in citrus. *Biol. Control* **2010**, *53*, 122–128. [CrossRef]
43. Leelasuphakul, W.; Hemmanee, P.; Chuenchitt, S. Growth inhibitory properties of *Bacillus subtilis* strains and their metabolites against the green mold pathogen (*Penicillium digitatum* Sacc.) of citrus fruit. *Postharvest Biol. Technol.* **2008**, *48*, 113–121. [CrossRef]
44. Yuan, J.; Raza, W.; Shen, Q.; Huang, Q. Antifungal activity of *Bacillus amyloliquefaciens* NJN-6 volatile compounds against *Fusarium oxysporum* f. sp. *cubense*. *Appl. Environ. Microbiol.* **2012**, *78*, 5942–5944. [CrossRef] [PubMed]
45. Khabbaz, S.E.; Zhang, L.; Cáceres, L.A.; Sumarah, M.; Wang, A.; Abbasi, P.A. Characterisation of antagonistic *Bacillus* and *Pseudomonas* strains for biocontrol potential and suppression of damping-off and root rot diseases. *Ann. Appl. Biol.* **2015**, *166*, 456–471. [CrossRef]
46. Sawant, S.S.; Song, J.; Seo, H.J. Characterization of *Bacillus velezensis* RDA1 as a biological control agent against white root rot disease caused by *Rosellinia necatrix*. *Plants* **2022**, *11*, 2486. [CrossRef]
47. Liu, W.; Mu, W.; Zhu, B.; Lui, F. Antifungal activities and components of VOCs produced by *Bacillus subtilis* G_8. *Curr. Res. Bacteriol.* **2008**, *1*, 28–34. [CrossRef]
48. Islam, M.R.; Jeong, Y.T.; Lee, Y.S.; Song, C.H. Isolation and identification of antifungal compounds from *Bacillus subtilis* C9 inhibiting the growth of plant pathogenic fungi. *Mycobiology* **2018**, *40*, 59–65. [CrossRef]
49. Giorgio, A.; De Stradis, A.; Lo Cantore, P.; Iacobellis, N.S. Biocide effects of volatile organic compounds produced by potential biocontrol rhizobacteria on *Sclerotinia sclerotiorum*. *Front. Microbiol.* **2015**, *6*, 1056. [CrossRef]
50. Gao, Z.; Zhang, B.; Liu, H.; Han, J.; Zhang, Y. Identification of endophytic *Bacillus velezensis* zsy-1 strain and antifungal activity of its volatile compounds against *Alternaria solani* and *Botrytis cinerea*. *Biol. Control* **2017**, *105*, 27–39. [CrossRef]
51. Lee, T.; Park, D.; Kim, K.; Lim, S.M.; Yu, N.H.; Kim, S.; Kim, H.Y.; Jung, K.S.; Jang, J.Y.; Park, J.C.; et al. Characterization of *Bacillus amyloliquefaciens* DA12 showing potent antifungal activity against mycotoxigenic *Fusarium* species. *Plant Pathol. J.* **2017**, *33*, 499–507. [CrossRef]
52. Mannaa, M.; Oh, J.Y.; Kim, K.D. Biocontrol activity of volatile-producing *Bacillus megaterium* and *Pseudomonas protegens* against *Aspergillus flavus* and aflatoxin production on stored rice grains. *Mycobiology* **2017**, *45*, 213–219. [CrossRef]
53. Hlebová, M.; Uzsáková, V.; Charousová, I.; Hleba, L. The in vitro antagonistic effects of some *Bacillus* spp. on the growth and mycotoxin production of toxigenic aspergilli. *J. Microbiol. Biotech. Food Sci.* **2021**, *11*, e5412. [CrossRef]
54. Lim, S.M.; Yoon, M.Y.; Choi, G.J.; Choi, Y.H.; Jang, K.S.; Shin, T.S.; Park, H.W.; Yu, N.H.; Kim, Y.H.; Kim, J.C. Diffusible and volatile antifungal compounds produced by an antagonistic *Bacillus velezensis* G341 against various phytopathogenic fungi. *Plant Pathol. J.* **2017**, *33*, 488–498. [CrossRef]
55. Myo, E.M.; Liu, B.; Ma, J.; Shi, L.; Jiang, M.; Zhang, K.; Ge, B. Evaluation of *Bacillus velezensis* NKG-2 for bio-control activities against fungal diseases and potential plant growth promotion. *Biol. Control* **2019**, *134*, 23–31. [CrossRef]
56. Liu, W.; Mu, W.; Zhu, B.; Du, Y.; Liu, F. Antagonistic activities of volatiles from four strains of *Bacillus* spp. and *Paenibacillus* spp. against soil-borne plant pathogens. *Agric. Sci. China* **2008**, *7*, 1104–1114. [CrossRef]
57. Massawe, V.C.; Hanif, A.; Farzand, A.; Mburu, D.K.; Ochola, S.O.; Wu, L.; Tahir, H.A.S.; Gu, Q.; Wu, H.; Gao, X. Volatile compounds of endophytic *Bacillus* spp. have biocontrol activity against *Sclerotinia sclerotiorum*. *Phytopathology* **2018**, *108*, 1373–1385. [CrossRef]
58. Monteiro, F.P.; Ferreira, L.C.; Pacheco, L.P.; Souza, P.E. Antagonism of *Bacillus subtilis* against *Sclerotinia sclerotiorum* on *Lactuca sativa*. *J. Agric. Sci.* **2013**, *5*, 214–223. [CrossRef]
59. Zhu, J.; Tan, T.; Shen, A.; Yang, X.; Yu, Y.; Gao, C.; Li, Z.; Cheng, Y.; Chen, J.; Guo, L.; et al. Biocontrol potential of *Bacillus subtilis* IBFCBF-4 against *Fusarium* wilt of watermelon. *J. Plant. Pathol.* **2020**, *102*, 433–441. [CrossRef]
60. Zhang, X.; Li, B.; Wang, Y.; Guo, Q.; Lu, X.; Li, S.; Ma, P. Lipopeptides, a Novel protein, and volatile compounds contribute to the antifungal activity of the biocontrol agent *Bacillus atrophaeus* CAB-1. *Appl. Microbiol. Biotechnol.* **2013**, *97*, 9525–9534. [CrossRef]

61. Mu, J.; Li, X.; Jiao, J.; Ji, G.; Wu, J.; Hu, F.; Li, H. Biocontrol potential of vermicompost through antifungal volatiles produced by indigenous bacteria. *Biol. Control* **2017**, *112*, 49–54. [CrossRef]
62. Toral, L.; Rodríguez, M.; Martínez-Checa, F.; Montaño, A.; Cortés-Delgado, A.; Smolinska, A.; Llamas, I.; Sampedro, I. Identification of volatile organic compounds in extremophilic bacteria and their effective use in biocontrol of postharvest fungal phytopathogens. *Front. Microbiol.* **2021**, *12*. [CrossRef] [PubMed]
63. Dhouib, H.; Zouari, I.; Abdallah, D.B.; Belbahri, L.; Taktak, W.; Triki, M.A.; Tounsi, S. Potential of a novel endophytic *Bacillus velezensis* in tomato growth promotion and protection against *Verticillium* wilt disease. *Biol. Control* **2019**, *139*, 104092. [CrossRef]
64. Zhang, L.; Wang, Y.; Lei, S.; Zhang, H.; Liu, Z.; Yang, J.; Niu, Q. Effect of volatile compounds produced by the cotton endophytic bacterial strain *Bacillus* sp. T6 against *Verticillium* Wilt. *BMC Microbiol.* **2023**, *23*, 8. [CrossRef]
65. Liu, C.; Yin, X.; Wang, Q.; Peng, Y.; Ma, Y.; Liu, P.; Shi, J. Antagonistic activities of volatiles produced by two *Bacillus* strains against *Monilinia fructicola* in peach fruit. *J. Sci. Food Agric.* **2018**, *98*, 5756–5763. [CrossRef]
66. Hu, J.; Dong, B.; Wang, D.; Meng, H.; Li, X.; Zhou, H. Genomic and metabolic features of *Bacillus cereus*, inhibiting the growth of *Sclerotinia sclerotiorum* by synthesizing secondary metabolites. *Arch. Microbiol.* **2023**, *205*, 8. [CrossRef]
67. de Ávila Santos, J.E.; de Brito, M.V.; Ávila Pimenta, A.T.Á.; da Silva, G.S.; Zocolo, G.J.; Muniz, C.R.; de Medeiros, S.C.; Grangeiro, T.B.; Lima, M.A.S.; da Silva, C.F.B. Antagonism of volatile organic compounds of the *Bacillus* sp. against *Fusarium kalimantanense*. *World J. Microbiol. Biotechnol.* **2023**, *39*, 60. [CrossRef]
68. Zhang, D.; Qiang, R.; Zhao, J.; Zhang, J.; Cheng, J.; Zhao, D.; Fan, Y.; Yang, Z.; Zhu, J. Mechanism of a volatile organic compound (6-methyl-2-heptanone) emitted from *Bacillus subtilis* ZD01 against *Alternaria solani* in potato. *Front. Microbiol.* **2022**, *12*, 808337. [CrossRef]
69. Wang, D.; Li, Y.; Yuan, Y.; Chu, D.; Cao, J.; Sun, G.; Ai, Y.; Cui, Z.; Zhang, Y.; Wang, F.; et al. Identification of non-volatile and volatile organic compounds produced by *Bacillus siamensis* LZ88 and their antifungal activity against *Alternaria alternata*. *Biol. Control* **2022**, *169*, 104901. [CrossRef]
70. Ren, L.; Zhou, J.; Yin, H.; Qin, N.; Yao, F.; Ma, D.; Zhao, X. Antifungal activity and control efficiency of endophytic *Bacillus velezensis* ZJ1 strain and its volatile compounds against *Alternaria solani* and *Botrytis cinerea*. *J. Plant Pathol.* **2022**, *104*, 575–589. [CrossRef]
71. Zhang, D.; Yu, S.; Yang, Y.; Zhang, J.; Zhao, D.; Pan, Y.; Fan, S.; Yang, Z.; Zhu, J. Antifungal effects of volatiles produced by *Bacillus subtilis* against *Alternaria solani* in potato. *Front. Microbiol.* **2020**, *11*, 1196. [CrossRef]
72. Ling, L.; Zhao, Y.; Tu, Y.; Yang, C.; Ma, W.; Feng, S.; Lu, L.; Zhang, J. The inhibitory effect of volatile organic compounds produced by *Bacillus subtilis* CL2 on pathogenic fungi of wolfberry. *J. Basic Microbiol.* **2021**, *61*, 110–121. [CrossRef]
73. Ling, L.; Luo, H.; Yang, C.; Wang, Y.; Cheng, W.; Pang, M.; Jiang, K. Volatile organic compounds produced by *Bacillus velezensis* L1 as a potential biocontrol agent against postharvest diseases of wolfberry. *Front. Microbiol.* **2022**, *13*, 987844. [CrossRef]
74. Kim, T.Y.; Hwang, S.H.; Noh, J.S.; Cho, J.Y.; Maung, C.E.H. Antifungal potential of *Bacillus velezensis* CE 100 for the control of different *Colletotrichum* species through isolation of active dipeptide, cyclo-(d-phenylalanyl-d-prolyl). *Int. J. Mol. Sci.* **2022**, *23*, 7786. [CrossRef]
75. Choub, V.; Won, S.J.; Ajuna, H.B.; Moon, J.H.; Choi, S.I.; Lim, H.I.; Ahn, Y.S. Antifungal activity of volatile organic compounds from *Bacillus velezensis* CE 100 against *Colletotrichum gloeosporioides*. *Horticulturae* **2022**, *8*, 557. [CrossRef]
76. Ghazala, I.; Chiab, N.; Saidi, M.N.; Gargouri-Bouzid, R. Volatile organic compounds from *Bacillus mojavensis* I4 promote plant growth and inhibit phytopathogens. *Physiol. Mol. Plant Pathol.* **2022**, *121*, 101887. [CrossRef]
77. Zhou, M.; Li, P.; Wu, S.; Zhao, P.; Gao, H. *Bacillus subtilis* CF-3 volatile organic compounds inhibit *Monilinia fructicola* growth in peach fruit. *Front. Microbiol.* **2019**, *10*, 1804. [CrossRef]
78. Yu, S.-M.; Oh, B.-T.; Lee, Y.H. Biocontrol of green and blue molds in postharvest satsuma mandarin using *Bacillus amyloliquefaciens* JBC36. *Biocontrol Sci. Technol.* **2012**, *22*, 1181–1197. [CrossRef]
79. You, W.; Ge, C.; Jiang, Z.; Chen, M.; Li, W.; Shao, Y. Screening of a broad-spectrum antagonist-*Bacillus siamensis*, and its possible mechanisms to control postharvest disease in tropical fruits. *Biol. Control* **2021**, *157*, 104584. [CrossRef]
80. Wang, W.-Y.; Kong, W.-L.; Liao, Y.-C.-Z.; Zhu, L.-H. Identification of *Bacillus velezensis* SBB and its antifungal effects against *Verticillium dahliae*. *J. Fungi* **2022**, *8*, 1021. [CrossRef]
81. Wu, J.J.; Huang, J.W.; Deng, W.L. Phenylacetic acid and methylphenyl acetate from the biocontrol bacterium *Bacillus mycoides* BM02 suppress spore germination in *Fusarium oxysporum* f. sp. *lycopersici*. *Front. Microbiol.* **2020**, *11*, 569263. [CrossRef] [PubMed]
82. Prakash, J.; Arora, N.K. Novel metabolites from *Bacillus safensis* and their antifungal property against *Alternaria alternata*. *Int. J. Gen. Mol. Microbiol.* **2021**, *114*, 1245–1258. [CrossRef] [PubMed]
83. Xie, S.; Liu, J.; Gu, S.; Chen, X.; Jiang, H.; Ding, T. Antifungal activity of volatile compounds produced by endophytic *Bacillus subtilis* DZSY21 against *Curvularia lunata*. *Ann. Microbiol.* **2020**, *70*, 2. [CrossRef]
84. Sharifi, R.; Ryu, C.M. Are bacterial volatile compounds poisonous odors to a fungal pathogen *Botrytis cinerea*, alarm signals to *Arabidopsis* seedlings for eliciting induced resistance, or both? *Front. Microbiol.* **2016**, *7*, 196. [CrossRef] [PubMed]
85. Castro, D.; Torres, M.; Sampedro, I.; Martínez-Checa, F.; Torres, B.; Béjar, V. Biological control of *Verticillium* wilt on olive trees by the salt-tolerant strain *Bacillus velezensis* XT1. *Microorganisms* **2020**, *8*, 1080. [CrossRef]
86. Cheffi Azabou, M.; Gharbi, Y.; Medhioub, I.; Ennouri, K.; Barham, H.; Tounsi, S.; Triki, M.A. The endophytic strain *Bacillus velezensis* OEE1: An efficient biocontrol agent against *Verticillium* wilt of olive and a potential plant growth promoting bacteria. *Biol. Control* **2020**, *142*, 104168. [CrossRef]

87. Syed-Ab-Rahman, S.F.; Carvalhais, L.C.; Chua, E.T.; Chung, F.Y.; Moyle, P.M.; Eltanahy, E.G.; Schenk, P.M. Soil bacterial diffusible and volatile organic compounds inhibit *Phytophthora capsici* and promote plant growth. *Sci. Total Environ.* **2019**, *692*, 267–280. [CrossRef]
88. Wang, K.; Qin, Z.; Wu, S.; Zhao, P.; Zhen, C.; Gao, H. Antifungal mechanism of volatile organic compounds produced by *Bacillus subtilis* CF-3 on *Colletotrichum gloeosporioides* assessed using omics technology. *J. Agric. Food Chem.* **2021**, *69*, 5267–5278. [CrossRef]
89. Zhao, P.; Li, P.; Wu, S.; Zhou, M.; Zhi, R.; Gao, H. Volatile organic compounds (VOCs) from *Bacillus subtilis* CF-3 reduce anthracnose and elicit active defense responses in harvested litchi fruits. *AMB Express* **2019**, *9*, 119. [CrossRef]
90. Wu, L.; Huang, Z.; Li, X.; Ma, L.; Gu, Q.; Wu, H.; Liu, J.; Borriss, R.; Wu, Z.; Gao, X. Stomatal closure and SA-, JA/ET-signaling pathways are essential for *Bacillus amyloliquefaciens* FZB42 to restrict leaf disease caused by *Phytophthora nicotianae* in *Nicotiana benthamiana*. *Front. Microbiol.* **2018**, *9*, 847. [CrossRef]
91. Jiang, C.H.; Liao, M.J.; Wang, H.K.; Zheng, M.Z.; Xu, J.J.; Guo, J.H. *Bacillus velezensis*, a potential and efficient biocontrol agent in control of pepper gray mold caused by *Botrytis cinerea*. *Biol. Control* **2018**, *126*, 147–157. [CrossRef]
92. Xie, Z.; Li, M.; Wang, D.; Wang, F.; Shen, H.; Sun, G.; Feng, C.; Wang, X.; Chen, D.; Sun, X. Biocontrol efficacy of *Bacillus siamensis* LZ88 against brown spot disease of tobacco caused by *Alternaria alternata*. *Biol. Control* **2021**, *154*, 104508. [CrossRef]
93. Lanisnik, R.T.; Wheeler, M.H. Melanin biosynthesis in the fungus *Curvularia lunata* (teleomorph: *Cochliobolus lunatus*). *Can. J. Microbiol.* **2003**, *49*, 110–119. [CrossRef]
94. Zheng, M.; Shi, J.; Shi, J.; Wang, Q.; Li, Y. Antimicrobial effects of volatiles produced by two antagonistic *Bacillus* strains on the anthracnose pathogen in postharvest mangos. *Biol. Control* **2013**, *65*, 200–206. [CrossRef]
95. Li, X.Y.; Mao, Z.C.; Wu, Y.X.; Ho, H.H.; He, Y.Q. Comprehensive volatile organic compounds profiling of *Bacillus* species with biocontrol properties by head space solid phase microextraction with gas chromatography-mass spectrometry. *Biocontrol Sci. Technol.* **2015**, *25*, 132–143. [CrossRef]
96. Wu, Y.; Zhou, J.; Li, C.; Ma, Y. Antifungal and plant growth promotion activity of volatile organic compounds produced by *Bacillus amyloliquefaciens*. *MicrobiologyOpen* **2019**, *8*, e00813. [CrossRef]
97. Ramírez, V.; Martínez, J.; Bustillos-Cristales, M.D.R.; Catañeda-Antonio, D.; Munive, J.A.; Baez, A. *Bacillus cereus* MH778713 elicits tomato plant protection against *Fusarium oxysporum*. *J. Appl. Microbiol.* **2022**, *132*, 470–482. [CrossRef]
98. Shifa, H.; Gopalakrishnan, C.; Velazhahan, R. Characterization of antifungal antibiotics produced by *Bacillus subtilis* G-1 antagonistic to *Sclerotium rolfsii*. *Biochem. Cell. Arch.* **2015**, *15*, 99–104.
99. Wu, Y.; Yuan, J.; Raza, W.; Shen, Q.; Huang, Q. Biocontrol traits and antagonistic potential of *Bacillus amyloliquefaciens* strain NJZJSB3 against *Sclerotinia sclerotiorum*, a causal agent of canola stem rot. *J. Microbiol. Biotechnol.* **2014**, *24*, 1327–1336. [CrossRef]
100. Zou, L.; Wang, Q.; Wu, R.; Zhang, Y.; Wu, Q.; Li, M.; Ye, K.; Dai, W.; Huang, J. Biocontrol and plant growth promotion potential of endophytic *Bacillus subtilis* JY-7-2L on *Aconitum carmichaelii* Debx. *Front. Microbiol.* **2023**, *13*, 1059549. [CrossRef]
101. Lahlali, R.; Aksissou, W.; Lyousfi, N.; Ezrari, S.; Blenzar, A.; Tahiri, A.; Ennahli, S.; Hrustić, J.; MacLean, D.; Amiri, S. Biocontrol activity and putative mechanism of *Bacillus amyloliquefaciens* (SF14 and SP10), *Alcaligenes faecalis* ACBC1, and *Pantoea agglomerans* ACBP1 against brown rot disease of fruit. *Microb. Pathog.* **2020**, *139*, 103914. [CrossRef] [PubMed]
102. Wu, S.; Zhen, C.; Wang, K.; Gao, H. Effects of *Bacillus subtilis* CF-3 VOCs combined with heat treatment on the control of *Monilinia fructicola* in peaches and *Colletotrichum gloeosporioides* in litchi fruit. *J. Food Sci.* **2019**, *84*, 3418–3428. [CrossRef]
103. Feng, B.; Chen, D.; Jin, R.; Li, E.; Li, P. Bioactivities evaluation of an endophytic bacterial strain *Bacillus velezensis* JRX-YG39 inhabiting wild grape. *BMC Microbiol.* **2022**, *22*, 170. [CrossRef] [PubMed]
104. Saleh, A.E.; Ul-Hassan, Z.; Zeidan, R.; Al-Shamary, N.; Al-Yafei, T.; Alnaimi, H.; Higazy, N.S.; Migheli, Q.; Jaoua, S. Biocontrol activity of *Bacillus megaterium* BM344-1 against toxigenic fungi. *ACS Omega* **2021**, *6*, 10984–10990. [CrossRef] [PubMed]
105. Ul Hassan, Z.; Al Thani, R.; Alnaimi, H.; Migheli, Q.; Jaoua, S. Investigation and application of *Bacillus licheniformis* volatile compounds for the biological control of toxigenic *Aspergillus* and *Penicillium* spp. *ACS Omega* **2019**, *4*, 17186–17193. [CrossRef]
106. He, C.N.; Ye, W.Q.; Zhu, Y.Y.; Zhou, W.W. Antifungal activity of volatile organic compounds produced by *Bacillus methylotrophicus* and *Bacillus thuringiensis* against five common spoilage fungi on loquats. *Molecules* **2020**, *25*, 3360. [CrossRef]
107. Kupper, K.C.; Moretto, R.K.; Fujimoto, A. Production of antifungal compounds by *Bacillus* spp. isolates and its capacity for controlling citrus black spot under field conditions. *World J. Microbiol. Biotechnol.* **2020**, *36*, 7. [CrossRef]
108. Surya, M.; Thiruvudainambi, S.; Ebenezar, E.G.; Vanniarajan, C.; Kumutha, K. GC-MS Analysis of antimicrobial compounds produced by *Bacillus* spp. against rice sheath rot pathogen *Sarocladium oryzae*. *J. Entomol. Zool. Stud.* **2020**, *8*, 1417–1423.
109. Awan, Z.A.; Shoaib, A.; Schenk, P.M.; Ahmad, A.; Alansi, S.; Paray, B.A. Antifungal potential of volatiles produced by *Bacillus subtilis* BS-01 against *Alternaria solani* in *Solanum lycopersicum*. *Front. Plant Sci.* **2023**, *13*, 1089562. [CrossRef]
110. Yuan, J.; Ruan, Y.; Wang, B.; Zhang, J.; Waseem, R.; Huang, Q.; Shen, Q. Plant growth-promoting rhizobacteria strain *Bacillus amyloliquefaciens* Njn-6-enriched bio-organic fertilizer suppressed *Fusarium* wilt and promoted the growth of banana plants. *J. Agric. Food Chem.* **2013**, *61*, 3774–3780. [CrossRef]
111. Wang, B.; Yuan, J.; Zhang, J.; Shen, Z.; Zhang, M.; Li, R.; Ruan, Y.; Shen, Q. Effects of novel bioorganic fertilizer produced by *Bacillus amyloliquefaciens* W19 on antagonism of *Fusarium* wilt of banana. *Biol. Fertil. Soils* **2013**, *49*, 435–446. [CrossRef]
112. Rangel-Montoya, E.A.; Delgado-Ramírez, C.S.; Sepulveda, E.; Hernández-Martínez, R. Biocontrol of *Macrophomina phaseolina* using *Bacillus amyloliquefaciens* strains in cowpea (*Vigna unguiculata* L.). *Agronomy* **2022**, *12*, 676. [CrossRef]
113. Aiello, D.; Leonardi, G.R.; Di Pietro, C.; Vitale, A.; Polizzi, G. A new strategy to improve management of citrus mal secco disease using bioformulates based on *Bacillus amyloliquefaciens* strains. *Plants* **2022**, *11*, 446. [CrossRef]

114. Cheffi, M.; Bouket, A.C.; Alenezi, F.N.; Luptakova, L.; Belka, M.; Vallat, A.; Rateb, M.E.; Tounsi, S.; Triki, M.A.; Belbahri, L. *Olea europaea* l. root endophyte *Bacillus velezensis* Oee1 counteracts oomycete and fungal harmful pathogens and harbours a large repertoire of secreted and volatile metabolites and beneficial functional genes. *Microorganisms* **2019**, *7*, 314. [CrossRef]
115. Calvo, H.; Mendiara, I.; Arias, E.; Gracia, A.P.; Blanco, D.; Venturini, M.E. Antifungal activity of the volatile organic compounds produced by *Bacillus velezensis* strains against postharvest fungal pathogens. *Postharvest Biol. Technol.* **2020**, *166*, 111208. [CrossRef]
116. Li, X.; Wang, X.; Shi, X.; Wang, B.; Li, M.; Wang, Q.; Zhang, S. Antifungal effect of volatile organic compounds from *Bacillus velezensis* CT32 against *Verticillium dahliae* and *Fusarium oxysporum*. *Processes* **2020**, *8*, 1674. [CrossRef]
117. Song, S.; Jeon, E.K.; Hwang, C.W. Characteristic analysis of soil-isolated *Bacillus velezensis* HY-3479 and its antifungal activity against phytopathogens. *Curr. Microbiol.* **2022**, *79*, 357. [CrossRef]
118. Roy, T.; Bandopadhyay, A.; Sonawane, P.J.; Majumdar, S.; Mahapatra, N.R.; Alam, S.; Das, N. Bio-effective disease control and plant growth promotion in lentil by two pesticide degrading strains of *Bacillus* sp. *Biol. Control* **2018**, *127*, 55–63. [CrossRef]
119. Chen, X.; Wang, Y.; Gao, Y.; Gao, T.; Zhang, D. Inhibitory abilities of *Bacillus* isolates and their culture filtrates against the gray mold caused by *Botrytis cinerea* on postharvest fruit. *Plant Pathol. J.* **2019**, *35*, 425–436. [CrossRef]
120. Altimira, F.; Godoy, S.; Arias-Aravena, M.; Araya, B.; Montes, C.; Castro, J.F.; Dardón, E.; Montenegro, E.; Pineda, W.; Viteri, I.; et al. Genomic and experimental analysis of the biostimulant and antagonistic properties of phytopathogens of *Bacillus safensis* and *Bacillus siamensis*. *Microorganisms* **2022**, *10*, 670. [CrossRef]
121. Guevara-Avendaño, E.; Bejarano-Bolívar, A.A.; Kiel-Martínez, A.L.; Ramírez-Vázquez, M.; Méndez-Bravo, A.; von Wobeser, E.A.; Sánchez-Rangel, D.; Guerrero-Analco, J.A.; Eskalen, A.; Reverchon, F. Avocado rhizobacteria emit volatile organic compounds with antifungal activity against *Fusarium solani*, *Fusarium* sp. associated with kuroshio shot hole borer, and *Colletotrichum gloeosporioides*. *Microbiol. Res.* **2019**, *219*, 74–83. [CrossRef] [PubMed]
122. Chaouachi, M.; Marzouk, T.; Jallouli, S.; Elkahoui, S.; Gentzbittel, L.; Ben, C.; Djébali, N. Activity assessment of tomato endophytic bacteria bioactive compounds for the postharvest biocontrol of *Botrytis cinerea*. *Postharvest Biol. Technol.* **2021**, *172*, 111389. [CrossRef]
123. Cavalcanti, V.P.; Araújo, N.A.F.; Machado, N.B.; Costa Júnior, P.S.P.; Pasqual, M.; Alves, E.; Schwan-Estrada, K.R.F.; Dória, J. Yeasts and *Bacillus* spp. as potential biocontrol agents of *Sclerotinia sclerotiorum* in garlic. *Sci. Hortic.* **2020**, *261*, 108931. [CrossRef]
124. Khalaf, E.M.; Raizada, M.N. Bacterial seed endophytes of domesticated cucurbits antagonize fungal and oomycete pathogens including powdery mildew. *Front. Microbiol.* **2018**, *9*, 42. [CrossRef]
125. Cao, H.; Jiao, Y.; Yin, N.; Li, Y.; Ling, J.; Mao, Z.; Yang, Y.; Xie, B. Analysis of the activity and biological control efficacy of the *Bacillus subtilis* strain Bs-1 against *Meloidogyne incognita*. *Crop Prot.* **2019**, *122*, 125–135. [CrossRef]
126. Luo, T.; Hou, S.; Yang, L.; Qi, G.; Zhao, X. Nematodes avoid and are killed by *Bacillus mycoides*-produced styrene. *J. Invertebr. Pathol.* **2018**, *159*, 129–136. [CrossRef]
127. Adam, M.; Heuer, H.; Hallmann, J. Bacterial antagonists of fungal pathogens also control root-knot nematodes by induced systemic resistance of tomato plants. *PLoS ONE* **2014**, *9*, e90402. [CrossRef]
128. Oka, Y.; Shuker, S.; Tkachi, N. Nematicidal efficacy of MCW-2, a new nematicide of the fluoroalkenyl group, against the root-knot nematode *Meloidogyne javanica*. *Pest Manag. Sci.* **2009**, *65*, 1082–1089. [CrossRef]
129. Huang, Y.; Xu, C.; Ma, L.; Zhang, K.; Duan, C.; Mo, M. Characterisation of Volatiles produced from *Bacillus megaterium* YFM3.25 and their nematicidal activity against *Meloidogyne incognita*. *Eur. J. Plant Pathol.* **2010**, *126*, 417–422. [CrossRef]
130. Yin, N.; Liu, R.; Zhao, J.L.; Khan, R.A.A.; Li, Y.; Ling, J.; Liu, W.; Yang, Y.H.; Xie, B.Y.; Mao, Z.C. Volatile organic compounds of *Bacillus cereus* strain Bc-Cm103 exhibit fumigation activity against *Meloidogyne incognita*. *Plant Dis.* **2021**, *105*, 904–911. [CrossRef]
131. Ayaz, M.; Ali, Q.; Farzand, A.; Khan, A.R.; Ling, H.; Gao, X. Nematicidal volatiles from *Bacillus atrophaeus* Gbsc56 promote growth and stimulate induced systemic resistance in tomato against *Meloidogyne incognita*. *Int. J. Mol. Sci.* **2021**, *22*, 5049. [CrossRef]
132. Du, J.; Gao, Q.; Ji, C.; Song, X.; Liu, Y.; Li, H.; Li, C.; Zhang, P.; Li, J.; Liu, X. *Bacillus licheniformis* JF-22 to control *Meloidogyne incognita* and its effect on tomato rhizosphere microbial community. *Front. Microbiol.* **2022**, *13*, 863341. [CrossRef]
133. Ye, L.; Wang, J.Y.; Liu, X.F.; Guan, Q.; Dou, N.X.; Li, J.; Zhang, Q.; Gao, Y.M.; Wang, M.; Li, J.S.; et al. Nematicidal activity of volatile organic compounds produced by *Bacillus altitudinis* AMCC 1040 against *Meloidogyne incognita*. *Arch. Microbiol.* **2022**, *204*, 521. [CrossRef]
134. Chen, W.; Wang, J.; Huang, D.; Cheng, W.; Shao, Z.; Cai, M.; Zheng, L.; Yu, Z.; Zhang, J. Volatile organic compounds from *Bacillus aryabhattai* MCCC 1K02966 with multiple modes against *Meloidogyne incognita*. *Molecules* **2021**, *27*, 103. [CrossRef]
135. Audrain, B.; Farag, M.A.; Ryu, C.-M.; Ghigo, J.-M. Role of bacterial volatile compounds in bacterial biology. *FEMS Microbiol. Rev.* **2015**, *39*, 222–233. [CrossRef]
136. Jousset, A.; Schmid, B.; Scheu, S.; Eisenhauer, N. Genotypic richness and dissimilarity opposingly affect ecosystem functioning. *Ecol. Lett.* **2011**, *14*, 537–545. [CrossRef]
137. de Boer, W.; Li, X.; Meisner, A.; Garbeva, P. Pathogen suppression by microbial volatile organic compounds in soils. *FEMS Microbiol. Ecol.* **2019**, *95*, fiz105. [CrossRef]
138. Caulier, S.; Nannan, C.; Gillis, A.; Licciardi, F.; Bragard, C.; Mahillon, J. Overview of the antimicrobial compounds produced by members of the *Bacillus subtilis* group. *Front. Microbiol.* **2019**, *10*, 302. [CrossRef]
139. Gómez-Tenorio, M.A.; Zanón, M.J.; de Cara, M.; Lupión, B.; Tello, J.C. Efficacy of dimethyl disulfide (DMDS) against *Meloidogyne* sp. and three formae speciales of *Fusarium oxysporum* under controlled conditions. *Crop Prot.* **2015**, *78*, 263–269. [CrossRef]

140. Papazlatani, C.; Rousidou, C.; Katsoula, A.; Kolyvas, M.; Genitsaris, S.; Papadopoulou, K.K.; Karpouzas, D.G. Assessment of the impact of the fumigant dimethyl disulfide on the dynamics of major fungal plant pathogens in greenhouse soils. *Eur. J. Plant Pathol.* **2016**, *146*, 391–400. [CrossRef]
141. Mulay, P.R.; Cavicchia, P.; Watkins, S.M.; Tovar-Aguilar, A.; Wiese, M.; Calvert, G.M. Acute illness associated with exposure to a new soil fumigant containing dimethyl disulfide—Hillsborough County, Florida, 2014. *J. Agromedicine* **2016**, *21*, 373–379. [CrossRef] [PubMed]

MDPI AG
Grosspeteranlage 5
4052 Basel
Switzerland
Tel.: +41 61 683 77 34

Antibiotics Editorial Office
E-mail: antibiotics@mdpi.com
www.mdpi.com/journal/antibiotics

www.ingramcontent.com/pod-product-compliance
Lightning Source LLC
Chambersburg PA
CBHW061600210926
51850CB00009B/2167
9783725860371